GASTROINTESTINAL AND HEPATIC PATHOLOGY DECENNIAL

1966–1975

SERIES EDITOR

SHELDON C. SOMMERS, M.D.

Director of Laboratories, Lenox Hill Hospital, New York, New York; Clinical Professor of Pathology, Columbia University College of Physicians and Surgeons, New York, New York; Clinical Professor of Pathology, University of Southern California School of Medicine, Los Angeles, California

GASTROINTESTINAL
AND HEPATIC
PATHOLOGY
DECENNIAL

1966-1975

APPLETON-CENTURY-CROFTS/New York
A Publishing Division of Prentice-Hall, Inc.

75   76   77   78   79/ 10   9   8   7   6   5   4   3   2   1

Library of Congress Catalog Card Number: 75–22635

Prentice-Hall International, Inc., London
Prentice-Hall of Australia, Pty. Ltd., Sydney
Prentice-Hall of India Private Limited, New Delhi
Prentice-Hall of Japan, Inc., Tokyo
Prentice-Hall of Southeast Asia (Pte.) Ltd., Singapore

PRINTED IN THE UNITED STATES OF AMERICA
0–8385–3092–3

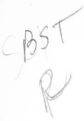

CONTRIBUTORS

Victor M. Areán, M.D.

Clinical Professor of Pathology, University of South Florida, Tampa, Florida

Bishnu Dutta, M.D.

Department of Histopathology, Royal Prince Alfred Hospital, Sydney, N.S.W., Australia

Giuseppe Grampa, M.D.

Professor of Morbid Anatomy, State University Medical School, Milan, Italy

George F. Gray, M.D.

Associate Professor of Pathology, New York Hospital—Cornell Medical Center, New York, New York

Parviz Haghighi, M.D.

Professor and Chairman, Department of Pathology, Pahlavi University School of Medicine, Shiraz, Iran

John Higginson, M.D., F.R.C.P.

Director, International Agency for Research on Cancer, Lyon, France

H. Edward MacMahon, M.D., M.R.C.P., Sc.D.

Visiting Professor of Pathology, University of Massachusetts Medical School, Worcester, Massachusetts

Robert W. McDivitt, M.D.

Professor and Chairman, Department of Surgical Pathology, University of Utah College of Medicine Medical Center, Salt Lake City, Utah

Vincent J. McGovern, M.D.

Director, Fairfax Institute of Pathology, Royal Prince Alfred Hospital, Sydney, N.S.W., Australia

Basil C. Morson, M.D., F.R.C.S., F.R.C.Path

Consultant Pathologist, St. Mark's Hospital, London, England

Richard M. Mulligan, M.D.

Professor of Pathology, The University of Colorado School of Medicine, Denver, Colorado

Khosrow Nasr, M.D.

Associate Professor of Medicine and Director, Nemazee Hospital, Pahlavi University, Shiraz, Iran

Sidney L. Saltzstein, M.D.

Associate Professor of Pathology, University of California, San Diego, School of Medicine, San Diego, California

Donald J. Svoboda, M.D.

Professor and Vice-Chairman, Department of Pathology and Oncology, University of Kansas Medical Center, Kansas City, Kansas

PREFACE

This year's *Pathology Annual 1975* is the tenth volume of the series begun in 1966. *Pathology Annuals* now have an established readership among practitioners of pathology. Since several volumes are out of print and the original plates have been preserved by the publisher, it was decided to collect the articles by organ systems and to republish them in seven decennial volumes. Not every article in the ten *Pathology Annuals* is included.

All authors were invited to prepare addenda updating their contributions to late 1974. About two-thirds were able to do so. One completely new essay was provided by Drs. Dixon and Cochrane for the *Kidney Pathology Decennial 1966–1975,* and Drs. Pierce and Abell rewrote their paper in the *Genital and Mammary Pathology Decennial 1966–1975.* The *Endocrine Pathology Decennial 1966–1975* differs from the others in that articles were included from the *Pathobiology Annuals* edited by Dr. Harry L. Ioachim and from other sources to provide a more complete coverage.

It is hoped that the *Pathology Decennial* volumes may appeal to clinical specialists as well as to pathologists. Better communication between clinician and pathologist in part involves a mutual familiarity with the special literature that each may read.

I would like to express my appreciation to the personnel at Appleton-Century-Crofts; David Stires, Doreen Berne, Berta Steiner Rosenberg, Laura Bird, and Joann Lindner, who have assisted me in the preparation and production of these volumes.

The seven volumes are as follows: *Kidney Pathology Decennial 1966–1975; Pulmonary Pathology Decennial 1966–1975; Gastrointestinal and Hepatic Pathology Decennial 1966–1975; Genital and Mammary Pathology Decennial 1966–1975; Hematologic and Lymphoid Pathology Decennial 1966–1975; Cardiovascular Pathology Decennial 1966–1975;* and *Endocrine Pathology Decennial 1966–1975.*

Sheldon C. Sommers

CONTENTS

GASTROINTESTINAL AND HEPATIC PATHOLOGY DECENNIAL

1966–1975

EXTRANODAL MALIGNANT LYMPHOMAS AND PSEUDOLYMPHOMAS

SIDNEY L. SALTZSTEIN *

Extranodal malignant lymphomas differ in their clinical behavior from those malignant lymphomas arising in the more usual sites. The prognosis, usually better than either that of malignant lymphomas in general or that of carcinomas of the particular organ, is related to cell type and to regional lymph node involvement. Treatment primarily is surgical; late deaths are uncommon.

The reported prognosis of extranodal lymphomas is further improved by the inclusion in many series of cases of benign "pseudolymphomas." These lesions, reactive in nature, must be separated by the pathologist from malignant lymphomas so that patients are not subjected unnecessarily to radical surgical procedures, radiotherapy, or chemotherapy. Counterbalancing this, many series of extranodal lymphomas contain examples of disseminated malignant lymphomas of the usual type, in which the first or most prominent clinical findings are related to some extranodal site. These too must be separated from the extranodal malignant lymphomas because of their poorer prognosis and because of the differences in appropriate therapy.

Definitions

An extranodal malignant lymphoma is defined as a malignant lymphoma of any cell type (lymphocytic, reticulum cell, or Hodgkin's) involving primarily an organ other than the lymph nodes, liver, spleen, bone marrows, thymus, or Waldeyer's ring.

* The assistance of Mr. Cramer Lewis, Department of Ilustration, Washington University School of Medicine, St. Louis, Missouri, and of Mr. Edward J. Peterson, Office of Learning Resources, UCSD School of Medicine, San Diego, California, in the preparation of the illustrations is gratefully acknowledged.

1

There must be no evidence of dissemination in that only the organ (or the organ and its immediately adjacent lymph nodes) is involved by the malignant lymphoma and the bone marrow and peripheral blood are free of the neoplasm. To exclude those cases of malignant lymphoma of the usual type in which dissemination already has occurred but is not apparent at the time of diagnosis, there must be no evidence of dissemination for at least three months after diagnosis. Also excluded will be cases in which the diagnosis of an extranodal lymphoma was made at autopsy only. Burkitt's lymphoma will not be included in this discussion.

A pseudolymphoma is a benign reactive process of known or unknown cause, usually forming a tumor, with sufficient proliferation of reticuloendothelial elements to be confused with a malignant lymphoma. In essence, a pseudolymphoma is the extranodal counterpart of a reactive lymph node.

Two terms will be avoided in this presentation as they have various conflicting meanings. The first of these is "lymphosarcoma" which, depending upon the author, can mean all malignant lymphomas, malignant lymphomas of both lymphocytic types, malignant lymphomas of the well-differentiated lymphocytic type, or even all lymphoid lesions including pseudolymphomas. The other term which will not be used is "follicle," as this can mean either nodules of tumor or lymphoid germinal centers. The words "nodule" and "germinal center" will be used instead.

Malignant lymphomas will be classified according to the system Rappaport[52] devised for lymph nodes, but for simplification, only the well-differentiated and poorly-differentiated lymphocytic types, the reticulum cell type, and the Hodgkin's type will be used (Table 1).

Table 1.   Classification: Malignant Lymphoma*

Malignant Lymphoma, Lymphocytic Type, Well Differentiated
Malignant Lymphoma, Lymphocytic Type, Poorly Differentiated
Malignant Lymphoma, Reticulum Cell Type
Malignant Lymphoma, Hodgkin's Type

* Modified after Rappaport, H., Winter, W.J., and Hicks, E.B. *Cancer,* 9:792, 1956.

Extranodal malignant lymphomas and pseudolymphomas have been described in virtually every organ of the human body. The most frequent sites are the lungs, stomach, small intestine, and large intestine. Extranodal malignant lymphomas and pseudolymphomas of these four sites will be discussed in detail separately. As a generalization, the observations pertaining to these lesions of these four sites can be extrapolated to the rest of the body.

Lung

Primary malignant lymphomas and pseudolymphomas of the lung are rare. As of 1963, only 102 reported cases were available for study.[56] A few scattered reports have appeared since.[16, 17, 26, 29, 31, 48, 51] Obviously, not all cases are reported; this writer has seen many in consultation since 1963. Compared to the estimate of 61,000 new cases of cancer of the lung in the United States alone each year,[3] malignant lymphomas and pseudolymphomas make up only an infinitesimal portion of primary lung tumors. Extrapolating from the American Cancer Society figures,[3] there must be at least 18,000 new cases of malignant lymphoma of all sites in the United States each year. Here again, malignant lymphomas which are primary in the lung represent only a very small fraction of all malignant lymphomas.

Presenting Symptoms. These tumors generally cause no symptoms and are detected on routine roentgenograms of the chest. Patients who do have symptoms complain of chills, fever, cough, chest pain, weakness, fatigue, and weight loss. Patients with malignant lymphomas of the reticulum cell type tend to be younger than those with malignant lymphomas of the lymphocytic type.

Radiologic Appearance. The radiologic picture is equally nonspecific; these lesions may present as large masses involving an entire lung, as small coin lesions, or as anything in between. The pseudolymphomas often demonstrate air bronchograms and only rarely show pleural effusion or lymphadenopathy.[31]

Gross Appearance. Operative findings reflect the gross appearance of these tumors. They may be firm masses occupying an entire lobe or lung, or they may be only a few centimeters in diameter. The tumors usually abut on the pleural surface. On section they are pink-white, fairly well demarcated, but not encapsulated (Figs. 1, 2). Pseudolymphomas and malignant lymphomas of the lymphocytic type are solid; malignant lymphomas of the reticulum and Hodgkin's types frequently are cystic (Fig. 2). Lymph nodes may be enlarged, but this does not invariably indicate involvement by tumor.

Microscopic Appearance. As seen under the microscope, the lesions are composed of masses of reticuloendothelial elements and remnants of the preexisting lung structure (Fig. 3). The pseudolymphomas and the lymphocytic type of malignant lymphoma tend to grow intraseptally about the periphery (Fig. 4); the reticulum cell and Hodgkin's types of malignant lymphoma tend to be more circumscribed. Necrosis is common in the reticulum cell type and accounts for the cystic gross appearance; pseudolymphomas and malignant lymphomas of the lymphocytic type show little, if any, necrosis. Growth beneath intact bronchial epithelium is frequent (Fig. 5). Vessel "invasion" can be found.

Differential Diagnosis. The diagnosis of a malignant lymphoma of the reticulum cell type is not difficult to establish if the characteristics of this neoplasm as it appears in lymph nodes are kept in mind. This tumor is composed of solid sheets of large, moderately pleomorphic cells without any suggestion of glandular or other differentiation. The individual cells have large, oval or bean-shaped nuclei with large nucleoli (Fig. 6). Large cell undifferentiated bronchogenic carcinoma, metastatic unpigmented malignant melanoma, metastatic renal adenocarcinoma, and metastatic seminoma are about the only sources of confusion. Eosinophilic granuloma of the lung conceivably could cause confusion.

Similarly, the diagnosis of malignant lymphoma, Hodgkin's type, is based on the finding of Reed-Sternberg cells, as it would be elsewhere in the body (Fig. 7). If one is strict in what he accepts as Reed-Sternberg cells and diligent in his search for them, he should neither overdiagnose or underdiagnose malignant lymphoma of the Hodgkin's type. This writer has not seen an example of this tumor arising in the lung in his personal experience but has had the opportunity to review the sections of four cases reported by Kern, et al.[38]

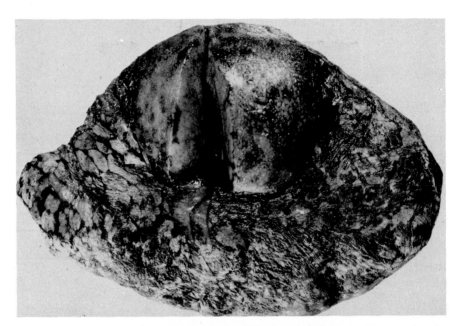

Fig. 1. This pulmonary malignant lymphoma of the lymphocytic type abuts on the pleura. The solid, well-demarcated nature of the lesion is seen. The gross appearance of a pseudo-lymphoma would be identical. W. U. III. #62-2534. (Reprinted from Saltzstein, S. L. *Cancer*, 16:928, 1963, with permission.)

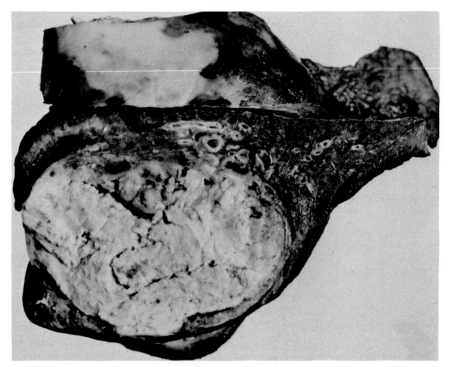

Fig. 2. Gross photograph of a malignant lymphoma, reticulum cell type, of the lung, showing the central necrosis and cyst formation. The lesion appears well demarcated. W. U. III. #55-3939. (Reprinted from Saltzstein, S. L. *Cancer*, 16:928, 1963, with permission.)

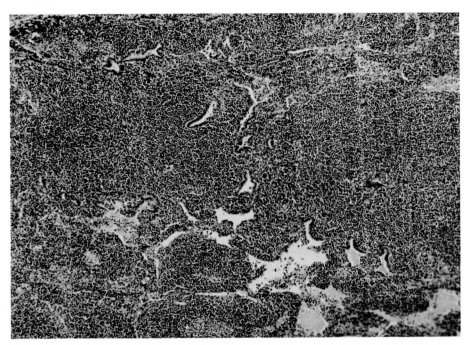

Fig. 3. The central portion of both malignant lymphomas and pseudolymphomas shows a dense infiltrate replacing the pulmonary parenchyma. A few remaining bronchioles and vessels can be identified. W. U. III. #61-1763. H&E. X93.

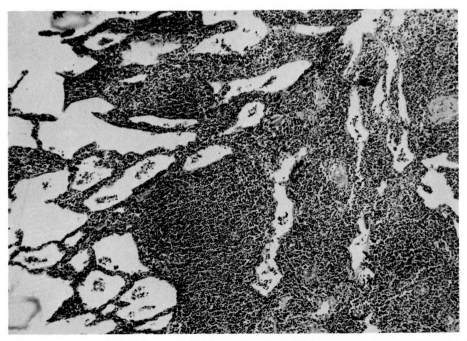

Fig. 4. Photomicrograph of the periphery of a pseudolymphoma showing the intraseptal growth seen in both malignant lymphomas of the lymphocytic type and pseudolymphomas. Other areas of this lesion showed many well-defined germinal centers. W. U. III. #62-224. H&E. X55.

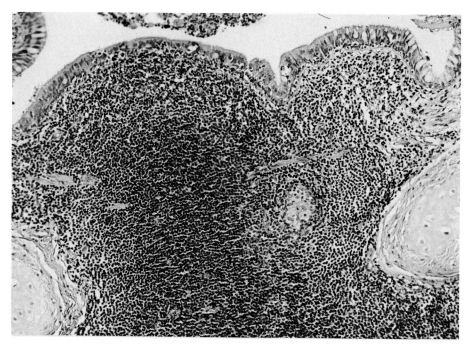

Fig. 5. Prominent endobronchial growth may be seen in either a malignant lymphoma or a pseudolymphoma. W. U. III. #61-1764. H&E. X170.

Malignant lymphomas of the lymphocytic type must be differentiated from "oat cell" carcinoma of the lung, on one hand, and from pseudolymphomas on the other. "Oat cell" carcinomas are large endobronchial tumors composed of pleomorphic, dark cells which are slightly larger than lymphocytes. These cells often are spindle-shaped and mitotic figures are seen frequently. Confusion between "oat cell" carcinoma and malignant lymphoma of the lymphocytic type has occurred in the cytologic evaluation of sputum specimens.

More germane to this discussion is the separation of a malignant lymphoma of the lymphocytic type from a pseudolymphoma. If one extends to the lung the criteria established by Rappaport, et al.[52] for distinguishing malignant lymphomas from reactive hyperplasia in lymph nodes, one usually can separate malignant lymphomas from pseudolymphomas (Table 2). Favoring pseudolymphoma are lym-

Table 2.   Differential Diagnosis

	PSEUDOLYMPHOMA	MALIGNANT LYMPHOMA
Germinal Centers	Usually Present	Absent
Infiltrate	Mixed, Mature	Uniform, Immature
Nodes	Never Involved	Often Involved

phoid germinal centers and a mixed cellular infiltrate of various inflammatory cells (Fig. 8). A uniform infiltrate of mature or immature lymphocytes without germinal centers rules for a diagnosis of malignant lymphoma; tumor in the regional lymph nodes obviously establishes the diagnosis of malignant lymphoma. Pleural seeding

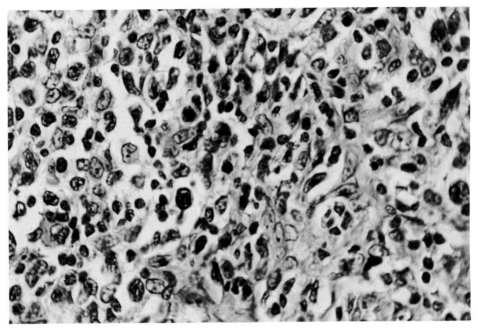

Fig. 6. The characteristic large cells with bean-shaped nuclei and prominent nucleoli of a malignant lymphoma, reticulum cell type, are seen in this pulmonary tumor. W. U. III. #62-3562. H&E. X600. (Reprinted from Saltzstein, S. L. Cancer, 16:928, 1963, with permission.)

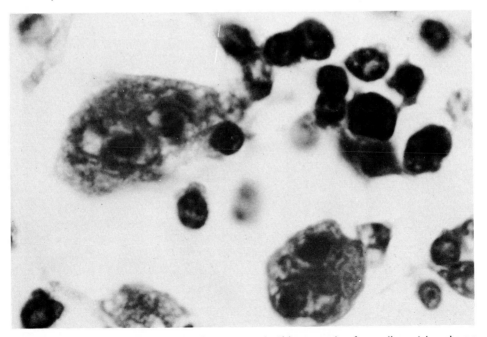

Fig. 7. Classical Reed-Sternberg cells are seen in this example of a malignant lymphoma of the Hodgkin's type arising in the lung. UCSD OLR. H&E. X400. (Original section obtained through the courtesy of Dr. William Kern and Dr. Jules Kernen, Los Angeles.)

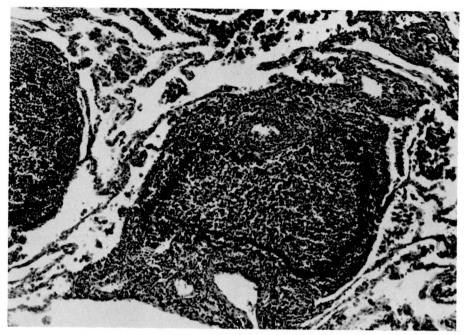

Fig. 8. Prominent germinal centers are seen in the intraseptal growth of this pulmonary pseudolymphoma. UCSD OLR. H&E. X25.

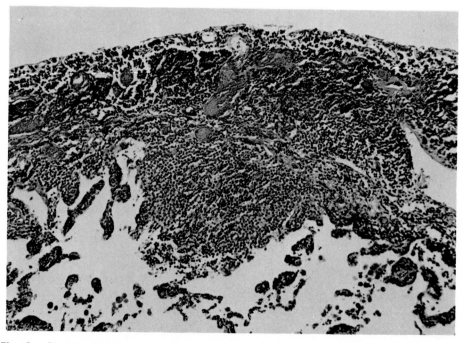

Fig. 9. Pleural seeding of the tumor, as seen here, favors a diagnosis of malignant lymphoma. W. U. Ill. #62-3560. H&E. X130.

strongly favors a diagnosis of malignancy (Fig. 9). As in the case with lymph nodes, occasionally one will be unable to separate pseudolymphoma from malignant lymphoma of the lymphocytic type.

Another non-neoplastic disease which may be difficult or even impossible to separate from malignant lymphomas arising in the lung is the lymphomatoid variant of the limited form of Wegener's granuloma.[40] In both there is diffuse proliferation of immature reticuloendothelial cells. Favoring the diagnosis of Wegener's granuloma are vasculitis, necrosis, and "plasmacytoid" cells in the infiltrate. Special stains for elastic tissue to demonstrate the destruction of vessels resulting from the vasculitis can be very helpful in separating these entities. The vascular changes may be easier to evaluate in the portions of the sections containing less of the reticuloendothelial cell infiltrate.

Treatment.　Complete surgical excision (lobectomy or even pneumonectomy) is the treatment of choice as it establishes the diagnosis, removes nonfunctioning lung tissue, and much of the time is sufficient to cure the patient. Radiotherapy should be reserved for those patients with involvement of regional lymph nodes or with evidence of recurrence. Very obviously, patients with pseudolymphomas do not require radiotherapy.

Prognosis.　If it is to happen, recurrence of the malignant lymphoma with progression to death occurs very rapidly. Virtually all patients who die from this condition died within 2½ years, although recurrences leading to the death of the patient have been reported at 5½ and 6¼ years.[17, 48] Nonfatal recurrences may occur later but respond well to radiotherapy or to surgical excision. Most of the reported nonfatal recurrences are very poorly documented; in only one instance was tissue excised and examined.

It is difficult to establish the prognosis of patients with malignant lymphomas of the lymphocytic type because of the admixture of cases of pseudolymphoma in all reports. Combining these two lesions, a relative five-year survival rate of 70 percent is reported. In an attempt to separate the mortality resulting from the lymphocytic type of malignant lymphoma from this combined group, it can be shown that only 20 percent of the patients in this combined group died of malignant lymphoma. The influence of nodal involvement is apparent: only one of 42 patients whose nodes were known to be free of tumor died of lymphoma, while almost 40 percent of the others died of lymphoma.

The five-year relative survival rate of patients with reticulum cell type of malignant lymphoma is only 53 percent. Here again, of six patients known to have no involvement of regional nodes by tumor, only one died of lymphoma, while over half of the other patients died of lymphoma.

The prognosis of malignant lymphoma, Hodgkin's type, of the lung is not known exactly but must be very poor. The total English language experience is only 23 cases.* Of these, only one[12] is reported to have lived more than five years and

---

* In addition to the cases cited and reported by Kern, et al.[38] in 1961, this author would add the one reported by Bass and Reibstein,[6] the second case of Robins,[53] Starkey's sixth and seventh cases,[66] Snyder's case,[64] and the first case of Meese, et al.,[43] Monahan's case,[45] Gregory, et al.'s first case,[24] and Joseph's first and fourth cases.[36] Contrary to Kern, et al., I would not accept the cases of Rubenfeld and Clark[54] and of Rubinovich,[55] as in both cases,

a second as long as three years.[21] Interestingly, one of the two had involvement of the regional lymph nodes and the other invasion of the pericardium.

Stomach

Gastric lymphomas are the commonest extranodal malignant lymphomas. Most series state that from 1 to 5 percent of all gastric cancers are malignant lymphomas.[42, 67, 69] Thus, the annual incidence of these tumors should be from 200 to 1,000 in the United States alone.[3] It is obvious that the great majority of gastric malignant lymphomas are not reported. Sperling summarized 17 series reported from 1939 to 1965 which included only 852 patients.[65] Many series include cases of malignant lymphoma not truly originating in the stomach, as well as many examples of pseudo-lymphoma, further diluting the data pertinent to primary malignant lymphomas of the stomach.

The stomach is also a common site of pseudolymphomas. Of the lymphoid tumors of the stomach, between one-fourth and one-half have been found to be pseudolymphomas.[7, 18, 33, 63] This undoubtedly is a reflection of the commonness of peptic ulcer, which is at least one cause of gastric pseudolymphomas (Fig. 10).[18] In spite of the histologic and clinical evidence that many gastric lymphoid lesions are pseudolymphomas rather than malignant lymphomas, not all authors have accepted completely the concept of pseudolymphomas.[73]

Presenting Symptoms. Unlike malignant lymphomas and pesudolymphomas of the lung, those of the stomach usually produce symptoms. Pain, often like that of peptic ulcer, is the commonest symptom.[21, 35, 46, 62, 70] Weight loss with or without anorexia is almost as common. Bleeding, nausea, and vomiting are described less often. The only physical sign of significance is a mass in the epigastrium; this is present in less than half of the patients. Laboratory studies may show an anemia if there has been sufficient blood loss. Achlorhydria is noted in only one-fourth of the patients.

Radiologic Appearance. Roentgenographic studies will establish the presence of a gastric lesion, but rarely will a specific diagnosis of lymphoma be offerred.[35, 62, 70, 73] Signs favoring malignant lymphoma over carcinoma of the stomach include a large superficial ulcer often on the posterior wall or lesser curvature, enlarged rugae close to a polypoid mass or ulcer, a thick, nonpliable wall, a large tumor with little change in the capacity and contour of the stomach, a smooth mucosal surface, and multiple polypoid masses or ulcers.[62] On the other hand, the findings noted with pseudolymphomas include ulcerating tumors, constricting or infiltrating lesions, isolated ulcer craters, and, least often, enlarged rugae.[50]

Gross Appearance. When the lesion is first seen, either by the surgeon or by

---

the histologic diagnosis was made at autopsy only. More recent cases to be excluded are Samuels, et al.'s third, fourth, and sixth,[59] Meese, et al.'s second, third, and fourth,[43] Joseph's third and fifth,[36] and both those reported by Gonpnathan and Sataline.[23] In all of these cases, the diagnosis of malignant lymphoma, Hodgkin's type, was made on nodal tissue. Although a "suggestive" diagnosis was made from tissue removed at bronchoscopy in Joseph's second case,[36] a supraclavicular lymph node excised only "a little later" showed malignant lymphoma, Hodgkin's type. The second and third cases of Gregory, et al.[24] arose in the thymus.

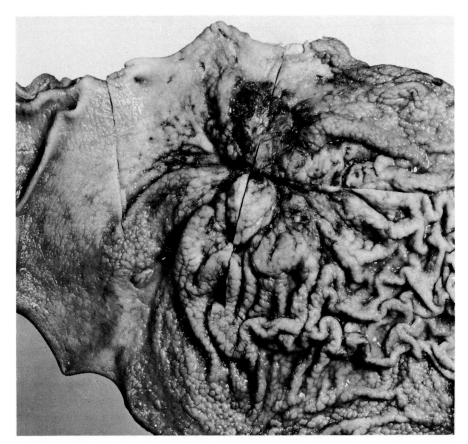

Fig. 10. Gross photograph of a gastric pseudolymphoma showing both an ulceration and a mass. The rugae are only slightly more prominent than normal. W. U. III. #55-4180. (Reprinted from Faris, T. D., and Saltzstein, S. L. *Cancer*, 17:207, 1964, with permission.)

the pathologist, the usual impression is that it is carcinoma. About one-half of the malignant lymphomas, as well as the pseudolymphomas, are ulcerated. Many others have one or more polypoid masses of tumor. Intramural growth is common. The frequently described large, brain-like rugae are seen only rarely and even then are not specific to lymphoma. Any combination of these various patterns may be present (Fig. 11).

Microscopic Appearance and Differential Diagnosis. The distinction between malignant lymphoma, pseudolymphoma, and carcinoma can be made only by thorough histologic examination. Whether this will entail biopsy of the tumor or of a lymph node, excision of an ulcerated lesion, or subtotal gastrectomy as an "excisional biopsy" will depend on the particular situation. Frozen section may be useful. Most carcinomas can be separated readily from the lymphomas, but an occasional carcinoma of the linitis plastica type may require demonstration of intracellular mucin production.

All of the malignant lymphomas and pseudolymphomas are characterized by a dense infiltrate composed of reticuloendothelial cells (Fig. 11). This may be

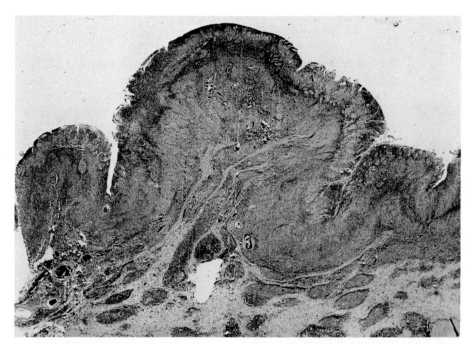

Fig. 11.   Low-power photomicrograph of a gastric pseudolymphoma showing the proliferation of reticuloendothelial elements to form a mass. W. U. III. #63-4328. H&E. X15. (Reprinted from Faris, T. D., and Saltzstein, S. L. *Cancer*, 17:207, 1964, with permission.)

limited to the mucosa, or may penetrate through the entire gastric wall (Figs. 12, 14, 15). As elsewhere, the diagnosis of malignant lymphoma of the reticulum cell and Hodgkin's types can be made if one is careful (Figs. 16, 17). Again, it is the distinction between malignant lymphoma of the well-differentiated lymphocytic type and pseudolymphoma that may be difficult and, at times, impossible.[37] Favoring the diagnosis of pseudolymphoma are a mixed infiltrate of various inflammatory cells, lymphoid germinal centers, and obviously, regional lymph nodes free of malignant lymphoma (Figs. 12, 13; Table 2). The opposite of each of these militates for a diagnosis of malignant lymphoma, i.e., a uniform monotonous infiltrate often of less-than-mature lymphocytes, no germinal centers in the lesion, and nodal involvement by malignant lymphoma (Figs. 14, 15).

   Treatment.   Virtually every author recommends surgical resection of gastric lymphomas if this can be done. This should include the regional lymph nodes in a manner analogous to procedures carried out for gastric carcinoma. The margins of grossly normal tissue about the primary tumor should be greater for a lymphoma than for a carcinoma because of the propensity of lymphomas to be large and to have multiple areas of tumor in the stomach.[42, 62] Although many five-year survivals are reported among those treated by surgical extirpation alone, most authors employ radiotherapy in the postoperative period. Long-term survivors, including some patients with unresectable tumors, are reported among the patients treated by radiotherapy alone. The placing of metal clips in the area of the tumor at operation to aid the radiotherapist is well worthwhile.

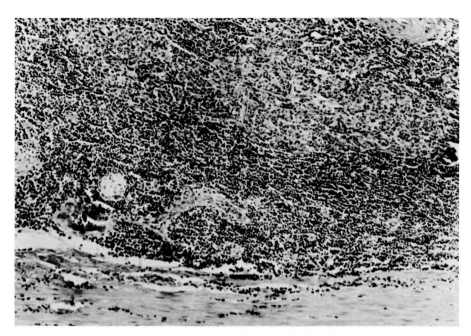

Fig. 12. The pleomorphic infiltrate of a gastric pseudolymphoma may extend to the muscular wall, as seen here, or even deeper. The depth of infiltration is no guide to the distinction between a malignant lymphoma and a pseudolymphoma. UCSD OLR. H&E. X25.

Fig. 13. Prominent lymphoid germinal centers, as seen just above the muscularis mucosæ in this gastric pseudolymphoma, are the most reliable basis for separating malignant lymphomas from pseudolymphomas. UCSD OLR. H&E. X25.

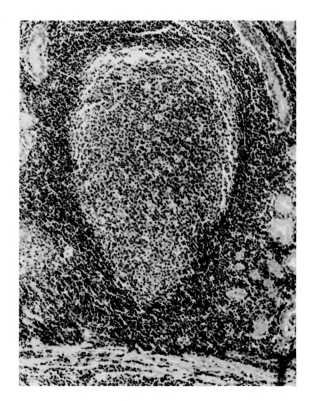

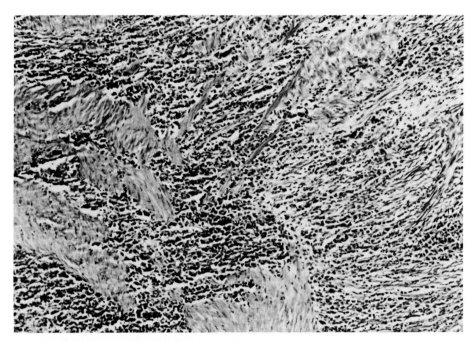

Fig. 14. Photomicrograph showing infiltration into the muscular wall of the stomach in a malignant lymphoma of the reticulum cell type. The distinction from a pseudolymphoma is made on the characteristics of the cells rather than on the depth of the infiltrate. UCSD OLR. H&E. X25.

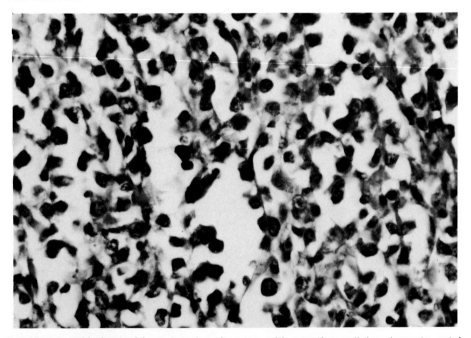

Fig. 15. A solid sheet of immature lymphocytes, with no other cellular elements, establishes the diagnosis of malignant lymphoma, lymphocytic type, poorly differentiated in this gastric lesion. UCSD OLR. H&E. X160.

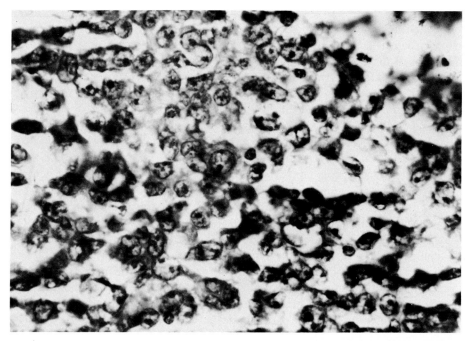

Fig. 16.   In the stomach as elsewhere, malignant lymphomas of the reticulum cell type are recognized by large cells with large, bean-shaped nuclei and prominent nucleoli. UCSD OLR. H&E. X160.

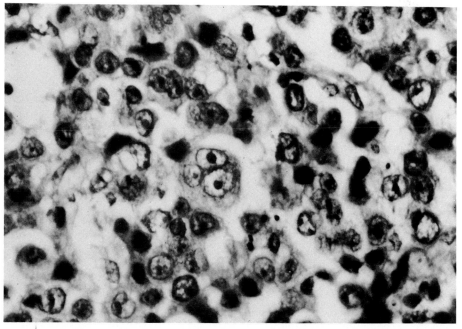

Fig. 17.   A typical Reed-Sternberg cell is seen in the center of this photomicrograph of a gastric malignant lymphoma of the Hodgkin's type. UCSD OLR. H&E. X160.

Prognosis. The five-year survival of all patients with malignant lymphomas of the stomach is about 34 percent.[65] This figure probably is inaccurate because many of the series included in Sperling's review mix together primary malignant lymphomas of the stomach, generalized malignant lymphomas secondarily involving the stomach, and pseudolymphomas. In the four series in which pseudolymphomas are separated out, the five-year survival of the remaining patients with primary malignant lymphomas of the stomach ranges from 7 to 70 percent.[7, 18, 33, 63] Three of these series are very small; in the fourth, 88 (67 percent) of 131 patients with primary gastric malignant lymphomas lived five years or more.

In contradistinction to primary pulmonary malignant lymphomas, late recurrences are reasonably common in gastric lymphomas. For this reason, ten-year survival figures may be more meaningful.

The influence of cell type on survival is well demonstrated. The five-year survival in patients with malignant lymphomas of the reticulum cell type ranges from 36 to 50 percent. In the same three series, the corresponding figures for patients with malignant lymphomas of the lymphocytic type range from 83 to 100 percent.[35, 43, 67] The ten-year survival rates are 30 percent and 77 percent, respectively. Most series do not contain many examples of malignant lymphomas of the Hodgkin's type arising in the stomach; Cornes reports 32 percent five-year and 5 percent ten-year survival rates in a group of 22 patients.[12] My personal experience exactly parallels the cited series.[57]

Nodal involvement by the malignant lymphoma cuts the five-year survival to about half of that in patients without nodal involvement.[2, 21, 35, 67] Larger tumors also carry poorer prognosis, as do those which invade deeply into the gastric wall.[35] A nodular pattern appears to improve the prognosis, similar to the situation in malignant lymphomas originating in lymph nodes.[35, 52, 77]

Small Intestine

In the small intestine, malignant lymphomas are relatively common. In various series, malignant lymphomas make up from one-sixth to one-third of all cancers of the small intestine.[34, 47, 60, 79] One author states that malignant lymphoma is the commonest malignant tumor of the small intestine.[1] This relative commonness of malignant lymphoma undoubtedly is only a reflection of the rarity of malignant tumors arising in the small intestine; the total number of reported malignant lymphomas of both the small and large intestine is less than 200.[15]

Pseudolymphomas are correspondingly rare in the small intestine. Weaver and Batsakis reported only three cases and were unable to find any earlier reports in the literature.[75] Over approximately the same time interval they reported ten malignant lymphomas of the small intestine.[74] Lymphoid hyperplasia of the terminal ileum as seen in children also warrants inclusion in the group of pseudolymphomas.[1, 68]

Presenting Symptoms. Symptoms of malignant lymphoma and pseudolymphoma in the small intestine, as elsewhere, do not allow distinction between the two. Abdominal pain, symptoms of intestinal obstruction, and changes in bowel habits are the commonest complaints.[8, 15, 19, 32, 44, 68, 74, 75, 76] A spruelike syndrome is being reported more and more frequently.[65] On examination, a palpable abdominal mass and evidence of weight loss are frequently noted. Occult blood may be present in the stool. Evidence of intestinal perforation is seen with some frequency. Other malignant tumors of the gastrointestinal tract have been reported in association with malignant lymphomas.[11]

Radiologic Appearance. Roentgenograms may show a discrete tumor, multiple tumors, thickened mucosal folds, or ulceration in addition to the findings of obstruction.[65] The separation from regional enteritis may be difficult.

Gross Appearance. Operative and gross pathologic findings are fundamentally those of a tumor arising in the submucosa of the small intestine. These tumors are variously described as annular, nodular, polypoid, ulcerative, or some combination of these.[8, 15, 19, 74] Lesions may be multiple;[9, 17] perforation is noted on occasion.[8] Involvement of regional lymph nodes is very common,[2, 8, 19, 20, 74] but enlargement of these nodes does not guarantee their involvement by tumor.[15] The tumors have the grey to pink appearance of lymphoid tumors elsewhere. They are more common in the ileum than elsewhere in the small intestine.

Microscopic Appearance and Differential Diagnosis. As in the other sites discussed, the distinction between malignant lymphoma and pseudolymphoma is made on histologic examination. Malignant lymphomas of the reticulum cell and Hodgkin's types should present no real diagnostic difficulties, although metastatic amelanotic malignant melanoma may be confused with the former. The features distinguishing pseudolymphomas from malignant lymphomas of the lymphocytic type again are the mixed infiltrate of mature cells, active phagocytosis (as might be seen in a germinal center), germinal centers, and regional lymph nodes free of tumor (Fig. 18; Table 2).[68, 75, 76]

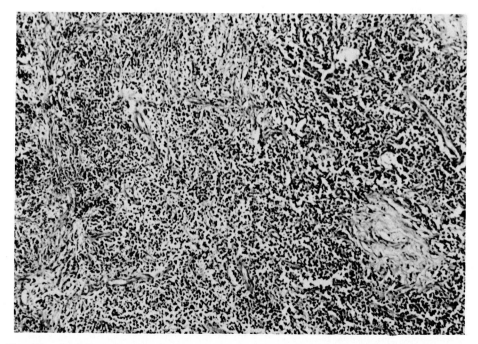

Fig. 18.   In this malignant lymphoma, lymphocytic type, well-differentiated, arising in the jejunum, solid sheets of small lymphocytes can be seen infiltrating the outer portion of the intestinal wall. UCSD OLR. H&E. X25.

Treatment. Surgical excision with wide margins of normal intestine and inclusion of regional lymph nodes is the standard treatment when feasible. Radiotherapy is generally given in addition, but it can be the only means of therapy.[10, 15]

Prognosis. For several reasons, it is most difficult to estimate accurately the prognosis of malignant lymphomas of the small intestine. Most series are quite small. Many series contain a mixture of primary malignant lymphomas of the small intestine along with disseminated disease involving the small intestine.[44] In other reports, primary malignant lymphomas are well separated from other malignant lymphomas, but small and large intestine are lumped together.[15, 78] Five-year survival rates range from 10 to 50 percent, depending on the particular tumor and therapy.[2, 4, 8, 10, 15, 19, 20, 74] A 33 percent average seems reasonable.[34] The influence of cell type and pattern is shown in that the survival for nodular malignant lymphoma is about 50 percent, while that of the diffuse lymphocytic type is 25 percent and that of the reticulum cell type is only 10 to 11 percent.[15, 74] Cornes had no five-year survivors with malignant lymphomas of the Hodgkin's type originating in the small intestine.[12] There is some indication that lymph node involvement decreases the prognosis; however, this is not as clear-cut as in the stomach or lung.[15, 20, 74] Certainly nodal involvement does not preclude long-term survival.[15] The poor prognosis in children reported by Mestel was not born out by Weaver and Batsakis.[44, 74] This probably reflects Mestel's inclusion of many cases not truly primary in the small intestine, as evidenced by death from dissemination in less than three months.

While a few recurrences have been noted in the period between five and ten years, none have been reported after ten years. Most patients who are to die from this condition will do so in the first two years.[15]

Large Intestine

The large intestine is the least common site in the gastrointestinal tract of malignant lymphomas. Woodruff and Skorneck estimate that only 0.5 percent of colonic malignancies are malignant lymphomas.[80] Glick and Soule in 1966 could find only 38 reported cases of primary appendiceal or colonic lymphomas, to which they, and later Wychulis, et al., added 50 more.[22, 82]

Pseudolymphomas, however, especially of the rectum, are very common. Individual series of 70 or 100 cases are not unusual.[13, 28] Of all of the pseudolymphomas of the gastrointestinal tract, the average pathologist has the most experience with those of the large intestine.[27, 30, 76]

Presenting Symptoms. Patients with malignant lymphomas of the large intestine complain of abdominal pain, weight loss, rectal bleeding, and changes in bowel habits.[22, 81, 82] There is an association with long-standing chronic ulcerative colitis.[15, 82] A mass is found on abdominal or rectal examination in at least two-thirds of these patients. Abdominal tenderness is almost as common. Lesions in the rectum can be visualized and may be polypoid.

Radiologic Appearance. Radiologic examination usually demonstrates either a filling defect or a mass; only rarely is no abnormality seen.[81] The specific diagnosis of malignant lymphoma usually is not made on roentgenographic study. Features favoring malignant lymphoma over carcinoma are a longer involved segment, a wide transition zone between the tumor and the normal intestine, a defect which is not annular, a mass out of proportion to the filling defect, dilation of the lesion, and flattening and obscuring of the mucosal changes by the contrast medium.[80, 81]

Gross Appearance.   Malignant lymphomas most often occur in the area about the cecum, to a lesser extent in the rectosigmoid area, and least often in the mid-portion of the large intestine.[22, 80, 82] The tumors usually are circumscribed, but diffuse involvement has been reported. The circumscribed tumors may project into the lumen or may form large intramural and extracolonic masses. Lesions may be multiple. Annular lesions are quite rare.[22, 82]

Pseudolymphomas of the colon present somewhat differently. Bleeding is the usual symptom, but prolapse, the presence of a mass, or abdominal pain also may occur.[13, 28, 30] Examination shows one or many polypoid lesions ranging in size from 2 mm to 5 cm. These "lymphoid polyps" usually are sessile but may be peduncu-lated. At times, the polypoid lesions may be so numerous as to mimic multiple polyposis; this variant has been named "pseudoleukemia."[14]

Microscopic Appearance and Differential Diagnosis.   Again, the final distinc-tion between malignant lymphoma and pseudolymphoma is based on the histologic appearance. The diagnosis of malignant lymphoma of the reticulum cell and Hodgkin's types should not be any more troublesome here than elsewhere. Pseudo-lymphoma differs from malignant lymphoma of the lymphocytic type in the char-acteristic presence of germinal centers, a mixed cellular infiltrate, and relatively little involvement of the attenuated overlying colonic epithelium (Figs. 19, 20, 21; Table 2).[13, 28] Only rarely does a pseudolymphoma involve the circular muscle of the colon.[13]

Treatment.   The usual treatment of a malignant lymphoma is surgical excision, as with a carcinoma. This may entail a segmental resection, a hemicolectomy, or even a total colectomy.[81] While some survivors have not received irradiation after operation, most patients have, and inclusion of this modality usually is recom-mended. This is true especially if there has been nodal involvement or extension to other organs.[82] Cook and Corbett reported two five-year survivors in ten patients with malignant lymphomas of the large intestine treated by irradiation alone.[10]

Prognosis.   Only from the recent reports from the Mayo Clinic may any con-clusions regarding prognosis be made.[22, 82] The five-year survival is 55 percent or better; the ten-year figure is 50 percent. Almost all of these patients had involve-ment of pericolic fat, and half had involvement of regional lymph nodes. Thus, the 55 percent five-year survival rate for malignant lymphoma exceeds the 50 percent five-year survival rate which could be expected with a similar group of colonic car-cinomas (one-half Dukes' "B" and one-half Dukes' "C").[30] The data are incon-clusive, but it appears that patients with lymphocytic type have a better chance of survival than those with the reticulum cell type. Only a few cases of the Hodgkin's type of malignant lymphoma originating in the large intestine have been reported. No meaningful estimate of prognosis can be made.[49, 61, 82]

As elsewhere, lymph node involvement worsens the prognosis. Wychulis, et al.[82] reported that 71 percent of their patients who died of recurrent malignant lym-phoma had regional lymph node involvement originally, while only 32 percent of the survivors did. Extension beyond the colon also has an ominous significance.[82]

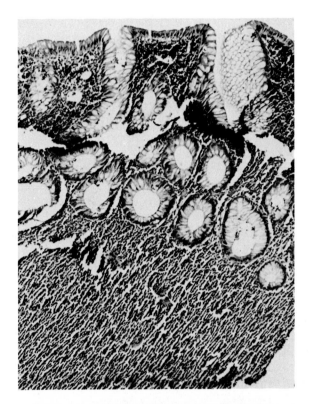

Fig. 19. This particular area seen in a malignant lymphoma, lymphocytic type, well-differentiated, arising in the rectum, would not allow distinction from a pseudolymphoma. A relatively small area of lymphocytes is not, in itself, a sufficient basis for a diagnosis of malignant lymphoma. See also Figures 20, 21. UCSD OLR. H&E. X25.

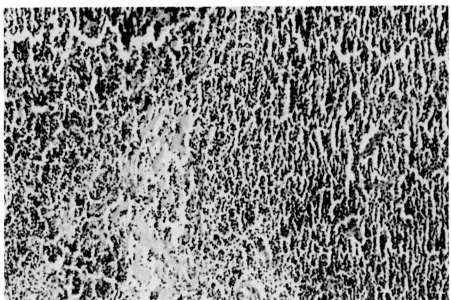

Fig. 20. In another area of the same tumor as illustrated in Figure 19, the monotonous infiltrate of small lymphocytes is seen again. Multiple areas like this, with no germinal centers, allow one to make a diagnosis of malignant lymphoma. See also Figures 19, 21. UCSD OLR. H&E. X25.

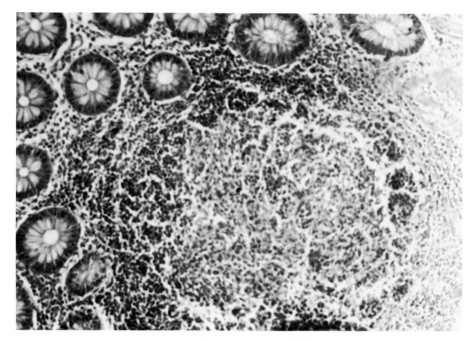

Fig. 21.   In this pseudolymphoma of the rectum ("lymphoid polyp"), prominent germinal centers allow separation from malignant lymphoma. Other areas were composed almost entirely of lymphocytes. Compare Figures 19, 20. UCSD OLR. H&E. X40.

Late recurrences are uncommon and apparently can be treated successfully by irradiation.[22, 82] Association with chronic ulcerative colitis indicates a poorer prognosis.[15, 82]

Discussion

The existence of both extranodal malignant lymphomas and pseudolymphomas is well established. The origin, etiology, and significance of these conditions merit further discussion.

The abundant lymphoid tissue in the submucosa of the gastrointestinal tract is the point of origin of malignant lymphomas in the stomach, small intestine, and large intestine. The lymphoid tissue which occurs regularly in the bronchial mucosa and in the fibrous tissue around the bronchial cartilages[41] can well explain the origin of malignant lymphomas in the lung. Primitive totipotential mesenchymal cells exist in the loose connective tissue everywhere, especially about blood vessels,[41] and can explain the development of malignant lymphomas anywhere in the body.

The etiology of extranodal malignant lymphomas is, like that of the usual malignant lymphomas, completely unknown. Only further study will determine if it is the same in all locations. It is of interest that chronic ulcerative colitis is associated with primary malignant lymphoma of the colon as well as with adenocarcinoma.[15, 82]

Extranodal malignant lymphomas have significance, and their separation from the usual malignant lymphoma is important because of their generally better prognosis and different therapy. For the first reason, separation from carcinoma also is important.

Pseudolymphomas are reactive lesions and, like other inflammatory lesions, can occur anywhere in the body. At times, every pathologist has seen dense lymphoid infiltrates, often with germinal centers, in almost every organ. In a sense, a pseudolymphoma is simply an extension of this and represents the extranodal counterpart of a reactive lymph node.

In the lungs, pseudolymphomas probably represent a form of chronic pneumonia in which lymphocytes predominate.[56] Pulmonary fibrous, xanthomatous, and plasma cell pseudotumors have been described as have lymphoid pseudotumors of the mediastinum.[9, 71, 72] The relationship to lymphoid interstitial pneumonia warrants intensive study.[40]

Gastric pseudolymphomas are generally part of the reaction to peptic ulcer (Fig. 22).[18] There is no reason why chronic gastritis alone could not lead to such a pseudolymphoma also.

Many of the pseudolymphomas of the small intestine are associated with regional enteritis and indeed may be only an extreme expression of that disease.[75] The pseudolymphomas of the very terminal ileum seen in young children are part of the generalized lymphoid hyperplasia characteristic of that age group.[1]

No specific factor can explain all of the colonic pseudolymphomas, but there

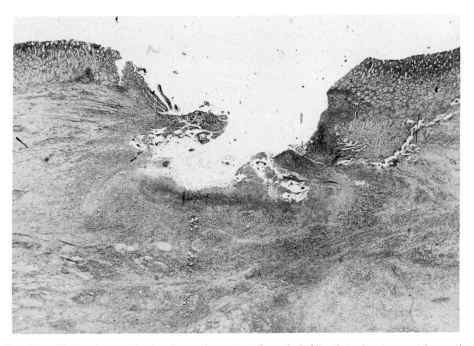

Fig. 22. Photomicrograph showing a dense lymphocytic infiltration about a gastric peptic ulcer. This is felt to be one origin of gastric pseudolymphomas. W. U. III. #63-4326. H&E. X15. (Reprinted from Faris, T.D., and Saltzstein, S. L. *Cancer*, 17:207, 1964, with permission.)

is general agreement that they are of inflammatory origin.[13, 28] We have seen one of the cecum resulting from anticonvulsant drug therapy.[57]

The significance of pseudolymphomas is obvious: they are benign lesions and do not require the extensive surgery, radiotherapy, or chemotherapy that true malignant lymphomas require. Similarly, the emotional impact of a diagnosis of cancer on a patient and his family can be avoided.

Endoscopic biopsy and exfoliative cytology are of little use in the differentiation of extranodal malignant lymphomas, especially of the lymphocytic types, from pseudolymphomas because in both lesions there may be large areas composed mainly of lymphocytes (Figs. 19, 20, 21). A piece of tissue is necessary, large enough to study the structure and to have a reasonable chance to find germinal centers. This often will mean excision of the entire lesion. The diagnosis of malignant lymphoma of the reticulum cell type can be made at times on gastric cytologic material,[39] and Reed-Sternberg cells can be identified in material from endoscopic biopsies. As pseudolymphomas of the rectum usually are small, excisional biopsy should be performed.

Summary

Malignant lymphomas of any cell type can originate in organs other than the lymph nodes, liver, spleen, bone marrow, thymus, or Waldeyer's ring. In these extranodal locations, the malignant lymphomas have a better prognosis than the usual malignant lymphomas or other malignant tumors of the specific organ.

Cell type and nodal involvement affect the prognosis. Surgical excision is the treatment of choice. Late recurrences and late deaths are uncommon.

In these same sites, benign reactive pseudolymphomas also can occur. These can be separated from malignant lymphomas by their mixed cellular infiltrate, the presence of lymphoid germinal centers, and the absence of involvement of lymph nodes.

References

1. Ackerman, L.V. Surgical Pathology, 3rd ed. St. Louis, C. V. Mosby Co., 1964, pp. 413-414, 418.
2. Allen, A.W., Donaldson, G., Sniffen, R.C., and Goodale, F. Primary malignant lymphoma of the gastrointestinal tract. Ann. Surg., 140:428, 1954.
3. Statistics on cancer. CA, 18:13, 1968.
4. Azzopardi, J.G., and Menzies, T. Primary malignant lymphoma of the alimentary tract. Brit. J. Surg., 47:358, 1960.
5. Barba, W.P. Benign lymphoid hyperplasia of the rectum. J. Pediat., 41:328, 1952.
6. Bass, H.E., and Reibstein, H.B. Hodgkin's disease of the lung. New York J. Med., 50:345, 1950.
7. Berry, G.R., and Mathews, W.H. Gastric lymphosarcoma and pseudolymphoma. Canad. Med. Ass. J., 96:1312, 1967.
8. Burman, S.O., and van Wyk, F.A.K. Lymphomas of small intestine and cecum. Ann. Surg., 143:349, 1956.
9. Castleman, B., Iverson, L., and Mendendez, V.P. Localized mediastinal lymph node hyperplasia resembling thymoma. Cancer, 9:822, 1956.

10. Cook, J.C., and Corbett, D.P. Roentgen therapy of primary gastrointestinal lymphoma. Radiology, 78:562, 1962.
11. Cornes, J.S. Multiple primary cancers: Primary malignant lymphomas and carcinomas of the intestinal tract in the same patient. J. Clin. Path., 13:483, 1960.
12 ―――― Hodgkin's disease of the gastrointestinal tract. Proc. Roy. Soc. Med., 60: 732, 1967.
13. ―――― Wallace, M.H., and Morson, B.C. Benign lymphomas of the rectum and anal canal: A study of 100 cases. J. Path. Bact., 82:371, 1961.
14. Cosens, G.S. Gastrointestinal pseudoleukemia: A case report. Ann. Surg., 148:129, 1958.
15. Dawson, J.M.P., Cornes, J.S., and Morson, B.C. Primary malignant lymphoid tumours of the intestinal tract. Brit. J. Surg., 49:80, 1961.
16. Ehrenstein, F. Primary puimonary lymphoma. J. Thorac. Cardiovasc. Surg., 52:31, 1966.
17. Ellison, R.G., Bailey, A.W., Yeh, T.J., Corpe, R.F., Liang, J., and Stergus, I. Primary lymphosarcoma of the lung. Amer. Surg., 30:737, 1964.
18. Faris, T.D., and Saltzstein, S.L. Gastric lymphoid hyperplasia: A lesion confused with lymphosarcoma. Cancer, 17:207, 1964.
19. Faulkner, J.W., and Dockerty, M.B. Lymphosarcoma of the small intestine. Surg. Gynec. Obstet., 95:76, 1952.
20. Frazer, J.W. Malignant lymphomas of the gastrointestinal tract. Surg. Gynec. Obstet., 108:182, 1959.
21. Friedman, A.I. Primary lymphosarcoma of the stomach: A clinical study of 75 cases. Amer. J. Med., 26:783, 1959.
22. Glick, D.D., and Soule, E.H. Primary malignant lymphoma of colon or appendix. Arch. Surg., 92:144, 1966.
23. Gonpnathan, H., and Sataline, L.R. Pulmonary Hodgkin's disease with cavitary lesion. Ohio Med. J., 62:238, 1966.
24. Gregory, J.J., Ribaudo, C.A., and Grace, W.J. Endobronchial Hodgkin's disease: Report of three cases. Ann. Intern. Med., 62:579, 1965.
25. Grismer, J.T., Raab, D.E., Dornbach, R., and Krafft, W. Primary lymphosarcoma: An interesting solitary lesion of the lung. Minn. Med., 49:242, 1966.
26. Havard, C.W.H., Nichols, J.B., and Stansfeld, A.G. Primary lymphosarcoma of the lung. Thorax, 17:190, 1962.
27. Hayes, H.T., Burr, H.B., and Pruit, L.T. Lymphoid tumors of the colon and rectum: Report of a case of simple lymphoma of rectum. Surgery, 7:540, 1940.
28. Helwig, E.B., and Hansen, J. Lymphoid polyps (benign lymphoma) and malignant lymphoma of the rectum and anus. Surg. Gynec. Obstet., 92:233, 1951.
29. Hilbun, B.M., and Chavez, C.M. Lymphoma of the lung. J. Thorac. Cardiovasc. Surg., 53:721, 1967.
30. Holtz, F., and Schmidt, L.A. Lymphoid polyps (benign lymphoma) of the rectum and anus. Surg. Gynec. Obstet., 106:639, 1958.
31. Hutchinson, W.B., Friedenberg, M.J., and Saltzstein, S. Primary pulmonary pseudolymphoma. Radiology, 82:48, 1964.
32. Jackson, P.P., and Coady, C.J. Primary lymphomas of the GI tract. Arch. Surg., 78:458, 1959.
33. Jacobs, D.S. Primary gastric malignant lymphoma and pseudolymphoma. Amer. J. Clin. Path., 40:379, 1963.
34. James, A.G. Cancer Prognosis Manual, 2nd ed. New York, American Cancer Society, 1966, pp. 51, 53.
35. Joseph, J.I., and Lattes, R. Gastric lymphosarcoma: Clinicopathologic analysis of 71 cases and its relation to disseminated lymphosarcoma. Amer. J. Clin. Path., 45:653, 1966.
36. Joseph, M. Hodgkin's disease of the lungs. Med. J. Aust., 1:795, 1965.
37. Kay, S. Lymphoid tumors of the stomach. Surg. Gynec. Obstet., 118:1059, 1964.

38. Kern, W.H., Crepeau, A.G., and Jones, J.C. Primary Hodgkin's disease of the lung: Report of four cases and review of the literature. Cancer, 14:1151, 1961.
39. Kernen, J.A., and Bales, C. Cytologic diagnosis of gastric cancer. Calif. Med., 108: 104, 1968.
40. Liebow, A.A. Personal communication, 1968.
41. Maximow, A.A., and Bloom, W. A Textbook of Histology, 7th ed. Philadelphia, W. B. Saunders Co., 1957, pp. 68-70, 437.
42. McNeer, G., and Berg, J. The clinical behavior and management of primary malignant lymphoma of the stomach. Surgery, 46:829, 1959.
43. Meese, E.H., Doohen, D.J., Elliott, R.C., and Timmes, J.J. Primary organ involvement in intrathoracic Hodgkin's disease. Dis. Chest., 46:699, 1964.
44. Mestel, A.L. Lymphosarcoma of the small intestine in infancy and childhood. Ann. Surg., 149:87, 1959.
45. Monahan, D.T. Hodgkin's disease of the lung. J. Thorac. Cardiovasc. Surg., 49:173, 1965.
46. Nicoloff, D.M., Haynes, L.B., and Wangensteen, O.H. Primary lymphosarcoma of the gastrointestinal tract. Surg. Gynec. Obstet., 117:433, 1963.
47. Pagtalunan, R.J.G., Mayo, C.W., and Dockerty, M.B. Primary malignant tumors of the small intestine. Amer. J. Surg., 108:13, 1964.
48. Papaionnou, A.N., and Watson, W.L. Primary lymphoma of the lung. An appraisal of its natural history and a comparison with other localized lymphomas. J. Thorac. Cardiovasc. Surg., 49:373, 1965.
49. Parkhurst, G.F., and MacMillan, S.F. Longevity in lymphomas of the lower intestinal tract. J.A.M.A. 179:351, 1967.
50. Perez, C.A., and Dorfman, R.F. Benign lymphoid hyperplasia of the stomach and duodenum. Radiology, 87:505, 1966.
51. Rabiah, F.A. Primary lymphocytic lymphoma (lymphosarcoma) of the lung. Amer. Surg., 34:275, 1968.
52. Rappaport, H., Winter, W.J., and Hicks, E.B. Follicular lymphoma. Cancer, 9:792, 1956.
53. Robbins, L.L. Roentgenological appearance of parenchymal involvement of lung by malignant lymphoma. Cancer, 6:80, 1953.
54. Rubenfeld, S., and Clark, E. An unusual case of Hodgkin's disease of lung. Radiology, 28:614, 1937.
55. Rubinovich, A.Z. A case of pulmonary lymphogranulomatosis. Klin. Med. (Moskva), 35:144, 1957. Abstracted in Abstr. Sov. Med., B-2:908, 1958.
56. Saltzstein, S.L. Pulmonary malignant lymphomas and pseudolymphomas: Classification, therapy, and prognosis. Cancer, 16:928, 1963.
57. ——— Unpublished data, Barnes Hospital, 1963.
58. ——— and Ackerman, L.V. Lymphadenopathy induced by anticonvulsant drugs and mimicking clinically and pathologically malignant lymphomas. Cancer, 12:164, 1959.
59. Samuels, M.L., Howe, C.D., Dodd, G.D., Jr., Fuller, L.M., Shullenberger, C.C., and Leary, W.L. Endobronchial malignant lymphoma: Report of five cases in adults. Amer. J. Roentgen., 85:87, 1961.
60. Schmutzer, K.J., Holleran, W.M., and Regan, J.F. Tumors of the small bowel. Amer. J. Surg., 108:270, 1964.
61. Shapiro, H.A. Primary Hodgkin's disease of the rectum. Arch. Intern. Med., 107: 270, 1961.
62. Sherrick, D.W., Hodgson, J.R., and Dockerty, M.B. The roentgenologic diagnosis of primary gastric lymphoma. Radiology, 84:925, 1965.
63. Smith, J.L., and Helwig, E.B. Malignant lymphoma of the stomach: Its diagnosis, distinction, and biologic behavior. Amer. J. Path., 34:553, 1958.
64. Snyder, J.M. Discussion. J. Thorac. Surg., 31:44, 1956.

65. Sperling, L. Malignant lymphoma of the gastrointestinal tract. Progr. Clin. Cancer, 2:338, 1966.
66. Starkey, G.W.B. Discussion. J. Thorac. Surg., 31:43, 1956.
67. Stobbe, J.A., Dockerty, M.B., and Bernatz, P.E. Primary gastric lymphoma and its grades of malignancy. Amer. J. Surg., 112:10, 1966.
68. Swartley, R.N., and Stayman, J.W. Lymphoid hyperplasia of the intestinal tract requiring surgical intervention. Ann. Surg., 155:238, 1962.
69. Thorbjarnson, B., Beal, J.M., and Pearce, J.M. Primary malignant lymphoid tumors of the stomach. Cancer, 9:712, 1956.
70. ——— Pearce, J.M. and Beal, J.M. Sarcoma of the stomach. Amer. J. Surg., 97:36, 1959.
71. Titus, J.L., Harrison, E.G., Clagett, O.T., Anderson, M.W., and Knaff, L.J. Xanthomatous and inflammatory pseudotumors of the lung. Cancer, 15:522, 1962.
72. Umiker, W.O., and Iverson, L. Postinflammatory "tumors" of the lung: Report of four cases simulating xanthoma, fibroma, or plasma cell tumor. J. Thorac. Surg., 28:55, 1954.
73. Valdes-Dapena, A., Affolter, H., and Vilardell, F. The gradient of malignancy in lymphoid lesions of the stomach. Gastroenterology, 50:382, 1966.
74. Weaver, D.K., and Batsakis, J.G. Primary lymphomas of the small intestine. Amer. J. Gastroenterol., 42:620, 1964.
75. ——— and Batsakis, J.G. Pseudolymphomas of the small intestine. Amer. J. Gastroenterol., 44:374, 1965.
76. ——— and Batsakis, J.G. Primary lymphomas and related benign lesions of the intestines. Amer. J. Proctol., 17:229, 1966.
77. Welborn, J.K., Ponka, J.L., and Rebuck, J.W. Lymphoma of the stomach: A diagnostic and therapeutic problem. Arch. Surg., 90:480, 1965.
78. ——— Rebuck, J.W., and Ponka, J.L. Intestinal lymphosarcoma. Arch. Surg., 94:717, 1967.
79. Wheelock, M.C., Atkinson, A.J., and Pizzo, A. Lymphosarcoma of the ileum. Gastroenterology, 15:158, 1950.
80. Wolf, B.S., and Marshak, R.H. Roentgen features of diffuse lymphosarcoma of the colon. Radiology, 75:733, 1960.
81. Woodruff, J.H., Jr., and Skorneck, A.B. Malignant lymphoma of the colon and rectum: Roentgen diagnosis. Calif. Med., 96:181, 1962.
82. Wychulis, A.R., Beahrs, O.H., and Woolner, L.B. Malignant lymphoma of the colon. Arch. Surg., 93:215, 1966.

Addendum

In the interval since 1968, the concept of pseudolymphoma has gained general acceptance. Case reports [1–3] continue to show the benign clinical course associated with these lesions and to point out the histologic criteria that enable one to separate these reactive processes from malignant lymphomas. In this author's personal experience, pathologists are having less and less trouble making this distinction. Endoscopic biopsies may prove useful.[3]

Much better survival for patients with gastric malignant lymphomas compared to those with gastric carcinomas continues to be reported.[4–10] Most authors show the influence of cell type and nodal involvement (or other staging technique) on the prognosis in gastric lymphomas, as has already been described. It is not possible to show any significant difference between the survival rate for patients with lymphomas of the small and large intestines compared to those with carcinomas of the same organs.[5] There continues to be a difference of opinion between the surgeons and the radiotherapists as to the best method of therapy. Two other controversies exist. The first is the role of cytology in the diagnosis of gastric lymphomas. Kline and Goldstein [11] have shown that they can separate malignant lymphomas from benign processes of the stomach by cytologic studies. Kobayashi et al described the benign significance of plasma cells in the gastric washings.[2] Nelson et al indicate a preference for gastroscopic biopsy.[3] This author would be more hesitant to accept a diagnosis of a differentiated lymphocytic lymphoma on the basis of cytologic studies alone. The other controversy centers about late recurrences. Isolated reports of fatal recurrences of gastric lymphomas after five years still show up.[4, 6] In the End Results Group study,[12] little difference could be shown between relative survival rates at 5 and at 10 years; these authors feel that the problem of late recurrence is overemphasized.

One of the more interesting syndromes which has been delineated over the past six years is the association of primary upper intestinal lymphomas, malabsorption, and immunologic abnormalities. This entity is frequently seen in the Mideast [12-15] but is not restricted to that part of the world.[8, 13, 16, 17] There is considerable variation in each of the three components of the syndrome. Not only are upper intestinal malignant lymphomas seen, but also malignant lymphomas apparently involving only the mesenteric lymph nodes,[15] carcinoma of the stomach or colon,[18, 19] benign nodular lymphoid hyperplasia of the gastrointestinal tract,[16-19] and plasma cell infiltrates in the total absence of any detectable malignancy.[15] Varying degrees of other histologic changes have been described in the intestinal villi.[14, 20] Malabsorption is not an inevitable accompaniment of upper small intestinal lymphoma, and the association appears to be age-dependent in part.[8] However, most authors imply that malabsorption is essential to the syndrome. In some instances there is a deficiency of immunoglobulins,[18, 19] but in others there is an increased production of immunoglobulins.[13-15, 17] Upper intestinal lymphoma and malabsorption have been described in the absence of reported immunologic abnormalities.[20, 21]

More questions than answers have been generated by these reports. Haghighi and Nasr [14] have pointed out the lack of knowledge of what represents "normal" intestinal villi in many of these populations. The syndrome differs around the world and may well be more than one entity. The association of intestinal parasites [18, 19] or viruses [13] needs much more study. Supporting the infectious origin concept are the reported responses to antibiotic therapy,[13, 14] but these responses are not uniform and may simply represent the treatment of a secondary complication. As previously shown, various authors disagree on which of the three features — upper intestinal lymphoma, malabsorption, immunologic abnormalities — are essential to the diagnosis and which is the primary lesion. Whether the plasma cell infiltrate emphasized by Rappaport et al [15] and described by others [14] is indicative of the fundamental underlying change, what its relationship to a possible preexisting immunologic abnormality in the patient may be, and whether the benign plasma cell proliferation may eventually become malignant are all problems for further study.

Some mention of the relationship of malignant lymphomas and pseudolymphomas to other disease entities should be made. Liebow et al [22] have described "lymphoid granulomatosis" of the lung. This certainly is a "pseudolymphoma." Some of their patients died with evidence of malignant lymphoma of one sort or another. While intestinal involvement occurred in only one of the 40 patients, lymphoid granulomatosis may be important as a model for studying the course of other lymphoproliferative diseases. Three of the 12 patients with the plasma cell type of giant lymph node hyperplasia reported by Keller et al [23] had mesenteric lymph node involvement and elevated serum globulins; some of these 12 had hypergammaglobulinemia. Steatorrhea was not described. The authors' histologic description of the lymph nodes is very reminiscent of the plasma cell infiltrate in the intestinal wall described by Rappaport et al.[15]

The current studies of B- and T-lymphocytes eventually may lead to much more understanding of the true nature of both pseudolymphomas and malignant lymphomas. So far, no studies of whether gastrointestinal lymphomas are of B-cell or T-cell type have been made.[24] Similarly, the relationship of pseudolymphomas to "immunoblastic lymphadenopathy" and "immunoblastic lymphoma" needs to be studied.

Four more examples of malignant lymphoma of the colon in patients with ulcerative colitis have been reported.[25] The presence of benign lymphoid polyposis of the colon in association with familial multiple polyposis and an incomplete Gardner's syndrome has been described.[26] Shaw is properly conservative in his interpretation of this association and of the significance of lymphoid polyposis in general. Finally, cases of familial multiple polyposis of the colon have been interpreted erroneously as lymphoid hyperplasia on roentgenologic studies.[27] This inability of any physician to separate the rare and obscure from the common and ordinary has been described best by Thurber.[28]

References

1. Hampson LG: Discussion of ref. 6 (following)
2. Kobayashi S, Prolla JC, Kirsner JB: Reactive lymphoreticular hyperplasia of the stomach. Arch Intern Med 125:1030, 1970
3. Nelson RS, Lanza FL, Bottiglieri NG: Lymphoreticular hyperplasia of the stomach (pseudolymphoma). Gastrointest Endosc 19:183, 1973
4. Bush RS, Ash CL: Primary lymphoma of the gastrointestinal tract. Radiology 92:1349, 1969
5. Freeman C, Berg JW, Cutler SJ: Occurrence and prognosis of extranodal lymphomas. Cancer 29:252, 1972
6. Hoerr SO, McCormack LJ, Hertzer NR: Prognosis in gastric lymphoma. Arch Surg 107:155, 1973
7. Jenkin RDT, Sonley MJ, Stephens CA, Darte JMM, Peters MV: Primary gastrointestinal tract lymphoma in childhood. Radiology 92:763, 1969
8. Kahn LB, Selzer G, Kaschula ROC: Primary gastrointestinal lymphoma: a clinicopathological study of 57 cases. Am J Dig Dis 17:219, 1972
9. Loehr WJ, Mujahed Z, Zahn FD, Gray GF, Thorbjarnarson B: Primary lymphoma of the gastrointestinal tract: a review of 100 cases. Ann Surg 170:232, 1969
10. Naqvi MS, Burrows L, Kark AE: Lymphoma of the gastrointestinal tract: prognostic guides based on 162 cases. Ann Surg 170:221, 1969
11. Kline TS, Goldstein F: Malignant lymphoma involving the stomach. Cancer 32:961, 1973

12. Al-Khateeb AK: Primary malignant lymphoma of the small intestine. Int Surg 54:295, 1970
13. Eidelman S: Abdominal lymphoma with malabsorption. JAMA 229: 1103, 1974
14. Haghighi P, Nasr K: Primary upper small intestinal lymphoma (so-called Mediterranean lymphoma). Pathol Annu 8:231, 1973
15. Rappaport H, Ramot B, Hulu N, Park JK: The pathology of so-called Mediterranean abdominal lymphoma with malabsorption. Cancer 29:1502, 1972
16. Davis SD, Eidelman S, Loop JW: Nodular lymphoid hyperplasia of the small intestine and sarcoidosis. Arch Intern Med 126:668, 1970
17. Kopec M, Swierczynska Z, Pazdur J, et al: Diffuse lymphoma of the intestines with a monoclonal gammopathy of IgG$_3$ kappa type. Am J Med 56:381, 1974
18. Hermans PE, Huizenga KA, Hoffman HN, Brown AL, Markowitz H: Dysgammaglobulinemia associated with nodular lymphoid hyperplasia of the small intestine. Am J Med 40:78, 1966
19. Hermans PE: Nodular lymphoid hyperplasia of the small intestine and hypogammaglobulinemia: theoretical and practical considerations. Fed Proc 26:1606, 1967
20. Brunt PW, Sircus W, Maclean N: Neoplasia and the coeliac syndrome in adults. Lancet 1:180, 1969
21. Spence WJE, Ritchie S: Lymphomas of the small bowel and their relationship to idiopathic steatorrhea. Can J Surg 12:207, 1969
22. Liebow AA, Carrington CRB, Friedman PJ: Lymphomatoid granulomatosis. Hum Pathol 3:457, 1972
23. Keller AR, Hochholzer L, Castleman B: Hyaline-vascular and plasma-cell types of giant lymph node hyperplasia of the mediastinum and other locations. Cancer 29:670, 1972
24. Lukes RJ: Personal communication, 1974
25. Nugent FW, Zuberi S, Bulan MB, Legg MA: Colonic lymphoma in ulcerative colitis: report of four cases. Lahey Clinic Foundation Bulletin 21:104, 1972
26. Shaw EB, Hennigar GR: Intestinal lymphoid polyposis. Am J Clin Pathol 61:417, 1974
27. Neitzschman HR, Genet E, Nice CM Jr: Two cases of familial polyposis simulating lymphoid hyperplasia. Am J Roentgenol Radium Ther Nucl Med 119:365, 1973
28. Thurber JG: The bear who let it alone. In: Fables for Our Time and Famous Poems Illustrated. New York, Harper, 1940 (reprinted 1954), pp 32–33

HISTOGENESIS AND BIOLOGIC BEHAVIOR OF GASTRIC CARCINOMA

R. M. MULLIGAN

The present paper might be entitled "Gastric Carcinoma Revisited." It includes a consideration of various aspects of the ultrastructure and regeneration of the cells of the gastric mucosa; their pathophysiology; the epidemiology of gastric carcinoma as related to pernicious anemia, intestinal cell metaplasia, and polyps; and a summation of the gastric carcinoma experience of Colorado General Hospital from 1927 through 1968. With few exceptions, the papers reviewed are those that have appeared since our paper in 1954.[1]

Gastric Mucosal Cells

Normal epithelial cells are concerned with secretion, except for the mucous neck cell, which acts mainly as a replenisher of the mucous cell. The mucous, chief, parietal, and pyloric and cardiac gland cells secrete directly into the lumen. The enterochromaffin and gastrin cells most likely secrete into the bloodstream. The only cell with an absorptive function is the metaplastic intestinal cell. This abnormal cell often coexists with acquired Paneth cells in the gastric crypts. Once formed, the chief cell, parietal cell, pyloric and cardiac gland cells, enterochromaffin cell, and the gastrin cell seem to have long lives, comparable to that of the liver cell.[2] Metaplastic intestinal epithelial cells are able to regenerate by mitosis. Paneth cells are an enigma, whether they appear normally in the small intestine or are acquired in the stomach.

Mucous Neck Cell

Salenius [3] was able to identify mucous neck cells in the gastric mucosa of 11- to 12-week-old embryos. Bélanger [4] studied 10-day-old rats by subcutaneous injection of ^{35}S in the form of weak sulfuric acid. One hour later the mucous neck cells were labeled, but 48 hours later they were not. He concluded that these cells produce a mucoprotein containing a sulfomucopolysaccharide. In young adult Long-Evans rats of both sexes given tritiated thymidine at 1 μc/g of body weight, at 7 hours the mucous neck cells were labeled primarily and the mucous cells secondarily. The label was still present in these cells at 6 days.[5] In the gastric mucosa of two men, 52 and 58 years old, with carcinomatosis, MacDonald, Trier, and Everett [6] found mucous neck cells labeled by injected tritiated thymidine and migration of these cells to the surface in 4 to 6 days. Teir and Räsänen [7] noted mitoses in the mucous neck cells of the noninvolved fundic and antral mucosa of patients with duodenal and gastric ulcer and gastric carcinoma. Clark and Baker [8] observed the highest level of mitoses in mucous neck cells at 8 AM and the lowest at midnight in young adult female Sprague-Dawley rats killed at 2-hour intervals. Hypophysectomy greatly depressed the levels of mitoses at 8 AM. Seen by electron microscopy, the bases of the mucous neck cells [9] are filled with many short, wide cisternae and particle-coated endoplasmic reticulum, among which are scattered mitochondria of medium size. Toward the apex of these cells, the amount of ribosomal material diminishes and light mucous granules appear.

Mucous Cell

The mucous cell is constantly replenished by the mitotic division and differentiation of the mucous neck cell. The mucous cell elaborates abundant mucin, a glycoprotein, to protect the gastric mucosa from autodigestion. Salenius [3] found mucous cells at 11 weeks of gestation in the human stomach on the lesser curvature of the antrum, and on the greater curvature at 13 to 15 weeks. Clark and Baker [8] found the highest level of mitoses in surface mucous cells at 4 AM and 8 AM and the lowest level at midnight in young female Sprague-Dawley rats sacrificed at 2-hour intervals. In the human, as seen by electron microscopy, mucous droplets are bunched in the apex of the mucous cell.[9] The droplets are unique membrane-enclosed granules, 0.7 to 1.3 μ in diameter, with a uniformly dotted or thread-like appearance. Golgi complexes, single mucous granules, and many small vesicles of smooth endoplasmic reticulum appear between the nucleus and the apical conglomerate of mucous granules. Beneath the nucleus the cytoplasm is filled with diffuse fibrillar material, some fine granules, a few clusters of mitochrondria about 0.2 μ in length, and relatively little ribosome-studded endoplasmic reticulum. The basal cell membrane is infolded at regular intervals of 800 Å near the basement membrane. The spaces between the cells are bridged by cytoplasmic processes of the same size. Helander and Ekholm observed similar ultrastructural features in the mucous cells of the mouse.[10] Intraperitoneal ethionine given to young adult rats in large doses failed to alter the mucous cells over a period of 41 days.[11] (See Figs. 36 and 37.)

In countries where there is a low risk of gastric carcinoma, such as the United States, the mucous cell is cancerized by whatever mechanisms are operative. The carcinoma cell so evolved might be amenable to treatment by glycoprotein identical to or closely similar to that synthesized by the normal mucous cell, as previously suggested for the glycoprotein thyroglobulin in the treatment of thyroid carcinoma.[12]

Chief Cell

In the stomach of the 12-week human embryo, Salenius [3] observed ribonucleic acid in morphologic chief cells as well as many black granules (with the Heidenhain iron hematoxylin stain). No labeling of chief cells of the stomachs of two men, 52 and 58 years old, with carcinomatosis was found [6] by giving them injections of tritiated thymidine and performing follow-up serial gastric biopsies for 4 to 6 days. Mitoses were not observed by Teir and Räsänen [7] in the chief cells of the nondiseased portions of the gastric mucosa of patients with duodenal and gastric ulcer and with gastric carcinoma.

By electron microscopy, the apex of the chief cell [9] contains numerous zymogen granules interspersed with mitochondria, a few oval 0.3-μ myelin figures, and various components of closely stacked, very dense endoplasmic reticulum. The 1- to 3-μ zymogen granules are light, finely granular, homogeneous, and encased in a smooth membrane, single around the larger granules. The subnuclear cytoplasm is filled with very long cisternae of particle-coated endoplasmic reticulum closely packed in parallel array. A few mitochondria are interposed. The surface plasma membrane is marked by uniform, short microvilli and a few invaginations along the lateral margins below the apical desmosomes. These characteristics appear in chief cells at all levels of the crypts. Helander and Ekholm [10] noted similar features in the chief cells of the gastric mucosa of the mouse.

More striking changes in the chief cell have been recorded in experiments than in any other normal cell of the stomach, as exemplified in the following four papers. In hypophysectomized young adult Sprague-Dawley and Long-Evans rats [13] observed for 3 to 108 days, the chief cells were reduced in size, cytoplasmic basophilia was lost, pepsinogen granules were depleted, mitochondria were decreased, and nuclei became pyknotic. These changes were maximal at 3 days and remained stable for 23 to 108 days. Gastric secretion and pepsin activity were decreased as these changes appeared. Young adult albino Wistar rats [11] given intraperitoneal ethionine, 25 and 50 mg every other day or 300 mg daily, exhibited selective ablation of the chief cells between 8 hours and 41 days, with failure of these cells to regenerate. The mitochondria and pepsinogen granules disappeared from the chief cells of adult white rats [14] killed 12 to 14 days after adrenalectomy. In acute experiments with rats and rabbits given calciferol or with rats on parathormone, hyperplasia of gastric chief cells was correlated with hypercalcemia.[15] A rise in the serum calcium level of 1.0 to 1.2 mg/100 ml resulted in a 20 percent increase of chief cells; a 5-mg rise was accompanied by a greater increase of the cells. The gastric mucosa also revealed hyperemia, hemorrhage, and calcification. The authors speculated that chief cell hyperplasia with attendant increased secretion of pepsinogen probably has a relation to the hypercalcemia of hyperparathyroidism. This mechanism could be operative in the syndrome of multiple endocrine adenomapeptic ulcer complex (MEA-PUC).[16]

Parietal Cell

In a 9-week human embryo, succinic dehydrogenase activity was seen at the bottom of fundic gastric crypts within apparent future parietal cells. These were definitely identified in the 11-week embryo as the first differentiated glandular cells of the gastric mucosa.[3] Nomura [17] examined by electron microscopy the fundic mucosa of human 3- to 10-month-old fetuses. He confirmed the parietal cell as the first differentiated cell recognizable at 10 weeks of gestation. Mitochondria were relatively sparse during the first stage studied but became more numerous with increased size of cell; their cristae became more closely packed, and they were almost as numerous at term as in adult parietal cells. Between the fourth and fifth month, the free cell surface invaginated into the cytoplasm with increasing penetration and complexity. From the fourth month onward, a system of flattened cisternae of agranular endoplasmic reticulum became increasingly complex with focal communication with the cell surface. Numerous basal infoldings were evident at term. MacDonald, Trier, and Everett [6] failed to find labeling of the parietal cells of the stomachs of two men, 52 and 58 years old, with carcinomatosis; the two patients were given injections of tritiated thymidine, and gastric biopsy specimens taken for 4 to 6 days were studied. No mitoses were found in the nondiseased portions of the fundic mucosa of patients with duodenal and gastric ulcer and gastric carcinoma.[7]

The parietal cell is very spectacular in reference to both ultrastructure and enzyme content. This is related to the elaboration of hydrochloric acid, a fundamental function involved in digestion of bits of bone and shell swallowed by mammals. The designation of "hydra-headed monster" is not exaggerated, as indicated by a composite summary of the ultrastructural features. The pyramidal shape is conspicuous, with the base resting on the basement membrane. The cytoplasm is packed with large, 0.7-μ, oval mitochondria with closely stacked cristae of the septate type. Numerous profiles of intracellular canaliculi form elongated oval structures with walls of interdigitated microvilli of irregular length and disposition and "unit membrane" appearance. The canaliculi are bordered by plump microvilli with clear centers. Many vacuoles appear throughout the cytoplasm, and surface microvilli are evident. This appearance has been described also as agranular endoplasmic reticulum in the form of branched, anastomosed tubules 200 to 500 Å in diameter. Ribosomes are scattered in the cytoplasm, but rough endoplasmic reticulum is scarce. The nucleus reveals a double membrane, with the outer portion marked by RNA granules. (See Ito,[18], Gusek,[19] and Lillibridge [9] for studies on man; Helander and Ekholm [10] for the mouse; and Lawn [20] for the rat.)

Hypophysectomized young adult rats [13] observed for 3 to 108 days developed smaller parietal cells with decreased but larger mitochondria. By stimulating the secretion of gastric hydrochloric acid in dogs with vagal nerve excitation, histamine, and insulin, Sedar and Friedman [21] observed (1) a greater concentration of profiles of smooth endoplasmic reticulum adjacent to the walls of intracellular canaliculi, or a great decrease of these profiles; (2) more extensively developed intracellular canaliculi with enlargement of surface area by increased, closely set, elongated microvilli or inconspicuous, nonpatent canaliculi with few associated profiles of endoplasmic reticulum; and (3) matrix of mitochondria less dense and cristae less closely set or absent. The authors interpreted these findings as indicative of varying secretion of hydrochloric acid in adjacent parietal cells.

Pylorocardiac Gland Cell

The least well understood cells of the gastric mucosa are those of the pyloric and cardiac glands. There appear to be few reports of ultrastructural studies of these cells. By light microscopy the cells are low columnar to cuboidal, pale acidophilic, vacuolated, and contain horizontal, compact, basal, ovoid nuclei seen with routine stains. They are intensely positive with the periodic acid-fuchsin-sulfurous acid method, sparingly mucinocarminophilic, and moderately positive with the Best carmine technique. These features carry over to the malignant cells of pylorocardiac gland cell carcinoma. The function of the pyloric and cardiac gland cells is also not well understood. Their close similarity to the cells of Brunner glands of the duodenum might indicate by analogy a function in the neutralization of hydrochloric acid. Salenius [3] observed that the pyloric and cardiac pits develop at 10 weeks of gestation, and that the pyloric glands are formed between 11 and 13 weeks. Teir and Räsänen [7] found no mitoses in these cells in the nondiseased portions of the stomachs of patients with duodenal and gastric ulcer and with gastric carcinoma. (See Fig. 35.)

Carvalheira, Welsch, and Pearse [22] and Pearse [23] placed the enterochromaffin cell (5-hydroxytryptamine) and the gastrin cell of the stomach in the APUD (amine and precursor uptake and decarboxylation) series. Pearse [23] also included the pituitary corticotroph and melanotroph; the pancreatic alpha, beta, and delta cells; and the C-cell of the thyroid, which secrete the polypeptides, corticotropin, melanotropin, glucagon, insulin, gastrin, and calcitonin, in this series.

Enterochromaffin Cell

The enterochromaffin or argentaffin cells are present throughout the gastric mucosa. They are characterized by the Masson-Hamperl, Bodian, and Davenport argyrophilic methods; positive by argentaffin, diazonium, and xanthydrol tests; blue-black to blue-violet with toluidine blue after hydrochloric acid; variably fluorescent when exposed to ultraviolet light after treatment with hydrochloric acid-pseudoisocyanin; and yellow fluorescent after formaldehyde fixation.[22, 24] By electron microscopy,[24] the enterochromaffin cell contains many irregular osmiophilic granules 150 to 400 μ, a well developed Golgi complex, free ribosomes, and a few profiles of endoplasmic reticulum near the nucleus. These cells are the source of carcinoid tumors.[25]

Gastrin Cell

The gastrin cells are localized mainly in the antral mucosa. They are red to violet with hydrochloric acid-toluidine blue and always fluoresce in ultraviolet light after hydrochloric acid-pseudoisocyanin.[24] They are also called cholinesterase cells because of their rich content of this enzyme, seen by the Bodian argyrophil reaction. The gastrin cell can pick up and decarboxylate parenterally injected dioxyphenyl-alanine and then demonstrate green fluorescence after freezing and exposure to formaldehyde vapor.[22] The cell is rich in nongranular E-600-resistant esterase and nonspecific cholinesterase, and is positive for carboxyl groups with toluidine blue metachromasia. Hydrochloric acid-toluidine blue plus the diazonium reaction differentially stains enterochromaffin cells black and gastrin cells red. Seen by electron microscopy,[24] the base of the gastrin cell is applied to the basement membrane of the pyloric glands. The gastrin cell contains variable infranuclear, rounded secretory granules enveloped by a thin membrane. The internal core of the granules is of low density and 150 to 300 μ in diameter. Endoplasmic reticulum is well developed, especially when granules are scarce. Supranuclear Golgi complexes are prominent. Mitochondria, lysosomes, and small vesicles are scattered throughout the cytoplasm. Tufts of microvilli project into the lumen of the pyloric glands. The granules of the gastrin cell represent gastrin (human I and II), a polypeptide with 17 amino acids, the C-terminal four of which are physiologically active.[26] The secretion of gastrin into the bloodstream activates intramural ganglionic cells, which regulate the elaboration of hydrochloric acid by the parietal cells.[27, 28] The gastrin or G cells may be identical to the D cells of the pancreatic islets [24] in man. If this hypothesis is correct, tumors of the D cells in the MEA-PUC syndrome [16] may be found in the pancreas or adjacent tissues, including the wall of the duodenum.

A consideration of the structure, function, and potential of the metaplastic intestinal epithelial cell appears under a separate heading in a later section.

Regeneration of Gastric Mucosa

Small wounds placed in the fundic mucosa of young adult female Sprague-Dawley rats were followed by migration of mucous neck cells from adjacent sound crypts, with numerous mitoses resulting in regeneration of mucous, chief, and parietal cells.[29] Specific stains were used to identify mucin, pepsinogenic granules, and succinic dehydrogenase in mucous, chief, and parietal cells. These microscopic findings were confirmed by others with tritiated thymidine labeling in animals that had similar mucosal defects.[29] Thus, the mucous neck cell is the stem cell of the gastric mucosa. Mucous cells are regenerated continuously and the chief and parietal cells are restored only under special circumstances. The renewal of pyloric and cardiac gland cells is still to be investigated. Probably, as is the case with chief and parietal cells, the pyloric and cardiac gland cells are long-lived in the normal animal.

Enzymes of Normal and Cancerous Cells of Gastric Mucosa

The enzymes of mucous neck and mucous cells display no special activity as compared to those of the chief and parietal cells. The enzymes of metaplastic intestinal cells are described in a subsequent section.

Chief Cell

Correia, Filipe, and Santos [30] and Ragins and Dittbrenner [31] found the chief cells positive for acid phosphatase, with the greatest activity in the apex. The first group [30] also noted diffuse activity for nonspecific esterases and 5-nucleotidase in the chief cells. The presence of pepsinogen in the granules of the chief cells is self-evident.

Parietal Cell

The parietal cell is supplied with a great variety of enzymes undoubtedly related to the secretion of hydrochloric acid. In adult albino Sprague-Dawley rats Villareal and Burgos [32] found succinic dehydrogenase in the parietal cells; this is an enzyme stimulated by acetyl-beta-methylcholine and depressed by an organic mercurial, presumably through combination of the metal with the sulfhydryl groups of the enzyme. Niemi, Siurala, and Sandberg [33] and Correia, Filipe, and Santos [30] confirmed the presence of this enzyme in the parietal cells. Lactic dehydrogenase,[33] diphosphopyridine nucleotide diaphorase,[30, 33] triphosphopyridine nucleotide diaphorase,[30] and nicotinamide adenine dinucleotide-reduced tetrazolium reductase [31] have been demonstrated in the parietal cells. The enzymes demonstrated were localized to the mitochondria of these cells [33] and were stimulated by histamine.[30]

Carcinoma Cells

Planteydt and Willighagen [34] found several enzymes in gastric carcinoma cells which were not identified as to type—i.e., mucous cell, pylorocardiac gland cell, or intestinal cell. These investigators observed no appreciable difference in the cells of the differentiated and undifferentiated gastric carcinomas. Acid phosphatase was present in 48 of 50 carcinomas; succinic and four other dehydrogenases in 29 of 32; lactic dehydrogenase in each of 32; and aminopeptidase in 17 of 50. One photomicrograph of intestinal cell carcinoma type 1 revealed malignant cells positive for aminopeptidase.[34]

Mast Cells

Räsänen [35] studied the gastric mucosa of male Wistar rats, 122 to 155 g and 3 to 4 months old, with one dose of 25 mg and seven doses of 25 mg of cortisone, and seven doses of 4 units of corticotropin; results showed progressively severe degranulation of the mast cells therein as compared to the mast cells of control rats. Somatotropin, seven doses of 20 tibia units, resulted in a tremendous increase in granules in mast cells of the gastric mucosa.

Cytology of Gastric Mucosa

For those interested in gastric cytology, Raskin, Palmer, and Kirsner [36] published a paper with 37 colored illustrations of esophagus, stomach, duodenum, and colon in various disease states, including pernicious anemia and gastric carcinoma.

Gastric Juice

The four constituents of gastric juice investigated relatively recently are mucin, carbohydrates, amino acids, and intrinsic factor. Substances with an influence on gastric function include glucagon, glucose, and fatty acids.

Mucin

Hoskins and Zamcheck [37] collected the gastric juice from fasted hospital patients and normal persons and processed the material to powder with a content of 65 percent protein and 35 percent carbohydrate. Epithelial mucins of this type are polymers of proteins bound to polysaccharides, which are very hygroscopic and highly viscous in solution. The polysaccharide portion includes hexoses, hexosamines, fucose, sialic acid, and a small amount of hexuronic acids. Sialic acid is a collective term for the natural derivatives of neuraminic acid: N-acetyl-, N-glycolyl-, and N,O-diacetyl-. The first predominates, with a pK of 2.6, occupies a probable terminal site in the polysaccharides, is easily hydrolyzed, and accounts for 2.1 percent of the powder analyzed. In such glycoproteins as gastric mucin, sialic acid occurs as the terminal portion of a disaccharide prosthetic group, N-acetylneuraminic acid and N-acetylgalactosamine linked by glutamic acid and aspartic acid at regular intervals along a protein core.[38] At a pH above 2.6, the carboxyl groups of sialic acid are largely dissociated and may be thought of as forming a loose shield of negative charges around a protein core.

In a 72-year-old man with mucinous adenocarcinoma of the stomach massively metastatic to the liver, Green and Bergman [39] found a unique serum protein precipitated by 3 percent acetic acid and containing the following (by percents): nitrogen 12, protein 55 (Biuret), hexose 7.1, hexosamine 1.8, sialic acid 5.4, and fucose 0.8. The inference in this case was that the mucin secreted by the neoplastic epithelial cells entered the blood in free form. The significant levels of hexose and sialic acid are confirmed by analysis of the gastric juice from patients with gastric carcinoma detailed in two papers cited in the following section.

Carbohydrates

Richmond, Caputto, and Wolf [40] studied the carbohydrate and protein composition of the gastric juice of normal persons and of patients with duodenal ulcer, gastric ulcer, gastric carcinoma, and pernicious anemia. By designating three groups—gastric carcinoma, pernicious anemia, and normal plus duodenal and gastric ulcer cases—their findings in approximate order of magnitude were as follows: total hexoses 80:60:30, hexosamines 50:70:35, fucose 3.0:3.0:1.2, sialic acid 20:20:10, and proteins 500:250:300. The values were expressed in average milligrams per 100 ml after passing dialyzed and lyophilized gastric juice through an Amberlite resin column. Masamune et al.[41] analyzed the carbohydrate content of the gastric carcinomas and adjacent uninvolved mucosa in an unstated number of cases in which the type of carcinoma was not identified. The percentages of various components in cancerous and noncancerous mucosa were, respectively, as follows: nitrogen 6.9 and 7.3, total hexosamine 26.4 and 25.0, galactose 21.8 and 26.7, fucose 6.7 and 10.9, and sialic acid 18.3 and 1.4. Schrager [42] studied the carbohydrate components of gastric polysaccharides in 36 control subjects and in 64 with duodenal ulcer, 16 with gastric ulcer, and 12 with gastric carcinoma. As compared with the other three groups, the patients with gastric carcinoma had greatly increased values for glucose and comparable or greatly reduced levels of galactose.

Amino Acids

In the gastric juice of 12 patients with peptic ulcer (six gastric, three duodenal, and three gastroduodenal), Shimizu [43] found 2+ levels of amino acids as follows: leucine in three, valine in three, and alanine in four. In 28 patients with gastric carcinoma and satisfactory data, he found 3+ levels of amino acids as follows: leucine in 19, valine in 17, and alanine in 11. Six other amino acids in this group were 3+ in three to seven patients. The level of hydrochloric acid and free amino acids did not correlate in this study. In six of eight cases of carcinoma after gastrectomy, the values of amino acids were 1+ as follows: leucine in two, valine in one, and alanine in three.

Oh-Uti and Awataguchi [44] studied the amino acids in the gastric juice of 68 patients with gastric carcinoma, 15 treated by total gastrectomy, 43 by subtotal gastrectomy, and 10 unresectable. Leucine, valine, alanine, serine plus glycine, and glutamic acid were strongly positive in 19 of 51 cases and positive in 17 of 49, depending upon which amino acid was tested. Positive values were found for proline, threonine, and a peptide in 33, 17, and 22 cases respectively. The presence of the amino acids was not related to the level of hydrochloric acid or to the histologic features of the tumor; it was equivocally related to the size of the tumor. Following resection in 43 cases, leucine, valine, alanine, serine plus glycine, and glutamic acid were strongly positive in only one to four cases; proline was positive in only three; and threonine and the peptide were absent.

Abasov [45] determined (in gammas per milliliters of gastric juice) the levels of alanine and leucine in: 25 normal persons, 5.6 and 7.1, respectively; 25 patients with chronic gastritis, 5.8 and 8.5; 55 with gastric ulcer, 6.4 and 8.4; 12 with gastric polyposis, 5.9 and 8.0; and 100 with gastric cancer, 13.8 and 19.6. In none of the five groups were hydrochloric acid values, the volume of gastric secretion, or the histologic type of carcinoma correlated with the levels of these amino acids. The chromatograms were most saturated, and alanine and leucine levels were the highest, with large gastric cancers. In six of these, serum amino acid nitrogen, alanine, and leucine were normal. The author interpreted the increased levels of alanine and leucine as reflecting metabolic products of neoplastic cells. After resection of the cancers in 17 patients, the levels of these two amino acids returned to normal; but in three with recurrent cancer following gastric resection, they again attained preoperative values.

Intrinsic Factor

Hoedemaeker et al.[46, 47] located the production of intrinsic factor in man as being in the parietal cell; they used radioactive vitamin B_{12} and observed by autoradiography the affinity of this substance for the parietal cell. Prevention of vitamin B_{12} uptake by the parietal cell was accomplished by incubating sections of fundic mucosa with human antibody to intrinsic factor. The cat, rabbit, guinea pig, rhesus monkey, and ox also produce intrinsic factor in the parietal cells, but in the rat and the mouse chief cells are the site of its formation, and in the hog the glandular cells of pylorus and duodenum elaborate this substance.

Gastric Secretion and Hyperglycemia

Solomon and Spiro [48] found that continuous intravenous infusion of glucagon consistently decreased the output of gastric acid and pepsin for several hours. Intravenous 10 percent glucose variably depressed the output of gastric acid and pepsin. Infused glucagon and glucose consistently raised gastric pH and lowered gastric pepsin concentration throughout the period of administration.

Dotevall [49] studied 1,218 diabetics, nine with duodenal ulcer (compared with an expected number of 33) and 13 with gastric ulcer (compared with 13 expected). He found that hyperglycemia was an effective suppressor of gastric secretion, and that diabetics secreted significantly less hydrochloric acid as compared to control subjects.

Gastric Absorption and Fatty Acids

In 11 subjects fed test meals of suspensions of potassium and sodium salts of saturated fatty acids, C-2 to C-18, acetic acid through decanoic acid (C-2 to C-10) were relatively ineffective in slowing emptying of the stomach. The C-2 to C-10 fatty acids are absorbed mainly into the portal blood with little duodenal esterification. Added sodium citrate did not change the results with C-2 to C-10 fatty acids. The C-12 to C-18 fatty acids were about four times more effective than the C-2 to C-10 compounds in slowing emptying of the stomach, with the salts of myristic acid or C-14 more active than those of C-12 or C-16. The C-12 to C-18 fatty acids are absorbed mostly by lymphatics. Sodium citrate at pH 8 increased the delayed gastric emptying induced by the C-12 to C-18 fatty acids.[50]

Pepsinogen and Uropepsin

Hoar and Browning [51] determined serum pepsinogen levels by the Mirsky method, which is based on the release of tyrosine residues from a hemoglobin substrate and measurement by a colorimetric procedure. The average results found in several persons (in tyrosine units per milligram of plasma) were as follows: 89 controls, 486; 74 duodenal ulcer patients, 689; 47 with subtotal gastrectomy, 314; 15 with gastric ulcer, 705; 5 with gastric carcinoma, 388 (652 in a sixth case and no correlation with type in any of the six); 5 with total gastrectomy, 147; and 33 with pernicious anemia, 132.

Bock et al.[52] determined serum pepsinogen levels in 100 normal persons, with the average of 196 units for men, 167 units for women, and 181 for both sexes. In 50 pernicious anemia patients, 47 to 88 years of age with a 1:3 male/female ratio, the range of serum pepsinogen was 30 to 90 units/ml (average 61 units/ml). Bock's group also studied serum pepsinogen levels in four other groups of persons as follows: normal 178 units/ml, superficial gastritis 140, atrophic gastritis 105, and gastric atrophy 65. The response to the secretion of hydrochloric acid stimulated by histamine was directly proportional to these decreasing serum pepsinogen values.

Uropepsin is a proteolytic enzyme found in the urine. It is elevated in persons with duodenal ulcer and low or absent in those with pernicious anemia; it tends to drop after partial gastrectomy and disappears after total gastrectomy.[51] The precursor of uropepsin and gastric pepsin is pepsinogen secreted by the chief cells.

In male students given injections of testosterone proprionate,[53] uropepsin became elevated in every case, from the control and placebo levels often to double the baseline values. Similar results were found in older indigent subjects.

Practical points gained from the preceding two sections are that screening tests to analyze gastric secretion should be performed in patients suspected of gastric carcinoma. If carcinoma is present, the tests would show: (1) elevated sialic acid, glucose, and fucose levels; and (2) increased free leucine, valine, and alanine concentrations. A correlation of these tests with the type of gastric carcinoma would be desirable. Screening patients with suspected gastric atrophy, with or without pernicious anemia, and patients with gastric polyps for serum or plasma pepsinogen might turn up intestinal cell carcinoma in these high-risk groups.

Epidemiology of Gastric Carcinoma

The frequency and trend of gastric carcinoma in the United States and other countries, some apparently significant features of etiology, and a familial tendency to gastric carcinoma are to be discussed in this section.

Frequency and Trend

Boles,[54] in a general review of gastric carcinoma, found the following incidence, as deaths per 100,000, in the United States: 28.9 in 1930, 26.5 in 1935, 22.5 in 1940, 20.0 in 1945, 16.0 in 1950, and 13.0 in 1955. In an extensive survey of the incidence and mortality from stomach cancer in the United States and other countries,[55] the figures given by Boles [54] essentially were confirmed. In the same study [55] the incidence of gastric cancer per 100,000 population in 1950 in several countries was found to be: Japan 67.5; Finland 65.5; Norway 42.1; Denmark 32.5; Sweden 31.7; United States—white 16.3, and nonwhite 23.6. In both groups in the United States, the male/female ratio was about 2:1. Higher rates were observed among lower socioeconomic groups; there were no clear-cut urban-rural differences, and higher rates occurred in northern latitudes. An astonishing feature of one rate distribution map was a rate of 130+ per 100,000 population in southeastern Colorado and northeastern New Mexico, a large portion accounted for by the San Luis Valley. This may have significance with regard to the clientele of the Colorado General Hospital, since many Spanish-American names appear in the records of patients with gastric carcinoma in this hospital, especially since 1954.[1]

In Iceland, Sigurjonsson [56] found the crude death rates for gastric carcinoma per 100,000 males to be 79.8 during the interval 1941–1945 and 55.6 during 1959–1963, a drop of 30 percent. During the same periods, the rates per 100,000 females were 53.6 and 33.7, respectively, a drop of 37 percent. Little change in mortality from all cancers combined occurred during these two time periods, and there was no increase in mortality from cancer of the digestive organs.

Etiology

In 1959 in Iceland, Dungal [57] saw 136 cancers of the alimentary tract, 16 of the esophagus, 89 of the stomach, 24 of the colon, and 7 of the rectum. He found a high level of polycyclic hydrocarbons in the diet—in smoked salmon, trout, and mutton—especially in Northwest Iceland. A tremendously high rate of 132 gastric cancers per 100,000 population was reported in the Westman Islands south of Iceland. The houses on these islands are heated with coal and oil and are supplied with water from rain that drips from the sooty roofs into barrels.

On a worldwide basis, Haenszel [55] found a higher gastric cancer risk among persons using rice as a staple, compared to those supplementing rice with other cereals. A lower risk was observed among users of soybean products, such as shoyu and miso. In the United States, he noted increased consumption of citrus fruits, tomato juice, and lettuce, which displaced cabbage as the main leafy vegetable, and decreased intake of potatoes and wheat flour. In persons with high income, intake of beef, milk, citrus fruits, and green vegetables was notable.

A possibly favorable effect on the incidence of gastric carcinoma in the United States is the increased ingestion of methylated purines such as the caffeine in coffee and cola drinks. The availability of these purines as building blocks for the repair of altered nucleic acids in the gastric mucosal cells should be considered.

Between 1951 and 1960 in Iceland, Sigurjonsson [58] found the following percentages of deaths from gastric cancer in five male occupational groups in the 35- to 64-year-old range: farmers 25.0, laborers 19.0, seamen 15.5, craftsmen 9.9, and white collar workers 8.4. In men 65 years of age and older the same trend was evident, with the first three groups being notably more often the victims of gastric cancer than the last two groups. This decrease of risk from gastric cancer was correlated with increasing economic status and with lesser consumption of home-smoked and singed foods by the last two groups. There was drastically reduced contact with 3,4-benzpyrene and other polycyclic hydrocarbons found in these foods. Sigurjonsson [58] attributed the downward trend in gastric cancer in Iceland from 1950 onward to the shift from farm-smoked to commercially smoked food, with a decreased intake of these carcinogens by the entire population.

Familial Tendency

Several papers concerning risk of gastric carcinoma in the relatives of patients with the disease have appeared. The most carefully controlled study was that by Videbaek and Mosbech,[59] who studied 198 men and 104 women who were the relatives of patients with gastric carcinoma and also had the disease. The incidence of gastric carcinoma among the male relatives was 5.0 percent and among the female relatives 4.0 percent, compared to 1.4 percent for males and 1.0 percent for females among the relatives of 390 healthy persons (219 men and 171 women). In the affected relatives of patients with gastric carcinoma, 41 percent of the cancers were primary in the stomach. In the affected relatives of the 390 healthy persons, 17 percent of the cancers were in the stomach. The authors indicated that the relatives (both male and female) of patients with gastric carcinoma were at a calculated risk four times that of the relatives of healthy persons. They concluded that hereditary disposition to gastric carcinoma may be a factor in the high frequency of the disease among relatives of afflicted patients.

A final point to be discussed under the pathology of gastric carcinoma, also pertaining to its epidemiology, is the apparent dominance of intestinal cell carcinoma in countries with a high risk of gastric carcinoma,[60-62] as compared to a high incidence of mucous cell carcinoma in countries with a low risk of gastric cancer.

Pernicious Anemia

The increased susceptibility of patients with pernicious anemia to gastric carcinoma has been known for many years. The most important precancerous condition is intestinal cell metaplasia of the gastric mucosa attendant upon atrophy of the chief and parietal cells. In some manner not yet elucidated, the mucous neck cells undergo a transformation into cells of intestinal epithelial type, rather than maturing normally to mucous cells. Several studies on pernicious anemia point to the direct cancerization of metaplastic intestinal epithelial cells in polyps or in the flat gastric mucosa.

Among 219 females and 82 males with pernicious anemia studied between 1928 and 1949, the disease was diagnosed at an average age of 57 years, and the average follow-up was 10.5 years.[63] During observation, 83 females and 32 males died (expected deaths: 89 females and 28 males). Eight females and six males died of gastric carcinoma established by radiography, operation, autopsy, or a combination of these methods, with six confirmed by microscopic study. A seventh male alive 6 months after operation was included. The total of 15 gastric carcinomas was nearly three times the expected figure of 5.2 cases. They were located as follows: pylorus five, body six, fundus two, and diffuse two.

Schell, Dockerty, and Comfort [64] credited H. E. Robertson with demonstrating that the flattened, atrophic mucosa of necropsied patients with pernicious anemia revealed microscopic intestinalization of the mucous cell elements, with subsequent hyperplasia of the metaplastic intestinal epithelial cells. Robertson contended that when treatment of the anemia would allow many patients to live into the "cancer age," a great increase of gastric carcinoma would occur. Schell's group found 94 gastric carcinomas associated with pernicious anemia between 1906 and 1950. The 94 patients included 67 men and 27 women (ratio 2.5: 1), whose age averaged 55.1 years when the pernicious anemia was recognized and 61.7 years at the diagnosis of carcinoma. Of these 94 patients, 48 had the gastric carcinoma excised and 46 had an exploratory laparotomy or no operation. Of the 49 surgical specimens, 39 (81.3 percent) were of the Borrmann I or II gross type. Of the 63 carcinomas in these 48 surgically excised cases, 61 were located as follows: antrum 13, fundus and cardia 41, and antrum and fundus 7. Among the 48, two primary carcinomas were discovered in 15 patients and one in 33. Microscopic foci of carcinoma in situ appeared in the mucosa away from the obvious carcinomas in several cases. Two carcinomas presented as an en plaque or superficial spreading lesions. Benign mucosal polyps were found in three patients. Of interest in the entire series of 94 cases was the following temporal distribution: 1906–1930, 8; 1931–1935, 18; 1936–1940, 20; 1941–1945, 21; and 1946–1950, 17. The authors concluded that gastric carcinoma in association with pernicious anemia tends to be late in producing symptoms; always is associated with achlorhydria; is often polypoid, fundic or cardiac, and multicentric; and is of a lower average histopathologic grade than most gastric carcinomas.

Between 1945 and 1950, Doehring [65] found eight of 432 patients with pernicious anemia also afflicted with gastric carcinoma, an incidence of 1.8 percent or six times the frequency of gastric carcinoma among the general population. Pernicious anemia was diagnosed at the average age of 56 years, and gastric carcinoma at 68 years. Between 1939 and 1948, autopsies on 13,554 persons over 40 years of age yielded 81 with pernicious anemia, of whom six (7.4 percent) had carcinoma of the stomach. The remaining 13,473 autopsied patients yielded 408 instances of the same cancer, an incidence of 3.0 percent.

Rubin [66] indicated that intestinal cell metaplasia in pernicious anemia was not reversible by treatment of the anemia and was the precursor of intestinal cell carcinoma in four cases, one in a 27-year-old mulatto. Electron and light micrographs of the intestinal epithelial cells supplied with microvilli supported his thesis that these cells are the precursors of intestinal cell carcinoma.

Siurala, Erämaa, and Tapiovaara [67] studied 69 patients with pernicious anemia (13 men and 56 women) whose average age was 66.7 years; six were untreated previously, two were in relapse, and 61 were in remission. The mean duration of the disease was 8.1 years, ranging from 6.5 years in those without tumor, to 11.7 years in those with gastric polyps, to 14.7 years in those with gastric carcinoma. The five patients with gastric carcinoma constituted 7.5 percent of the entire group, and those with polyps 6.0 percent. One of the patients with pernicious anemia and gastric carcinoma was free of disease 8 years after gastric resection. In 1954 in Finland among persons past the age of 60 years, the incidence of gastric carcinoma was 0.34 percent, but in those with pernicious anemia it was 9.8 percent. In a series of 405 patients with a mean age of 66 years and a minimum age of 55 years, 12 diagnoses of gastric carcinoma (1.2 percent) were established by radiography and gastroscopy. Twelve of 963 relatives of 60 patients with pernicious anemia had gastric carcinoma; one was suspected of gastric carcinoma, and one had esophageal cancer. Four of 911 relatives of 54 patients without pernicious anemia had gastric carcinoma; one was suspected of the same cancer, and one had esophageal cancer.

Of 53 patients with atrophic gastritis (31 men and 22 women), with a mean age of 50.8 years and observed for 5.8 years, 11 died—four apparently of gastric carcinoma, two of cardiovascular disease, three of apoplexy, and two of marasmus senilis.[68] Reexamination of 33 available remaining patients of the original series of 53 disclosed one with signs of gastric carcinoma and one with an established gastric polyp. Among 166 control patients (95 men and 71 women), with a mean age of 49.4 years and followed for 6 years, 15 died, but none from gastric carcinoma. Cardiovascular disease was the cause of death in nine, pulmonary cancer in two, breast cancer in two, malignant melanoma in one, and rectal cancer in one.

Grable et al.[69] determined the longest average nuclear diameter of gastric epithelial cells as follows: 24 normal, 6.98μ; 32 pernicious anemia, 9.08μ; and 15 carcinoma, 9.11μ.

Joske, Finckh, and Wood [70] secured two pieces of mucosa from the body of the stomach in 726 patients. In 536 (73.8 percent) the microscopic features were very similar, but in 190 (26.2 percent) there were significant differences. The findings in 1,000 gastric biopsy specimens were as follows: normal 167, slight superficial gastritis 178, moderate to severe gastritis 253, superficial gastritis with atrophy 125, atrophic gastritis 128, severe atrophic gastritis 93, and gastric atrophy 56. Among the 56 cases of gastric atrophy, the fundic mucosa resembled the mucosa of the intestine, averaged 0.42 mm thick, and was often villous. The epithelial cells of the surface and pits were almost all goblet cells, and the crypts often contained Paneth cells. Some specimens had many plasma cells in the lamina propria. Of 100 biopsy specimens from patients with pernicious anemia, 35 had severe atrophic gastritis and 40 had gastric atrophy.

Megaloblastic bone marrow developed in 11 patients—six with gastric adenocarcinoma; two with gastric ulcer; and one each with esophageal varices, hypertrophic gastritis, and esophagitis—who had undergone total gastrectomy for their diseases, had had no prophylaxis for pernicious anemia, and who had survived more than 3 years after operation.[71] Megaloblastic anemia developing after total gastrectomy responds to parenteral vitamin B_{12}.

Intestinal Cell Metaplasia

No more fascinating transformation can be imagined than that observed in the conversion of the stem cell of the gastric mucosa—the mucous neck cell. Normally it is concerned with regeneration of the mucous cell, which has an exclusively secretory function. It becomes so completely changed, however, as to provide a cell that is wholly absorptive.

In his study of the noncancerous mucosa in three cases of gastric carcinoma and one of gastric ulcer, Schmidt [72] was a pioneer in recognizing that gastric mu-

cosal atrophy associated with chronic inflammation may be accompanied by transformation of the gastric epithelium to intestinal epithelium. He was uncertain
as to the genesis and physiologic significance of this change. Ragins and Dittbrenner [31] found high activity for thiamine pyrophosphatase in the Golgi complexes of
metaplastic intestinal epithelial cells.

Klein, Sleisenger, and Weiser [73] studied the antral mucosa of normal persons
and those with intestinalization with regard to three enzymes and glucose-U-^{14}C
uptake. The average unit values in normal and intestinalized mucosa, respectively,
were: sucrase 0.2 and 2.6, maltase 0.4 and 5.6, and leucine aminopeptidase 8.8
and 70.6. The intestinalized mucosa took up significantly more glucose-U-^{14}C compared to normal mucosa.

A patient with pernicious anemia was studied by serial gastric biopsy before
and after administration of three types of high-fat meals given after an 18-hour
fast. Rubin et al.[74] observed in this patient no lipid in the metaplastic intestinal
epithelial cells, but abundant lipid in the subjacent lamina propria in the pre-
prandial biopsy specimen. Two hours after the meals, abundant lipid was present
also in the intestinal epithelial cells, more at the surface of the mucosa than in the
crypts. Lipid was absent or scarce in the mucous epithelial cells and in the subjacent lamina propria. These findings were interpreted as indicative of migration
of lipid from the apex into the base of the intestinal epithelial cells and then into
the lamina propria. The intestinal epithelial cells of the stomach are believed similar to normal jejunal epithelial cells in their physiologic properties. What an ideal
situation for the absorption of fat-soluble carcinogens in the genesis of intestinal
cell carcinoma! Also what possibilities for absorption of such carcinogens into the
lamina propria to bathe pyloric and cardiac gland cells, since intestinal cell metaplasia commonly occurs in the mucosa of the stomach in all three major types of
gastric carcinoma.

The work of Rubin et al.[74] summarized in the preceding paragraph may explain the xanthelasma of the gastric mucosa observed by Kimura, Hiramoto, and
Buncher [75] in 113 (58 percent) of 193 necropsies in Kyoto, Japan. The gross
lesion was 1 to 2 mm and either flat or elevated. Histiocytes in the lamina propria
contained cholesterol esters or neutral fat. The lesion increased in frequency and
severity with age, was more common in men, and often was seen in association
with intestinal cell metaplasia. The authors explained the xanthelasma as due to
transport of lipid by metaplastic intestinal epithelial cells into the histiocytes of the
lamina propria.

Rubin et al.[76] studied, by electron microscopy, the metaplastic intestinal
epithelial cell of the fundic mucosa of the stomach of five fasting patients with
pernicious anemia and compared the features of this cell to those of the jejunal
mucosa in normal persons and in patients with lactase deficiency. The fine structure
of both types of cell was similar, but a careful correlation between light and electron microscopy was not made. Two types of metaplastic intestinal cells were
described. The first was the villous epithelial cell with well developed microvilli and
a terminal bar, lateral interdigitations with adjacent cells, many ribosome-studded
profiles of endoplasmic reticulum, several Golgi complexes, sausage-shaped mitochondria, lysosomes stuffed with ribosomal membranes, many basal villous

processes extending into intervillous spaces, and fewer subnuclear than apical organelles. The second was the crypt epithelial cell with shorter, wider, and less numerous microvilli, no developed terminal web, many more free ribosomes, fewer profiles of endoplasmic reticulum, notable mitoses, membrane-bound secretory apical granules, and straight lateral cell membranes. The orderly migration of the crypt epithelial cells to the surface of the mucosa was clearly suggested. The authors also detailed the fine structure of goblet cells, Paneth cells, and argentaffin cells. (See Figs. 32–34.)

Geissendorfer [77] studied the stomach in 10 cases of gastric carcinoma and three of gastric ulcer. He concluded: (1) Intestinal glands or intestinal cell metaplasia of the gastric mucosa are a postfetal phenomenon increasing with age. (2) Intestinal cell metaplasia is a focal alteration of the gastric mucosa and not a heterotopia of intestinal epithelium. (3) The site of predilection for intestinal cell metaplasia is the "Magenstrasse" (gastric street) in the antrum and lesser curvature, with less involvement of the greater curvature and fundus. (4) Intestinal cell metaplasia is as frequent and as well developed in gastric ulcer as in carcinoma, but may be lacking in both diseases. (5) Intestinal cell metaplasia has a parallel occurrence with carcinoma and is manifest as a benign process by itself and as a malignant process in the direction of carcinoma.

Järvi and Lauren [78] studied 184 carcinomas and six gastric papillomas occurring in 122 men and 67 women. They found the periodic acid-fuchsin-sulfurous acid (PA-F-SA) stain useful in demonstrating the striated border of epithelial cells. This striated border occurred in five of six papillomas, seven of ten papillary carcinomas, 62 of 81 adenocarcinomas, 11 of 27 "colloid" carcinomas, five out of 23 solid carcinomas, and five of 43 scirrhous carcinomas. Their detailed analysis of these groups by mucicarmine and Best carmine stains was difficult to follow. The striated border of the cells shown by the PA-F-SA method, as well as by electron microscopy, most likely was related to the presence of microvilli at the free margin of the neoplastic metaplastic intestinal epithelial cells. The high frequency of this phenomenon in the papillomas, papillary carcinomas, and adenocarcinomas would strengthen the interpretation that the striated border seen by light microscopy was characteristic of metaplastic intestinal epithelial cells.

Morson [79] found the incidence of intestinal metaplasia greatest in stomachs containing carcinoma, next highest in stomachs bearing ulcers, and least in portions of stomachs removed for duodenal ulcer. In cancerous stomachs the incidence of intestinal cell metaplasia was 4.5 percent at 50 to 59 years and 5.1 percent at 60+ years, compared to 1.9 and 1.6 percent, respectively, for those same age groups in noncancerous stomachs. In stomachs removed for carcinoma, the incidence and severity of intestinal cell metaplasia was greatest at the pylorus, and there was less evidence of metaplasia in the mucosa of the lesser and greater curvatures. Teir and Räsänen [7] found intestinal-type glands in the antral mucosa: 78 percent in 17 gastric cancer cases, 60 percent in 35 gastric ulcer cases, and 25 percent in 32 duodenal ulcer cases, compared to 43, 40, and 6 percent, respectively, in the fundal mucosa.

Several investigators [1, 60-62, 80-83] have traced satisfactorily the origin of intestinal cell carcinoma of the stomach from metaplastic intestinal epithelial cells.

Polyps and Gastric Carcinoma

Some students of gastric carcinoma [1, 84, 85] recognized that gastric polyps, whether single or multiple, must display a preponderant intestinal cell metaplasia to be significant in the genesis of gastric carcinoma. Paradoxically, polyps composed mainly of mucous epithelial cells are seldom progenitors of carcinoma of the mucous cell type. Rather, the setting of mucous cell carcinoma is the flat gastric mucosa cancerized at many points by malignant mucous epithelial cells. Some authors failed to realize that malignant change in gastric polyps is overwhelmingly a feature of those containing a high proportion of metaplastic intestinal epithelial cells.

In 1950 the author's study of 20 cases of gastric polyps at the Armed Forces Institute of Pathology drove home the points emphasized in the preceding paragraph. Of particular interest was the case of a man 52 years old with a sleeve resection of the stomach for three polyps of intestinal cell type, the largest measuring 75 mm. He died 12 years later with a primary carcinoma of intestinal cell type in the remaining portion of the stomach. The carcinoma extended to the line of the previous gastrojejunostomy and metastasized to regional, abdominal, and mediastinal lymph nodes, to liver, and to the lungs.

Following our emphasis on the significant frequency of the development of intestinal cell carcinoma from both the polypoid and flat intestinalized gastric mucosa, Morson [84] examined 12 gastric polyps, five composed of metaplastic intestinal epithelium and arising in mucosa affected by intestinal cell metaplasia. Of 107 carcinomas of the stomach, Morson [82] concluded that five revealed an origin from metaplastic intestinal epithelium. He pointed to evidence in the literature suggesting that 30 percent of gastric carcinomas arise in metaplastic epithelium, and that in patients with pernicious anemia this lesion is more common in the fundus than in the antrum.[64]

Berg [85] examined 106 gastric polyps in 45 patients with the following distribution: 11 patients with independent primary gastric cancers had 19 polyps; 15 patients with multiple gastric polyps had 68 polyps; and 19 patients had single polyps. The cases confirmed that intestinalization was common in cases of cancer, but Berg thought that the association between cancer and polyps containing metaplastic intestinal epithelium was indefinite. Despite this opinion, he found: (1) Intestinalization was a major component in nine of 106 polyps and a minor component in three others. (2) Nine of these 12 polyps contained cancer. (3) In all five patients with intestinalization of polyps, independent primary gastric cancers were present.

Monroe, Boughton, and Sommers [86] found a statistically significant association between epithelial hyperplasia of foveolar and glandular types in the stomachs of patients with gastric cancer.

Pathology of Gastric Carcinoma

The author's classification of gastric carcinoma into mucous cell, pylorocardiac gland cell, and intestinal cell types was thought to be unique in 1954, until acquisition of a little-read book on neoplasia and laboratory technique by Masson.[81] The material therein indicated that Masson, a master anatomic pathologist, had defined the microscopic types of gastric carcinoma, even though he made no correlation with gross features and biologic behavior, with or without various types of gastrectomy. Acknowledgment of this signal but ignored contribution was made in a paper on the comparative pathology of cancer in man and the dog.[87] Masson [81] distinguished by ordinary and mucicarmine-stained sections the following types of gastric carcinoma: *épithéliomas atypiques muqueux*—mucous cell carcinoma; *épithéliomas gastriques à cellules claires et à cellules cubiques*—pylorocardiac gland cell carcinoma; *épithéliomas gastriques à forme intestinale*—intestinal cell carcinoma type 1; and *épithéliomas gastriques à cellules basophiles*—intestinal cell carcinoma type 2.

The precise description of the first case of carcinoma in the mucous cells of the stomach—for convenience including the mucous neck and mucous cells—is lost in antiquity. This elusive and devastating neoplasm presents in several anatomic forms, related to the variable synthesis of mucin by the neoplastic mucous epithelial cells and the usually notable productive fibrosis—evidently a defense mechanism of the host. Such terms as scirrhous, linitis plastica, gelatinous or colloid, and undifferentiated have been used to designate the various forms this type of gastric carcinoma can take.

Apparently the first cases of pylorocardiac gland cell carcinoma were described by McPeak and Warren.[88] Our own material [1] abundantly confirmed this as a valid histologic type, with findings indicative of a more favorable prognosis after surgery than for mucous cell carcinoma. The usual localization of this type of gastric carcinoma to the pyloric and cardiac glands of the stomach also has been confirmed in this laboratory. The wider recognition of pylorocardiac gland cell carcinoma may come eventually through further study of microscopic sections, including special stains, of ultrastructural features of the normal and cancerous pyloric and cardiac gland cells, and by identification of the secretions and enzymes elaborated by these cells.

Until proved otherwise, the amply illustrated description of Gosset and Masson [80] may be accepted as the first documented example of intestinal cell carcinoma type 1. In like manner, the blue cell carcinoma of the stomach [89] is the first clinicopathologic correlation of intestinal cell carcinoma type 2 originally recognized by Masson.[81]

During the past decade, descriptions of intestinal cell carcinoma have emanated from three countries—Finland,[60] Japan,[61] and Colombia [62]—where there is a high risk of gastric carcinoma. These investigations have confirmed the significance of this type of gastric carcinoma. Contrary to a former preconceived notion that mucous cell carcinoma was most common in high risk countries, intestinal cell carcinoma is not only seemingly the most common,[90, 91] but postoperative follow-up figures tend to confirm a better prognosis for this type after gastrectomy.[91]

As indicated in the section on polyps and carcinoma of the stomach, Morson [82] was impressed by the origin of some gastric carcinomas from metaplastic intestinal epithelium.

In Japan [90] the incidence of gastric carcinoma per 100,000 population was 42.3 in 1935 and 47.9 in 1951. In a large autopsy series, the peak incidence for the disease was at 50 to 59 years, with 522 men and 279 women represented. The locations of the primary tumors were as follows (in percent): pylorus 66.7, lesser curvature 13.9, cardia 10.4, and greater curvature 9.0. Of the total series, cylindrical cell or adenomatous cancer accounted for 50.0 percent and gland cell cancer or carcinoma simplex for 39.6 percent. This indicated that intestinal cell carcinoma was the most frequent in this series.

The total experience of Colorado General Hospital with gastric carcinoma from 1927 through 1968 is detailed and illustrated in the next section. Confirmation of previous findings [1] is evident.

Ringertz [91] recognized intestinal cell carcinoma as a valid histologic type with a resemblance to adenocarcinoma of the large intestine. He emphasized that intestinal cell metaplasia is the preneoplastic lesion.

As already summarized in the section on intestinal cell metaplasia, Järvi and Laurén [78] established that the histologic structure of gastric carcinoma often displays features of intestinal mucosa. They claimed that in at least 50 percent of their cases gastric carcinomas arose from intestinal cell metaplasia of the gastric mucosa. On the basis of their and other published observations, the term "intestinal-type gastric carcinoma" has been used increasingly in the literature. Laurén [60] studied the surgical pathology specimens of 1,344 patients with gastric carcinoma between 1945 and 1964; a battery of special stains was used in 309. On this basis 715 (53 percent) were classified as intestinal-type carcinoma, 441 (33 percent) as diffuse carcinoma, and 188 (14 percent) as heterogeneous carcinoma. The 715 patients with intestinal cell carcinoma included 465 men (65 percent) and 250 women (35 percent). The mean age was 55.4 years, with a peak in the decade 60 to 69, and 55 percent of patients being more than 60 years of age. The gross appearance was polypoid or fungated in 215 of 361 cases (60 percent), excavated in 91 (25 percent), and infiltrative in 55 (15 percent). In 356 cases, mucosal intestinal cell metaplasia adjacent to the carcinoma was moderate to severe.

The microscopic features included the following: (1) glandular structures with papillary folds or distinct epithelial tracts; (2) cells larger, more clearly defined, and more variable than those of the diffuse type of gastric carcinoma; (3) nuclei large, of variable shape, and often mitotic; (4) cells columnar and fairly well polarized, with the apical surface continuous from one cell to the next; (5) well developed brush border in 146 of 176 cases (83 percent) of intestinal cell carcinoma and in 146 of 152 cases (92 percent) of those forming glands; (6) margins of tumor distinct and parallel spread in the mucosa and stomach wall; (7) frequently medullary type of growth with profuse inflammatory cell infiltration at advanced margins of the tumor; and (8) little productive fibrosis, even though surface ulceration occurred in some cases.

Kuru and Ryozo [61] classified 150 gastric carcinomas confined to the mucosa or submucosa into five groups. The first was distinguished by cancerous transformation of the polypoid-glandular mucosa into carcinoma of the intestinal cell type. In the second group the great majority of lesions were ulcerated and displayed undifferentiated features, suggesting that most were mucous cell carcinomas. In the third group the lesions were labeled superficial spreading carcinomas with ulceration, a later stage of the second group. The fourth group included superficial carcinomas in situ of intestinal cell type, lacking polypoid or ulcerative features and associated with intestinal metaplasia of the adjacent mucosa. The fifth group included carcinomas with miscellaneous features.

In Cali, Columbia,[62] the incidence of gastric carcinoma in males was 50.88 per 100,000 population and in females 21.05. Of 191 cases examined, 99 (51.8 percent) were intestinal cell type, 75 (34 percent) diffuse type, and 27 (14.1 percent) nonspecific type by the Laurén classification. Intestinal metaplasia was thought to be an important precancerous lesion in the first group.

Nakamura, Sugano, and Tagaki [83] studied 31 resected stomachs containing 33 foci of primary carcinoma less than 5 mm in diameter which were regarded as an early phase of the development of overt carcinoma. In 28 foci (84.8 percent) the origin of the carcinoma was traced to metaplastic intestinal epithelium; in four foci (12.1 percent) the origin of the carcinoma was ascribed to the mucous epithelial cells; and in one focus (3.0 percent) the lesion was an ulcer-cancer.

Kori et al.[93] assessed the growth of human gastric carcinoma in vivo via tritiated thymidine. They found that the normal gastric epithelial cells between the surface and crypt epithelium were labeled at a level of 40 percent, compared to 20 to 25 percent for the carcinoma cells, type unspecified. They also observed that desoxyribonucleic acid synthesis times in the carcinoma cells were 24 to 32 hours and the cell generation times were 12.0 to 12.3 days; both phenomena were two to three times longer than for the normal epithelial cells. The same growth rates were found in early and late carcinomas. An atlas of colored illustrations of early gastric carcinoma has been published in Japan.[94]

Treatment

The paucity of sound contributions to the pathology of gastric carcinoma is nowhere more evident than in the United States. Many valuable contributions to the diagnosis, treatment, and prognosis have been vitiated by the failure of many pathologists to furnish sound guidance in classification. Such guidance is much more evident and well understood for mammary, bronchial, testicular, and thyroid carcinomas. The better results of surgery for gastric carcinoma in Japan strongly suggest the high frequency of intestinal cell carcinoma there, compared to the dismal results in the United States with its clear prevalence of mucous cell carcinoma.

A thorough study was made of a large series of gastric carcinomas by Katami.[91] During a period of 11 years and 8 months he found 976 patients with gastric cancer. Of 959 operated upon, 687 (71.6 percent) had gastrectomy—76 total and 611 ordinary and subtotal. Of the latter 611 cases—subtracting 79 postoperative deaths, 81 eliminated for no evident reason, and 16 with information unobtainable—435 remained for detailed analysis. The age distribution was as follows: under 40 years, 55 (13 percent); 41 to 50 years, 122 (28 percent); and 51+ years, 258 (59 percent). The 5-year survival by sex was: male 33.6 percent, female 21.8 percent. The 5-year survival by age was: under 40 years (16.7 percent), 41 to 50 years (28.3 percent), and 51+ years (32.8 percent). The 5-year survival related to Borrmann gross types of 430 cases was: types I (22) and II (282), 36.2 percent, and types III (91) and IV (35), 12.3 percent. The 5-year survival by histologic type was: carcinoma adenomatosum 37.5 percent, and carcinoma solidum 23.1 percent. The 5-year survival by penetration in 435 cases was: submucosal (23) plus muscle coats (73), 56.0 percent; spread to serosa (339), 21.0 percent.

Experience of Colorado General Hospital with Gastric Carcinoma, 1927–1968

Material and Methods

Of the 268 cases studied, the minimal criteria for inclusion in the series were as follows: sufficient tissue sections of primary tumor obtained at autopsy or partial or complete gastric resection with regional lymph node dissection of variable efficacy, adequate preservation of primary tumor and metastases, satisfactory description of primary tumor and metastases, and proof of primary origin in the stomach. Five cases included were excepted from these criteria because adequate radiographic and operative information and satisfactory biopsy specimens of the primary tumor were available in three cases and abdominal metastases in two. Reasons for rejection of other cases included too small biopsy specimens of primary tumor or metastases, inadequate gross description, poorly preserved autopsy tissues, and adequate gross description but skimpy sampling of tumor for microscopic study.

Techniques for tissue processing in the original 138 cases were described.[1] Four percent formaldehyde fixation, dehydration in graded ethyl or isopropyl

Table 1. Gastric Carcinoma, Relation to Sex

Carcinoma type	Cases, males		Cases, females		Cases, total		Male/female ratio
	No.	%	No.	%	No.	%	
Mucous cell	83	68.6	38	31.4	121	46.7	2.18:1.00
Pylorocardiac gland cell	62	80.5	15	19.5	77	29.7	4.13:1.00
Intestinal cell	46	75.4	15	24.6	61	23.6	3.07:1.00
Total	191	–	68	–	259	–	2.81:1.00

Table 2. Gastric Carcinoma, Relation to Age

Carcinoma type	Cases (No.)	Age (years)		
		Minimum	Maximum	Average
All classified cases	259	32	95	65.4
Mucous cell	121	32	87	62.0
Pylorocardiac gland cell	77	43	95	68.5
Intestinal cell*	61	41	85	68.2

*Two primary carcinomas in five cases and three primary carcinomas in one case.

Table 3. Gastric Carcinoma, Relation to Age by Decades

Carcinoma type	Cases (No.)	31 to 40		41 to 50		51 to 60		61 to 70		71 to 80		81 to 90		91 to 100	
		No.	%	No.	%	No.	%	No.	%	No.	%	No.	%	No.	%
Mucous cell	121	11	9.1	11	9.1	27	22.3	39	32.2	27	22.3	6	5.0	0	0
Pylorocardiac gland cell	77	0	0	3	3.7	15	19.5	25	32.5	25	32.5	7	9.1	2	2.6
Intestinal cell	61	0	0	2	3.3	14	23.0	19	31.3	16	26.2	10	16.4	0	0

Table 4. Gastric Carcinoma, Relation to Sex and Age by Decades

Carcinoma type	Cases (No.)	31 to 40 years	41 to 50 years	51 to 60 years	61 to 70 years	71 to 80 years	81 to 90 years	91 to 100 years
Mucous cell								
M	83	5	7	17	29	21	4	0
F	38	6	4	10	10	6	2	0
Pylorocardiac gland cell								
M	62	0	1	13	19	21	6	2
F	15	0	2	2	6	4	1	0
Intestinal cell								
M	46	0	2	11	13	12	8	0
F	15	0	0	3	6	4	2	0
Total		11	16	56	83	68	23	2
Percent		4.2	6.2	21.6	32.0	26.3	8.8	0.8

alcohol, clearing in butyl acetate or xylene, cutting of sections at 6 to 8 μ, and staining with hematoxylin and eosin were followed for the second series of 130 cases. Periodic acid-fuchsin-sulfurous acid and mucicarmine stains were applied in selected cases of the second series, usually on surgical specimens.

Observations and Comment

CARCINOMA TYPES. Of the 268 gastric carcinomas, 121 were classified as mucous cell, 77 as pylorocardiac gland cell, and 61 as intestinal cell. Actually, five patients with intestinal cell carcinoma had two primary tumors each and one had three primary tumors, making a total of 68 carcinomas of this type. The remaining nine cases of the 268 total were unclassified.

SEX AND AGE. The data for sex and age coincident with first tissue diagnosis of gastric carcinoma of the 259 patients with 266 histologically classified carcinomas are summarized in Tables 1 through 4.

The overall male/female ratio of 2.81 is practically identical to that (2.95) for 257 autopsied patients with assorted cancers who were 70 years of age or older,[95] and it is more representative than the 3.75 in our first series.[1] The male/female ratio of 2.18 for mucous cell carcinoma and of 3.07 for intestinal cell carcinoma is within the range of nonsignificance compared to that for the entire series. The 4.13 male/female ratio for pylorocardiac gland cell carcinoma is probably significant and may be related to the possible hormonal etiology of this type of carcinoma referred to below.

Table 3 indicates that 18 percent of mucous cell carcinomas occurred before the age of 50 years as contrasted with about 3.5 percent for the other two cancer types, which displayed a later onset and decline than the mucous cell carcinoma. The almost equal frequency of all three types during the seventh decade is of interest.

The surface position of mucous neck and mucous epithelial cells would allow the topical application of carcinogens to play a role in the development of malignant changes in them. The ability of these cells to concentrate radioisotopes—e.g., those of iodine—also could operate as a carcinogenic factor. The protected position of the pyloric and cardiac gland epithelial cells deep in the gastric mucosa suggests that hematogenous stimuli—e.g., steroid hormones—may be factors in the development of carcinomas involving them. Since metaplastic intestinal epithelial cells occur most frequently with advancing age and are primarily absorptive, carcinogens dissolved in lipids could well be responsible for the malignant changes in them.

The differences for age and sex are shown in Table 4.

The male/female ratio of 2.81 for the 259 cases of gastric carcinoma approximates the 3:1 to 4:1 ratio given for most series reported from large centers. The occurrence of 80 percent of the cases between 50 and 80 years of age is close to the 70 or 80 percent given in other studies. In 1947 the male/female ratio for gastric cancer in 10 metropolitan areas of the United States was 1.9:1.0. The figures for 1957 and 1967 are said to be forthcoming. In 1968 estimated gastric cancer deaths in the United States were 10,300 males and 6,800 females with a ratio

Table 5. Gastric Carcinoma, Site

Carcinoma type	Antrum No.*	%	Fundus No.	%	Cardia No.	%	Entire stomach No.	%
Mucous cell	68[5]	56.2	22	18.2	8	6.6	23	19.0
Pylorocardiac gland cell	50[2]	65.0	12	15.6	13	17.0	2	2.6
Intestinal cell†	43[1]	63.2	18	26.5	6	8.8	1	1.5

*Superscript figures indicate the number of carcinomas that extended also in the fundus.
†There were 68 carcinomas in 61 cases—two in five cases and three in one case.

of 1.5:1.0.[96] In the same compilation, during 1962–1963 the male/female ratio in the United States was 10.80:5.48 based on death rates per 100,000 population as contrasted to 68:36 in Japan, or 2.0 and 1.9, respectively.

SITE.   The microscopic structures of the mucosa of the stomach, rather than the gross divisions often employed, are used here in the localization of the 266 classified gastric carcinomas. The normal mucous neck and mucous epithelial cells lining the entire surface and the orifices of the crypts of the mucosa of the stomach, the normal specialized epithelial cells of the pyloric and cardiac glands deep in the mucosa of antrum and cardia, and metaplastic intestinal epithelial cells found with increasing frequency with age throughout the gastric mucosa have been established in this laboratory as sources for most gastric carcinomas.

The occurrence of the majority of carcinomas in this series within the gastric antrum supports previous observations. Mucous cell carcinoma (Table 5) involved the stomach diffusely nearly 10 times more frequently than the other two types of carcinoma. Pylorocardiac gland cell carcinoma was about twice as common at the cardia as the other two types. Intestinal cell carcinoma maintained top ranking in the fundus.

In the entire series, naturally occurring pernicious anemia affected four patients with intestinal cell carcinoma, two with mucous cell carcinoma, and one with pylorocardiac gland cell carcinoma. An additional patient, mentioned below, survived total gastrectomy for mucous cell carcinoma; she developed pernicious anemia 5 years later and was treated successfully for this complication.

SIZE.   In Table 6 are listed the sizes or greatest diameters of the 266 classified gastric carcinomas. Size usually was directly proportional to the amount of extension and the number of metastases. In a study of the diameter of 682 gastric carcinomas [97] 23.2 percent were less than 4 cm in diameter and 76.8 percent were

Table 6. Gastric Carcinoma, Size

Carcinoma type	2 to 5 cm No.	%	5 to 10 cm No.	%	10 cm or larger No.	%
Mucous cell	21	17.4	43	35.5	57	47.1
Pylorocardiac gland cell	25	32.5	36	46.8	16	20.8
Intestinal cell	21	30.9	35	51.5	12	17.6

Table 7. Gastric Carcinoma, Stage

Carcinoma type	Stage I		Stage II		Stage III		Stage IV	
	No.	%	No.	%	No.	%	No.	%
Mucous cell	1	0.9	2	1.7	6	5.0	112	92.6
Pylorocardiac gland cell	1	1.3	3	4.0	13	16.9	60	78.0
Intestinal cell	4	6.0	7	10.3	17	25.0	40	58.8

4 cm or larger. It was thought that any gastric mucosal lesion should be suspect for cancer when it was more than 4 cm in diameter, until it proved to the contrary. The observations that 67 (25 percent) of the carcinomas in the present series of 266 total primary tumors were less than 5 cm in diameter and 189 (75 percent) were larger than 5 cm are in close agreement.

In the same study [97] the diameters of 638 gastric ulcers were also measured, with 92.3 percent being less than 25 mm and none larger than 40 mm. Unusually high figures for allegedly benign gastric ulcers later proved by pathologic analysis to be carcinoma were found in two series: 13 percent [98] and nearly 20 percent.[99] During the past 20 years at the Colorado General Hospital, this figure was estimated at less than 2 percent. Certainly, any gastric lesion 5 cm or larger should be strongly suspect of cancer, carcinoma, or another malignant tumor until proved otherwise. A direct correlation was made between the size of gastric carcinoma and the presence or absence of metastases to regional lymph nodes following radical gastrectomy.[100]

STAGE. A slight modification of the method used by Dochat and Gray [101] based upon the Dukes classification [102] was employed in the staging of 266 classified gastric carcinomas (Table 7). They obtained a much sharper determination of 5-year survival after gastric resection with the Dukes staging than with the Broders microscopic grading. In the present study the microscopic extension of the carcinoma within and beyond the stomach established the following four stages: I, limited to the mucosa; II, extended into the muscle coats; III, extended into the serosa; and IV, extended into adjacent structures and/or metastasized.

Table 8. Gastric Carcinoma, Size and Stage Correlated

Carcinoma type	2 to 5 cm		5 to 10 cm		10 cm and larger	
	No.	%	No.	%	No.	%
Mucous cell						
Stage I–III	3	2.5	4	3.3	2	1.7
Stage IV	18	14.9	39	32.2	55	45.4
Pylorocardiac gland cell						
Stage I–III	8	10.4	5	6.5	4	5.2
Stage IV	17	22.1	31	40.2	12	15.6
Intestinal cell						
Stage I–III	10	14.7	15	22.1	3	4.3
Stage IV	11	16.2	20	29.4	9	13.2

Table 9. Gastric Carcinoma: Extensions of Primary Tumors

Extension site	Mucous cell	Pylorocardiac gland cell	Intestinal cell
Pancreas	27	14	4
Duodenum	20	9	0
Esophagus	19	8	11
Liver	5	4	1
Bile duct	3	6	0
Colon	3	3	1
Diaphragm	2	2	0
Spleen	0	2	0
Portal or splenic veins	0	1	2
Kidney	1	0	0
Adrenal	1	0	0
Jejunum	1	0	0
Total extensions	82	49	19
Total patients	55	29	13

The relatively more aggressive behavior of mucous cell carcinoma of the stomach is readily apparent, compared with that of the other two types. Only 7.6 percent of mucous cell carcinomas were confined to the stomach, compared to 22.2 percent of pylorocardiac gland cell carcinomas and 41.3 percent of intestinal cell carcinomas. The more favorable figures for the last two types are correlated with prognosis in a later section. Stout [103] studied 143 cases of gastric carcinoma, 10.5 percent of which were confined to the stomach. Harding and Harkins [104] recorded a figure of 28 percent in 158 autopsies. Walther [105] found 25 percent of 711 carcinomas limited to the stomach. The figure in the present series of 266 carcinomas is 20.3 percent.

A striking parallel between percentages for stage IV recorded in Table 7 and prognosis as discussed below is evident. Size and stage have been correlated in Table 8 by contrasting the size of carcinomas confined to the stomach—stages I, II, and III—with the size of those spread beyond the stomach. The figures confirm the foregoing remarks.

EXTENSION. The extension was ascertained for all cases according to the three following groups: autopsy only, surgery followed by autopsy, or surgery followed by death without autopsy. In the last group, the assumption was made conservatively that the patient died of gastric carcinoma during the immediate postoperative period of 2 months or at varying intervals thereafter, unless strong proof to the contrary was included in the clinical findings, adequate physical examination, and supportive laboratory tests, such as radiographic study of the stomach. The number of extensions is given in Table 9. Had all patients subjected to operation with later clinical signs of recurrent carcinoma and death been autopsied, the number of extensions undoubtedly would have increased.

In Table 10 the number of primary tumors with extension, the number of extensions, and the number of carcinomas of each of the three major types are given.

Table 10. Gastric Carcinoma: Extensions of Primary Tumors

Carcinoma type	Primary tumors extended	No. of extensions	Total No. of primary tumors	Extension index (Ie)*
Mucous cell	55	82	121	0.68
Pylorocardiac gland cell	29	49	77	0.64
Intestinal cell	13	19	68	0.28

*Total number of extensions divided by the total number of carcinomas.

By dividing the total number of extensions by the number of carcinomas in each group, a figure called the extension index (Ie) is obtained. The original findings are confirmed: The tendency of intestinal cell carcinoma to invade locally is relatively small—about 40 percent of that for pylorocardiac gland cell carcinoma or mucous cell carcinoma—and both of these types have about equal propensities to extend beyond the stomach.

METASTASIS. The metastases of 266 carcinomas—121 mucous cell, 77 pylorocardiac gland cell, and 68 intestinal cell—are listed in Tables 11 through 13. The patients dying of recurrent carcinoma after operation but not autopsied surely would have added to the totals given if postmortem examination had been made in all cases. Regional lymph nodes [100, 104, 106-108] include those of the superior gastric, inferior gastric, greater omental, lesser omental, subpyloric, paracardial, and pan-

Table 11. Gastric Carcinoma Metastases: Mucous Cell Type

Metastatic site	No.	Metastatic site	No.
Regional lymph nodes	78	Pericardium	4
Peritoneum	69	Prostate	4
Abdominal lymph nodes	45	Appendix	4
Lungs	27	Pancreas	4
Thoracic lymph nodes	27	Heart	3
Liver	25	Tubes	2
Small intestine	24	Thymus	2
Pleura	17	Scrotum	2
Adrenals	16	Meninges	2
Ovaries	13	Seminal vesicles	2
Bones	12	Ureters	2
Colon	10	Spleen	2
Gallbladder	7	Common bile duct	1
Uterus	7	Duodenum	1
Diaphragm	6	Vagina	1
Kidneys	6	Thyroid	1
Bladder	5	Pituitary	1
Skin	5	Larynx	1
Esophagus	5	Skeletal muscle	1
Peripheral lymph nodes	4		

$$\text{Metastatic index (Im)} = \frac{448 \text{ total metastases}}{121 \text{ total carcinomas}} = 3.70$$

Table 12. Gastric Carcinoma Metastases: Pylorocardiac Gland Cell Type

Metastatic site	No.	Metastatic site	No.
Regional lymph nodes	41	Colon	2
Liver	20	Peripheral lymph nodes	2
Peritoneum	17	Spleen	1
Abdominal lymph nodes	16	Ovaries	1
Thoracic lymph nodes	4	Diaphragm	1
Lungs	4	Bones	1
Pleura	4	Common bile duct	1
Small intestine	4	Bladder	1
Adrenals	3	Ureters	1
Pancreas	3	Gallbladder	1

$$\text{Metastatic index (Im)} = \frac{128 \text{ total metastases}}{77 \text{ total carcinomas}} = 1.66$$

creaticolienal groups within the abdomen. The mucous cell carcinomas followed a pattern of metastasis like that recorded by others [103-105, 109-111] in autopsied cases of gastric carcinoma.

Included in each table is the metastatic index obtained by taking the total number of metastases and dividing them by the number of carcinomas in each group. This index and the extension index help quantitate the biologic behavior of the three types of gastric carcinoma. Mucous cell carcinoma exhibited a twice greater propensity to metastasize than the pylorocardiac gland cell carcinoma and about three times that of intestinal cell carcinoma. If two patients with intestinal cell carcinoma dying at 10 and 46 months after operation and accounting for 23 metastases are eliminated, the metastatic index for the remaining 66 carcinomas of this type is 0.91.

Table 13. Gastric Carcinoma Metastases: Intestinal Cell Type

Metastatic site	No.	Metastatic site	No.
Regional lymph nodes	34	Kidneys	2
Liver	10	Bones	1
Abdominal lymph nodes	9	Cervical stump	1
Peritoneum	5	Pleura	1
Thoracic lymph nodes	4	Diaphragm	1
Lungs	4	Thyroid	1
Adrenals	3	Heart	1
Small intestine	2	Ovaries	1
Bladder	2	Colon	1

$$\text{Metastatic index (Im)} = \frac{83^* \text{ total metastases}}{68 \text{ total carcinomas}} = 1.22$$

*Of these, 23 are accounted for by two carcinomas with autopsies 10 and 46 months post gastrectomy. Im in remaining 66 carcinomas is 0.91.

Moore and coworkers [106] found in patients treated by radical gastrectomy for carcinoma a 5.3 percent 5-year survival for those with metastases to regional lymph nodes compared to 45 percent for those without such metastases. When the carcinomas of these patients were typed by the Borrmann method, those with types 1 and 2 had an 18.7 percent 5-year survival, and those with types 3 and 4 a 10.9 percent survival. In their experience, the presence or absence of metastases to regional lymph nodes was a more accurate indicator of prognosis than the Borrmann method of typing.

PROGNOSIS. For each type of carcinoma, three groups of patients were delineated: (1) death without operation, usually within a brief period following admission; (2) operation, simple gastrostomy to radical total gastrectomy, and death from disease at variable intervals afterward with or without autopsy; and (3) operation designed to be curative, and either survival free of disease or death from other causes including second primary carcinomas in the remnant of stomach, proved at autopsy or by critical clinical assessment. A few cases of incidental carcinoma found at autopsy are included in the third group.

The 121 cases of mucous cell carcinoma included 37 dead without operation, 78 dead from disease after operation, and six in the salvage group. Of these six (5 percent), three did not stand the test of a 5-year follow-up—one because the patient could not be traced; and two due to the short interval of follow-up. Of the three remaining, one patient died at 18 months without clinical recurrence; one with a superficial ulcerated carcinoma died at 12 years 8 months of a heart attack without clinical recurrence; and one was alive and free of disease at 17 years 3 months when a carcinoma of the common bile duct was resected by the Whipple procedure, with death from clinical spread of this second cancer 29 months later.

The 77 patients with pylorocardiac gland cell carcinoma include all 14 dead without operation, 51 dead from disease after operation, and 12 in the salvage group (15 percent). Of the 12 in the salvage group, six died of other causes without residual carcinoma at autopsy; the carcinomas of two were incidental and confined to the stomach at autopsy; two percent were alive and free of disease at 6 years 2 months and 8 years 8 months, respectively, after operation; one died of other causes without clinical recurrence; and one was alive and free of disease at 5 years 8 months. In the last patient at a second operation 9 years 4 months after resection of the first primary tumor a second primary tumor in the gastric remnant extended to the colon, small intestine, liver, spleen, and peritoneum.

The 61 patients with intestinal cell carcinoma include six dead without operation, 31 dead from disease after operation, and 23 in the salvage group (38 percent), since one additional patient was not traced after operation. Of the 23 patients traced in the salvage group, seven died of other causes with no residual carcinoma at autopsy; six were alive and free of disease at 19 months, 53 months, 7 years 6 months, 8 years 8 months, 11 years 8 months, and 18 years, respectively, after operation; five died of other causes without clinical recurrence; four were special cases, detailed below; and one patient had an incidental carcinoma limited to the stomach at autopsy. The four special cases of intestinal cell carcinoma are as follows:

Case 115—patient was alive and free of disease at 42 months, but death occurred at 6 years 6 months from a clinical second primary carcinoma in the gastric remnant.

Case 246—death occurred from bronchopneumonia 79 months after resection of the first primary carcinoma of the antrum and 6 months after resection of the second primary carcinoma of the cardia, without residual carcinoma at autopsy.

Case 252—death occurred 14.5 months after resection of carcinoma limited to the stomach and 15.5 months after resection of adenocarcinoma of the sigmoid colon. The latter caused death by spread throughout the abdomen after initial resected sigmoid colon with metastases in regional lymph nodes.

Case 261—patient was alive and free of disease 5 years after resection of first gastric carcinoma and died 6 years after the first operation when laparotomy disclosed a second primary carcinoma in the remnant of stomach; the cancer extended to esophagus, liver, and pancreas.

As has been noted for this series, the salvage of mucous cell carcinoma is 5 percent, pylorocardiac gland cell carcinoma 15 percent, and intestinal cell carcinoma 38 percent. Conversely, lethality for these three types is 95, 85, and 62 percent, respectively, not too far from our original estimates of 98, 75, and 60 percent.[1] Better results than these surely can be achieved by putting in the first surgical team for every case of gastric carcinoma.

GROSS AND MICROSCOPIC FEATURES.   By assessing the entire experience with 266 classified gastric carcinomas, the microscopic features of the three major types have become so stereotyped in this laboratory that feeding the essential characteristics of each into a computer would result in close to a 100 percent correct diagnosis. Repetition of one statement in our original paper [1] is appropriate: "Undoubtedly study of 138 or more cases will vastly improve our attempts to evaluate the biologic behavior of gastric carcinoma by histologic pattern, as has already been accomplished for other cancers; namely, thyroid, mammary, bronchial, and testicular." In Table 14 is summarized the histologic spectrum of 266 gastric carcinomas. Figures 1 through 3 depict some of the features of mucous cell carcinoma; Figures 4 through 17, of pylorocardiac gland cell carcinoma; Figure 18, of intestinal cell metaplasia; and Figures 19 through 31, of intestinal cell carcinoma.

Mucous Cell Carcinoma.   A summary of the salient features is as follows:
1. Grossly diffuse and nondelimited involvement of mucosa and other coats
2. Barely perceptible and irregular transformation of mucous neck and mucous cells of the surface of the gastric mucosa and the orifices of the crypts into carcinoma cells
3. Alternate cancerization of mucosa with persistence of noncancerous or compressed noncancerous mucosa
4. Cytoplasm of polyhedral carcinoma cells pale acidophilic to amphophilic; nuclei enlarged, rounded, chromatin heavily stippled; nucleoli minute or small (Fig. 1)
5. Mitoses rare
6. Droplets of light basophilic secretion appearing in cytoplasm with coalescence into large globules displacing and flattening the nucleus to the periphery of the cell, the "signet ring" cell or the hallmark of mucous cell carcinoma (Fig. 3)

Table 14. Gastric Carcinoma: Histologic Spectrum of 266 Primary Tumors

Carcinoma type	Cases (No.)	Undifferentiated	Small glands	Signet ring cells	Mucus*	Focal large glands	Large glands
Mucous cell	121	111	70	106	101	16	5
Pylorocardiac gland cell	77	14	74	4	71	4	69
Intestinal cell							
IC-1	33	9	29	0	1	1	29
IC-2	35	32	30	0	1	7	0

*More appropriately called "secretion" for pylorocardiac gland cell carcinoma.

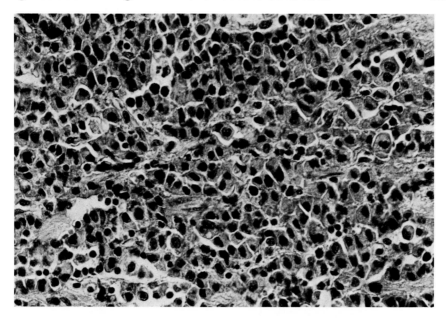

Fig. 1. Case 52 (male, 66): mucous cell carcinoma. Tumor: more than 10 cm, fundus, stage IV. Undifferentiated features, small gland pattern, signet ring cells, and mucin. Tumor originating diffusely from gastric mucosa with barely perceptible origin from mucous epithelial cells and formation of small cords and tubules. H&E. × 400.

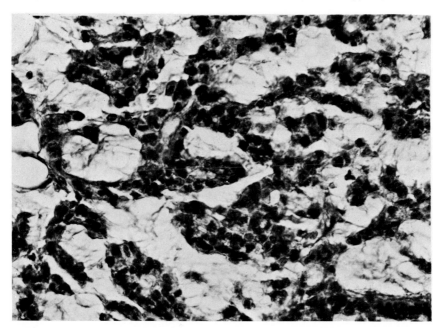

Fig. 2. Case 49 (male, 75): mucous cell carcinoma. Tumor: 6 cm, antrum, stage IV. Undifferentiated features, small gland pattern, signet ring cells, mucin, and focal large gland pattern with metastases to regional lymph nodes. Portion of serosa with imperfectly formed small glands suspended in mucin. H&E. × 400.

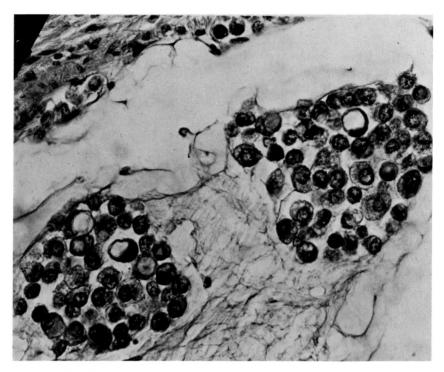

Fig. 3. Case 40 (male, 75): mucous cell carcinoma. Tumor: 6 cm, antrum, stage IV. Undifferentiated features, small gland pattern, signet ring cells, mucin, and focal large gland pattern. Muscle coats flooded by clusters of partly to completely formed signet ring cells containing and surrounded by mucin. H&E. × 400.

7. Spotty or diffuse formation of signet ring cells often suspended in mucin
8. Arrangement of carcinoma cells in solid cords and small tubular structures on the persistent reticular framework of the mucosa (Fig. 1)
9. Infrequent formation of relatively complete large and small glands in mucosa lined by cuboidal and cylindrical mucous epithelial cells blending in submucosa, muscle coats, and serosa (Fig. 2) with carcinoma cells already described
10. Brilliant staining of normal mucous neck and mucous cells and many of their cancerous counterparts by the periodic acid-fuchsin-sulfurous acid method and the mucicarmine stain (see Table 17 of original paper [1])
11. Carcinomatous flooding of the connective tissue of the submucosa, muscle coats, and serosa of the stomach (Fig. 3), with displacement of bundles of smooth muscle fibers, cuffing of small blood vessels and nerves, and invasion of lymphatics with dispersal of carcinoma cells in loose aggregates, clusters, cords, or singly, and with incitation of a variable fibrous connective tissue reaction and relatively few lymphoid cells
12. The more mucin elaborated by the undifferentiated carcinoma cells, the less the connective tissue reaction; the less mucin formed, the greater the productive fibrosis

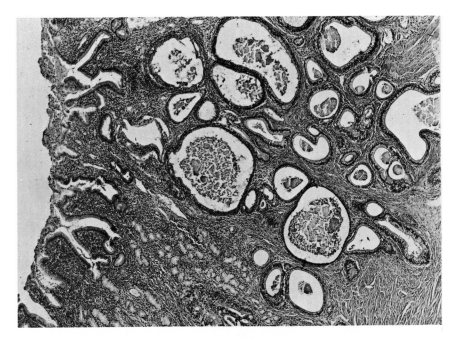

Fig. 4. Case 95 (male, 59): pylorocardiac gland cell carcinoma. Tumor: 7 cm, antrum, stage II. Lumen at left. Slightly autolyzed mucosa at surface. Neoplastic glands deep in mucosa, frequently dilated, lined by flattened epithelium and extending into submucosa. H&E. × 35.

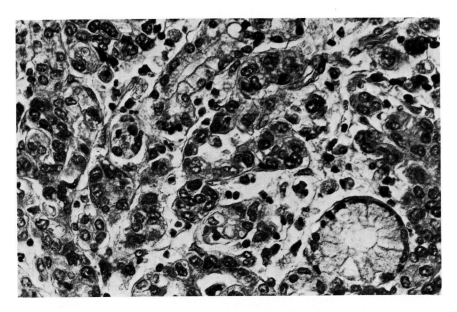

Fig. 5. Case 70 (male, 63): pylorocardiac gland cell carcinoma. Tumor: 5 cm, antrum, stage IV. Small and large gland patterns with metastases to regional lymph nodes. Partly cancerous glands in upper middle and lower right corner. Anaplastic glands in remainder of field. H&E. × 400.

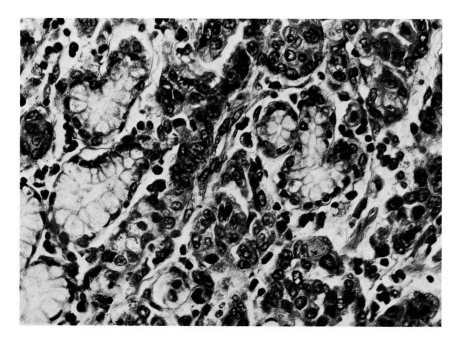

Fig. 6. Case 70: pylorocardiac gland cell carcinoma. See legend for Figure 5. Note the few noncancerous epithelial cells in glands in lower left corner. Anaplastic epithelial cells in glands in rest of field. H&E. × 400.

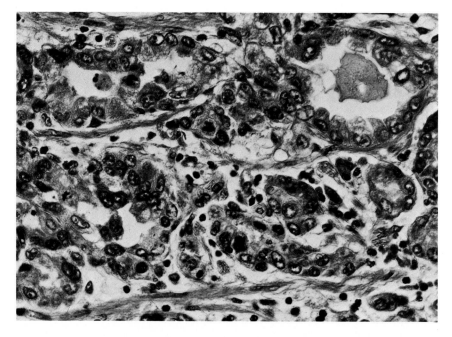

Fig. 7. Case 70: pylorocardiac gland cell carcinoma. See legend for Figure 5. Malignant epithelial cells in all glands depicted. Compare with Figures 5 and 6. H&E. × 400.

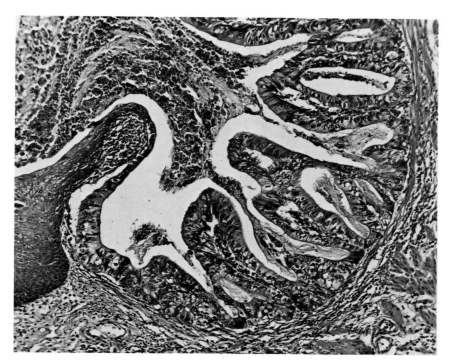

Fig. 8. Case 92 (male, 64): pylorocardiac gland cell carcinoma. Tumor: 6 cm, cardia, stage III. Small and large gland patterns. At left, junction between lower border of stratified squamous epithelium of esophagus and carcinoma. Pseudostratification, finely foamy cytoplasm, and frequently basal nuclei in tumor cells. H&E. × 100.

13. Productive fibrosis much more frequent and extensive in the extramucosal invasion of mucous cell carcinoma than in pylorocardiac gland cell carcinoma or intestinal cell carcinoma; peptic digestion found in an occasional case of any of the three types excepted

14. Growth of the carcinoma cells in solid, interlocked ribbons punctuated by small rounded spaces and abortive signet ring cells

15. Anastomosed, coiled cords of carcinoma cells forming incomplete small glands and suspended in mucin (Fig. 2)

16. Microscopic foci of cancerized mucosa in the grossly intact mucosa bordering the main carcinoma

Pylorocardiac Gland Cell Carcinoma.   A summary of the salient features is as follows:

1. Usual delimited growth fungated into lumen or sometimes widely ulcerated and fibrosed

2. Infrequent satellite foci adjacent to the main carcinoma as compared to mucous cell carcinoma or intestinal cell carcinoma

3. Origin of the neoplastic cells in the pyloric and cardiac glands with invasion of submucosa, muscle coats, and serosa, and spread toward the surface of the mucosa along the crypts to displace partly or completely the mucous neck cells and mucous cells (Figs. 4 through 17)

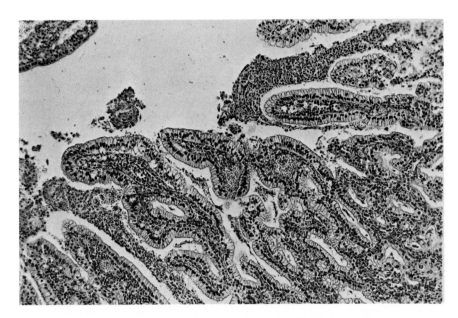

Fig. 9. Case 90 (male, 66): pylorocardiac gland cell carcinoma. Tumor: 4 cm, antrum, stage IV. Small and large gland patterns with metastases to regional lymph nodes. Striking vacuolation and glandular differentiation of carcinoma cells. H&E. × 100.

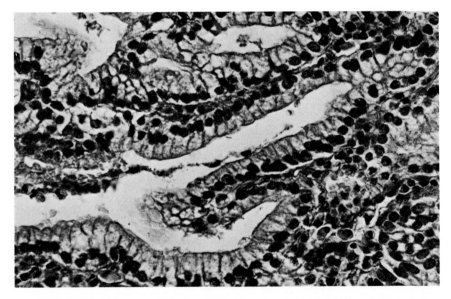

Fig. 10. Case 90: pylorocardiac gland cell carcinoma. Enlargement of middle portion of Figure 9. Tumor involving all coats of stomach. Cells marked by finely foamy cytoplasm, basal nuclei, and orientation in a single layer. Focal stratification in other fields. Appearance reminiscent of secretory endometrial glands. Lumen of glands often filled with purulent exudate. H&E. × 400.

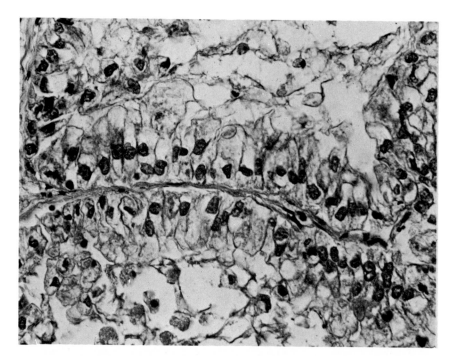

Fig. 11. Case 77 (female, 64): pylorocardiac gland cell carcinoma. Tumor: 4 cm, antrum, stage IV. Small and large gland patterns. Cells finely foamy to partly clear; nuclei usually basal, local stratification. Appearance of this metastasis in the liver reminiscent of gestational endometrial glands. H&E. × 400.

4. Formation of complete small and large glandular structures with variably stratified or singly oriented carcinoma cells of low to tall cylindrical shape

5. *With predominant cell stratification,* finely granular and acidophilic to partly clear cytoplasm; central, parabasal or basal, ovoid or rounded nuclei containing lightly to heavily stippled chromatin and small nucleoli (Figs. 4 through 8, 13, 15, and 17), sometimes clear zones above and below central or parabasal nuclei, relatively numerous abnormal mitotic figures, formation of small glands within or at the borders of large glands

6. *With cells oriented mainly in a single layer,* vacuolated, partly clear to almost entirely clear cytoplasm; rounded or ovoid nuclei with abundant, finely stippled chromatin, small nucleoli, and relatively infrequent abnormal mitoses (Figs. 9 through 12, 14, and 16)

7. Basal nuclei of some cells flattened perpendicularly to the long axis of the cell (Fig. 12) to mimic normal pyloric and cardiac gland cells

8. Transitions between stratified and simple columnar patterns in the same and in different tumors

9. Arrangement of epithelial cells in undulated or papillary folds, especially in the stratified pattern (Fig. 8)

10. With or without stratification of the epithelial cells, occurrence of flattening of the cells by inspissated secretion (Fig. 4), with rounded spaces formed to

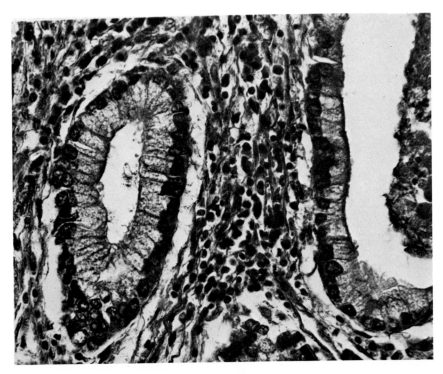

Fig. 12. Case 89 (male, 78): pylorocardiac gland cell carcinoma. Tumor: 3 cm; anterior wall, antrum; stage IV. Small and large gland patterns with metastases limited to regional lymph nodes at autopsy. Muscle coats containing neoplastic glands lined by columnar epithelial cells with finely granular cytoplasm and basal nuclei. H&E. × 400.

mimic spaces lined by endothelial or mesothelial cells, a pattern confusing in metastases

11. With periodic acid-fuchsin-sulfurous acid routine, cytoplasm of singly oriented cells containing more abundant positive material than the more granular or less clear stratified cells

12. Mucicarmine stain infrequently positive or at most moderately positive for intracellular material whether cells are stratified or singly oriented

13. Normal pyloric and cardiac gland cells stained brilliantly with periodic acid-fuchsin-sulfurous acid routine, but only moderately with mucicarmine stain, indicating close parallels between normal and cancerized pyloric and cardiac gland cells

14. Cells of an occasional carcinoma staining well with Best carmine, even after routine formaldehyde fixation and routine processing

15. Material in lumens of neoplastic glands strongly positive with periodic acid-fuchsin-sulfurous acid and mucicarmine stains with similar material surrounding neoplastic glands in a few cases

16. Desquamation of carcinoma cells into the lumens of some glands, attainment of a rounded contour, intracellular demonstration of periodic acid-fuchsin-

sulfurous acid-positive material, and designation thereby as pseudosignet ring cells

17. Interplay between stratification and single orientation of the carcinoma cells in a single tumor or from tumor to tumor, suggesting a parallel between the growth of this type of carcinoma and that of the endometrial glands in the proliferative and secretory phases of the menstrual cycle

18. Invasion of the carcinoma into the submucosa, muscle coats, and serosa, accompanied by relatively little productive fibrosis, except when the tumor occasionally becomes ulcerated and peptically digested

19. Strong tendency to invade submucosal veins

Intestinal Cell Carcinoma.   A summary of the salient features of intestinal cell (IC) carcinoma is as follows:

1. Gross presentation of the primary carcinoma as a delimited, polypoid, fungated, or relatively flat, nodular growth

2. High frequency of origin in the metaplastic intestinal epithelial cells of polyps or of flat mucosa

3. Frequent multiple foci of carcinoma in situ [83] adjacent to the border of the main carcinoma(s)

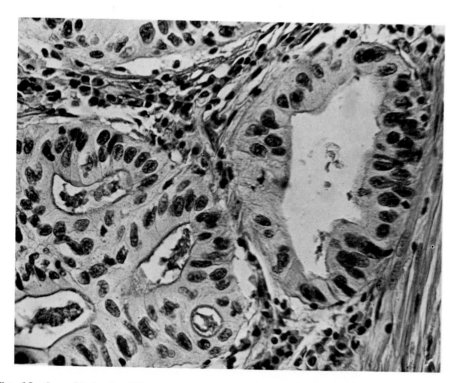

Fig. 13. Case 85 (male, 72): pylorocardiac gland cell carcinoma. Tumor: 7 cm, antrum, stage III. Small and large gland patterns. Cells finely granular to foamy, nuclei basal or parabasal. H&E. × 400.

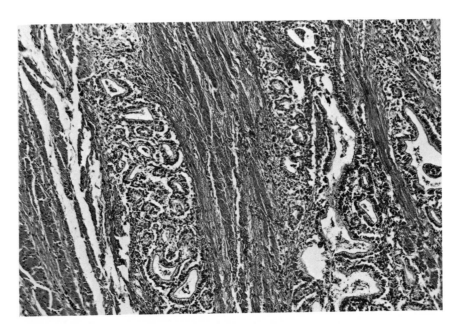

Fig. 14. Case 100 (male, 76): pylorocardiac gland cell carcinoma. Tumor: 7.5 cm, cardia, stage III. Small and large gland patterns. Neoplastic gland structures have invaded muscle coats. H&E. × 100.

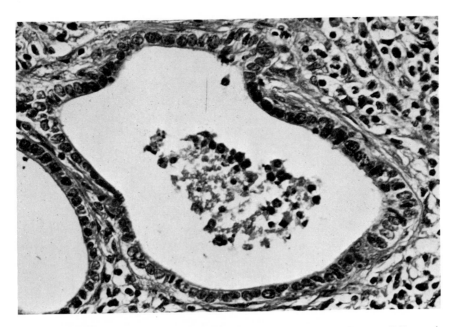

Fig. 15. Case 97 (male, 66): pylorocardiac gland cell carcinoma. Tumor: 2.5 cm; lesser curvature, antrum; stage II. Small and large gland patterns. Neoplastic glands in submucosa. H&E. × 400.

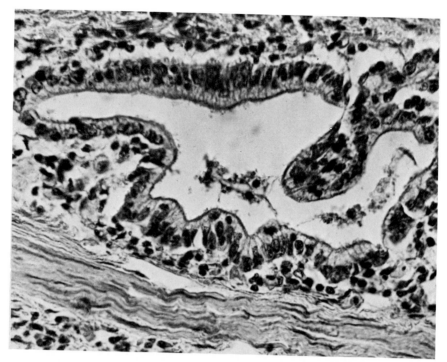

Fig. 16. Case 97: pylorocardiac gland cell carcinoma. See legend for Figure 15. Appearance of neoplastic glands reminiscent of secretory endometrial glands. H&E. × 400.

4. Association with one or more glandular polyps, usually of the intestinal cell type
5. Significant frequency of double or triple synchronous or metachronous primary carcinomas in a significant number of cases [1, 64]
6. Origin of the carcinoma in metaplastic intestinal epithelium comparable to the development of adenocarcinoma from the hyperplastic epithelial cells of glandular polyps of the large intestine
7. The growth of the carcinoma in small and large glands of the IC-1 pattern, or as undifferentiated, large, anastomosed aggregates of carcinoma cells marked by small glands of the IC-2 pattern, associated with abundant lymphoid tissue and relatively little connective tissue reaction
8. Crossover between the two patterns in a single tumor or in two tumors in a single case regardless of gross presentation; indicative of the fundamental identity of the cell of both patterns as an anaplastic derivative of the metaplastic intestinal epithelial cell
9. Metaplastic intestinal epithelial cells of a polyp or replacing the normal cells of the surface and crypts of the gastric mucosa; of low to tall cylindrical shape with cytoplasm relatively homogeneous and amphophilic; nuclei ovoid, basal, and marked by finely stippled chromatin and small nucleoli
10. Single nuclei or nuclei in several adjacent metaplastic epithelial cells enlarged,

rounded, disoriented, marked by peripherally shifted chromatin, and distinguished by more prominent nuclei, features indicating atypicality

11.   Metaplastic intestinal epithelial cells stratified or singly oriented (Fig. 18)

12.   Material in the lumens of these metaplastic glands and the cytoplasm of a few cells moderately positive with periodic acid-fuchsin-sulfurous acid and mucicarmine stains; Best carmine stain completely negative

13.   *Features of IC-1 pattern*

    a.   Increased stratification; flagrant dyspolarity of cells; amphophilic to basophilic cytoplasm; progressively enlarged, rounded nuclei with irregular chromatin pattern, large nucleoli, abnormal mitoses, and focal growth in small solid aggregates—features typifying the transformation of metaplastic intestinal epithelial cells into carcinoma cells (Figs. 19 through 25, 27 and 29)

    b.   Large glands revealing stratified or singly oriented cylindrical carcinoma cells with flattening of the cells in the more dilated glands

    c.   Formation of secondary small glands within or at the margins of the large glands

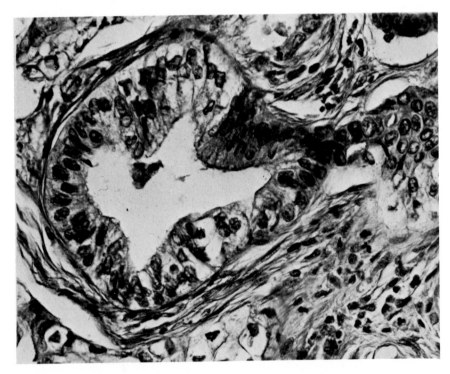

Fig. 17. Case 87 (male, 59): pylorocardiac gland cell carcinoma. Tumor: 4 cm, antrum, stage IV. Small and large gland patterns. Many neoplastic epithelial cells containing supra- and subnuclear vacuoles. H&E. × 400.

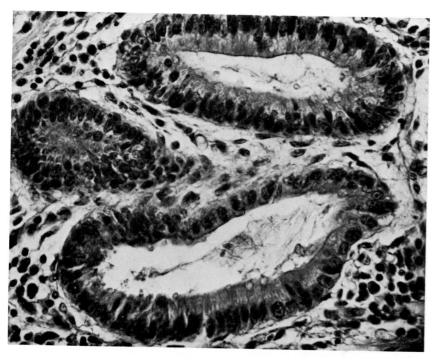

Fig. 18. Case 115 (male, 70): intestinal cell metaplasia. Patient had known pernicious anemia for 10 years before subtotal gastrectomy for polypoid carcinoma of intestinal cell type 1: 5 cm; anterior wall, fundus. Small and large gland patterns. Metaplastic intestinal epithelial cells lining crypts at base of tumor. Many nuclei atypical, basal or parabasal. Cytoplasm finely granular and amphophilic. H&E. × 400.

    d. Small glands proliferated by themselves reproducing a sinuous tubular arrangement with low columnar, cuboidal, or flattened cells

    e. Clusters of segmented neutrophils found in lumens of small and large glands

    f. Lymphoid tissue relatively sparse in mucosa of polypoid or flat lesions, but often increased as carcinoma invades submucosa, muscle coats, and serosa, especially when the tumor is superficially eroded

    g. Material in the lumens of anaplastic glands moderately positive with periodic acid-fuchsin-sulfurous acid routine and negative or slightly positive with mucicarmine stain, but cytoplasm of neoplastic cells negative with both these methods

    h. Best carmine stain entirely negative

    i. Same remarks for these stains applicable for lumens of small glands and cells of the IC-2 pattern

14. *Characteristics of IC-2 pattern*

    a. Carcinoma cells disposed in compact to loose, large aggregates with small gland spaces interspersed, but with abundant intermingled lymphoid tissue (Figs. 24, 26, 28, 30, and 31)

   b.   Polyhedral cells with amphophilic or basophilic cytoplasm; enlarged, rounded or ovoid nuclei with heavily stippled, marginated chromatin, thick membranes, large nucleoli, and many abnormal mitotic figures (Figs. 26, 30, and 31)

   c.   Interplay between both large and small glands of IC-1 pattern and the undifferentiated large aggregates of carcinoma cells of the IC-2 pattern, the punctuation of these undifferentiated large aggregates of cells by small glands, and focal undifferentiated portions in the IC-1 pattern—all indicative of a single carcinoma cell capable of growing as described and with growth characteristics comparable to those of adenocarcinoma of the large intestine

   d.   Abrupt transition of mucosa transformed by metaplastic intestinal epithelial cells to carcinoma also observed in the development of adenocarcinoma of the large intestine

14.   Equally favorable prognosis for IC-1 or IC-2 patterns

15.   Strong tendency to invade submucosal veins

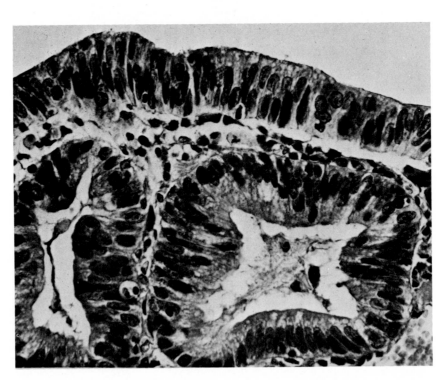

Fig. 19. Case 115: intestinal cell carcinoma type 1. See legend for Figure 18. Details of partly atypical and partly cancerous epithelium at surface and lining glands of carcinoma. Left gland depicting enlarged hyperchromatic nuclei in stratified, disorderly epithelial cells. In other fields at base of tumor, anaplastic glands merged with large aggregates of carcinoma cells in type 2 pattern and suggestively invaded the submucosa. H&E. × 400.

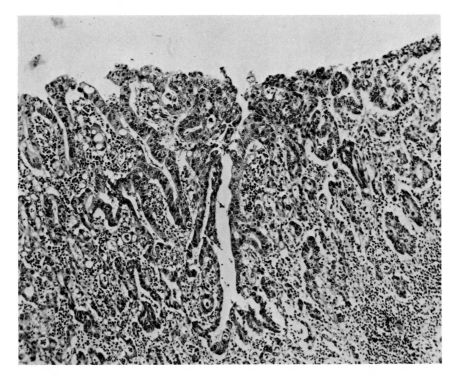

Fig. 20. Case 106 (female, 64): intestinal cell carcinoma type 1. Tumor; 35 mm; lesser curvature, antrum; stage II. Small and large gland patterns. Radical subtotal gastrectomy probably would have cured this patient. Cancerous metaplastic intestinal epithelial cells at surface and in crypts of mucosa. H&E. × 100.

A quantitative summary of the histologic features, seen with the hematoxylin and eosin stain, of all three types of carcinoma appears in Table 14.

SPECIAL STAINS. In selected carcinomas in the second series of 130 cases studied, periodic acid-fuchsin-sulfurous acid and mucicarmine stains were employed. The results confirmed those given in Table 17 of our original paper [1] and are woven into the histologic features detailed above.

FREE HYDROCHLORIC ACID. Special attention was paid to the level of free hydrochloric acid in the gastric juice of the 126 patients in the second series with classified carcinomas. Values were recorded in 24 of these 126 patients (about 20 percent—10 with mucous cell carcinoma: nine with zero values and one with 34° of hydrochloric acid; eight with pylorocardiac gland cell carcinoma: seven with zero values and one with 62° of hydrochloric acid; and six with intestinal cell carcinoma: three with zero values and three with 24, 66, and 88° of hydrochloric acid). Those with elevated levels of free hydrochloric acid revealed striking ulceration and destruction of their carcinomas and extensive fibrosis of the submucosa, muscle coats, and serosa directly beneath the ulcers; there was relatively little or at most slight superficial necrosis of the carcinomas in patients with zero values.

PERNICIOUS ANEMIA. Among the total series of 259 patients with classified carcinomas, pernicious anemia was found in four with the intestinal cell type, in

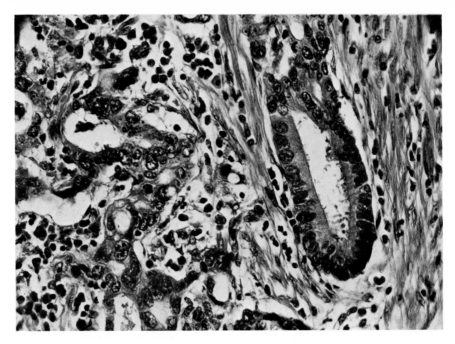

Fig. 21. Case 106: intestinal cell carcinoma type 1. See legend for Figure 20. In gland at right, transition of atypical metaplastic epithelial cells to carcinoma cells; at left, anastomosed neoplastic glandular structures. H&E. × 325.

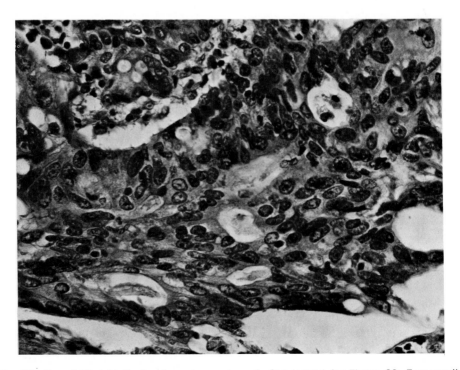

Fig. 22. Case 106: intestinal cell carcinoma type 1. See legend for Figure 20. Few small glands and anastomosed solid aggregates of carcinoma cells in mucosa. H&E. × 325.

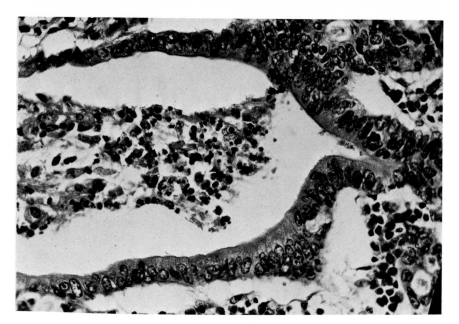

Fig. 23. Case 106: intestinal cell carcinoma type 1. See legend for Figure 20. Detail of carcinoma cells lining neoplastic gland of mucosa. H&E. × 325.

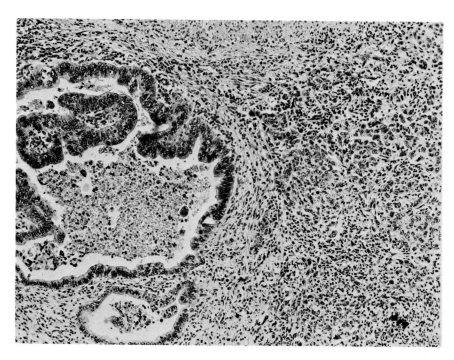

Fig. 24. Case 104 (male, 78): intestinal cell carcinoma with types 1 and 2 patterns. Tumor: 4 cm; lesser curvature, antrum found at autopsy; stage IV. Undifferentiated features, small and large gland patterns, and origin from glandular polyp. Mucosa of stomach marked by multiple glandular polyps. Large gland pattern (left half of figure); undifferentiated pattern and prominent lymphoid admixture (right half). H&E. × 100.

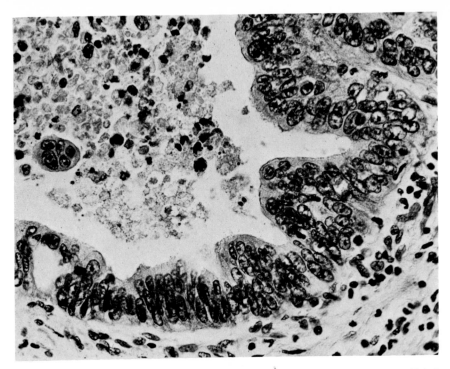

Fig. 25. Case 104: intestinal cell carcinoma with types 1 and 2 patterns. Detail of large gland pattern seen in Figure 24. Enlarged, hyperchromatic nuclei in stratified, disorderly, columnar epithelial cells in undulated folds. H&E. × 400.

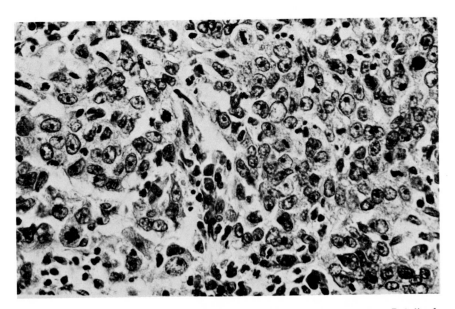

Fig. 26. Case 104: intestinal cell carcinoma with types 1 and 2 patterns. Detail of undifferentiated portion seen in Figure 24. Cells in loose aggregates intermingled with lymphocytes. Nuclei enlarged, rounded, chromatin marginated, nucleoli prominent, abnormal mitoses. H&E. × 400.

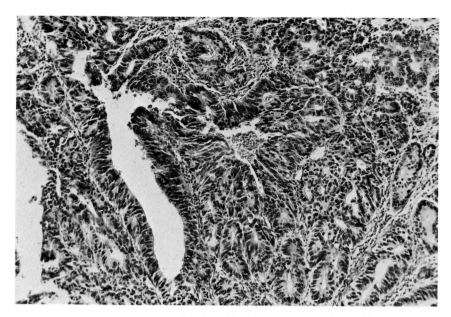

Fig. 27. Case 113 (male, 65): intestinal cell carcinoma type 1. First tumor: 95 mm; posterior wall, fundus; stage IV. Small and large gland patterns. Only metastasis in a superior gastric lymph node. Large gland at left with many secondary glands. Small glands at right. H&E. × 100.

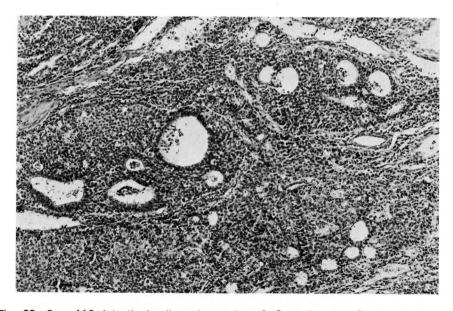

Fig. 28. Case 113: intestinal cell carcinoma type 2. Second tumor; 9 cm; anterior wall, fundus; stage IV. Diffusely confluent aggregates of carcinoma cells punctuated by small glands and surrounded by abundant lymphoid tissue. H&E. × 100.

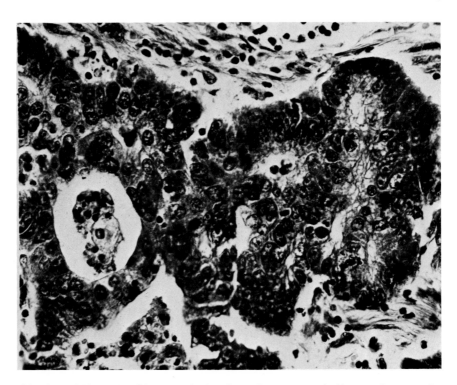

Fig. 29. Case 111 (male, 81): intestinal cell carcinoma type 1. Tumor: 3 cm, antrum, stage IV. Small and large gland patterns. Suggestive origin from a glandular polyp. Merging of small gland pattern with solid aggregates of carcinoma cells. H&E. × 400.

three with the mucous cell type (one related to prior total gastrectomy 5 years before the anemia became manifest), and two with the pylorocardiac gland cell type.

Intestinal Cell Metaplasia.   With the much greater frequency of routine sampling of grossly noncancerized mucosa in the 126 patients in the second series with classified carcinomas, more adequate comment regarding intestinal cell metaplasia previously referred to as atrophy can be made. Of 56 patients with mucous cell carcinoma, 21 had intestinal cell metaplasia of the gastric mucosa (37.5 percent); of 42 with pylorocardiac gland cell carcinoma, 18 (43 percent); and of 28 with intestinal cell carcinoma, 22 (80 percent). Intestinal cell metaplasia was not only more common but more severe in the grossly noncancerized mucosa of patients with intestinal cell carcinoma than in those with the other two types of carcinoma.

Contributory Causes of Death.   Among 165 autopsied patients with classified carcinoma—92 mucous cell, 49 pylorocardiac gland cell, and 24 intestinal cell—the following important contributory causes of death were observed: pneumonia 25, peritonitis 16, hemorrhage 8, pulmonary embolism 7, fatty metamorphosis of the liver 7, myocardial infarction due to arteriosclerosis of coronary arteries with stenosis or thrombosis 6, severe ulcerative esophagitis 6, active tuberculosis of lungs and bronchial lymph nodes 4, septicemia 4, cerebral hemorrhage 2,

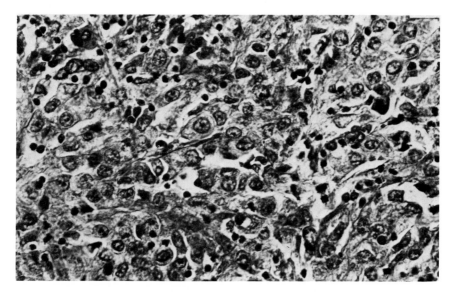

Fig. 30. Case 131 (male, 41): intestinal cell carcinoma type 2. Tumor: 8 cm; lesser curvature, fundus; stage III. Undifferentiated features, small glands, and abundant lymphoid tissue. H&E. × 400.

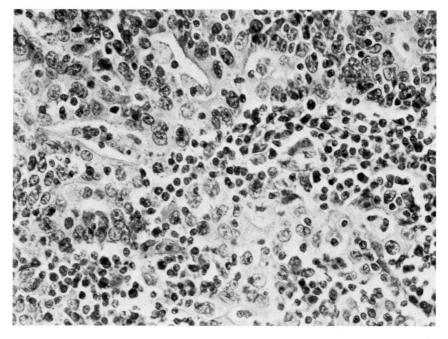

Fig. 31. Case 129 (male, 71): intestinal cell carcinoma type 2. Tumor: 8 cm, antrum, stage III. Undifferentiated features in this field and spotty small gland pattern in others not depicted. Histologic features identical with those in Figure 26. H&E. × 400.

mediastinitis 2, portal cirrhosis 2, pancreatitis 2, and collapse of lung due to massive hydrothorax, cerebral infarction, and rheumatic heart disease 1 each.

TUMORS COEXISTENT WITH GASTRIC CARCINOMA. Table 15 presents a listing of the benign and malignant tumors coexistent with gastric carcinoma. Those with the greatest pertinence are adenocarcinoma of the large intestine, four; polyps of the large intestine, three; polyps of the stomach, three; independent carcinoma in situ of the stomach, one. Of passing note are the following: four adenocarcinomas of the prostate, often coincident with other carcinomas,[95] and one case each of squamous cell carcinoma of the bladder, lymphocytic lymphosarcoma, adenocarcinoma of the common bile duct, malignant melanoma of the skin, and infiltrative duct carcinoma of the breast.

Table 15. Tumors Coexistent with Gastric Carcinoma*

Case 7 — Male 60; MC; 15-mm rectal polyp

Case 69 — Male 74; PGC; pancreatic heterotopia, wall of stomach

Case 71 — Male 60; PGC; localized squamous cell carcinoma of bladder

Case 101 — Female 72; IC; polyp 1 cm, antrum, stomach

Case 104 — Male 78; IC; multiple polyps, stomach

Case 114 — Male 75; IC; adenocarcinoma, prostate

Case 141 — Male 71; MC; carcinoma in situ, vocal cords

Case 145 — Male 72; MC; lymphocytic lymphosarcoma; carcinoid tumor, duodenum

Case 165 — Female 72; MC; adenocarcinoma, common bile duct

Case 177 — Female 33; MC; malignant melanoma, skin, back, widely metastatic

Case 180 — Female 56; MC; carcinoma in situ, cervix

Case 182 — Female 57; MC; leiomyoma 4 cm, broad ligament

Case 188 — Male 74; MC; small leiomyoma, stomach

Case 191 — Female 75; MC; fibroadenoma, right breast

Case 193 — Female 60; MC; infiltrative duct carcinoma, left breast

Case 195 — Male 84; PGC; adenocarcinoma, rectum, localized; leiomyoma, ileum

Case 198 — Female 74; PGC; basal cell carcinoma, skin, neck

Case 199 — Male 67; PGC; cortical adenoma 4 cm, right adrenal

Case 205 — Male 79; PGC; polyp 1 cm, transverse colon

Case 213 — Male 74; PGC; two small leiomyomas, stomach

Case 215 — Male 67; PGC; adenocarcinoma, prostate

Case 219 — Female 69; PGC; mucous cell carcinoma in situ; 8-mm polyp, antrum; two carcinomas in situ, IC type, mucosa antrum; pancreatic heterotopia, duodenum

Case 220 — Female 60; PGC; bronchial cyst 14 mm, distal esophagus

Case 221 — Male 95; PGC; adenocarcinoma, prostate

Case 223 — Male 81; PGC; cystadenoma 1 cm, kidney

Case 244 — Male 83; IC; two basal cell carcinomas, skin, face

Case 252 — Male 78; IC; adenocarcinoma, sigmoid colon, metastatic to regional lymph nodes

Case 261 — Male 72; IC; adenocarcinoma, cecum, localized

Case 262 — Male 84; IC; polyp, intestinal cell type 3 cm, antrum; nodular hyperplasia, prostate; adenocarcinoma, rectum, localized; adenocarcinoma, prostate; polyp, small, descending colon

*The type of carcinoma is identified in each case as follows: MC, mucous cell; PGC, pylorocardiac gland cell; IC, intestinal cell.

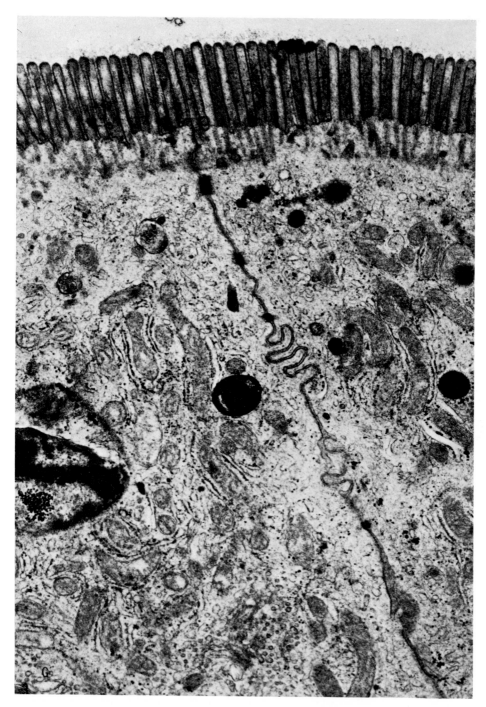

Fig. 32. Metaplastic intestinal epithelial cell of mucosa, human stomach. Prominent micro-villi, interdigitation with adjacent cells, numerous profiles of ribosome-studded endoplasmic reticulum, sausage-shaped mitochondria, and lysosome containing ribosomal membranes. From Rubin, Ross, Jeffries, and Sleisenger. Lab. Invest., 15:1024–1049, 1966. Courtesy of The Williams & Wilkins Co.

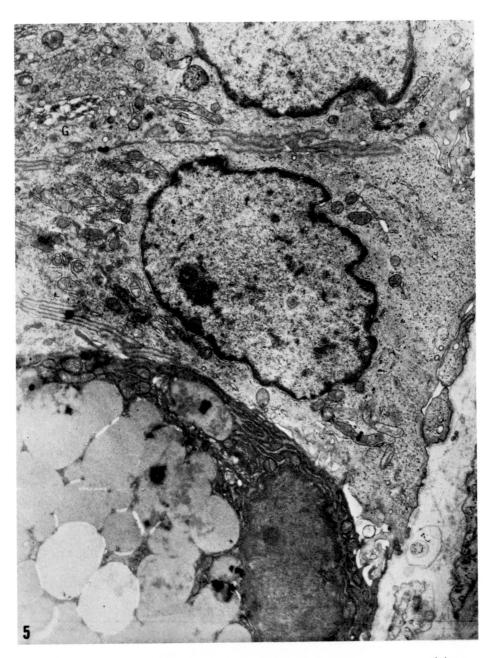

Fig. 33. Two metaplastic intestinal epithelial cells, middle and top, mucosa of human stomach. Mitochondria and endoplasmic reticulum at left, base of middle cell at right. Portion of mucous cell at bottom. From Rubin, Ross, Jeffries, and Sleisenger. Lab. Invest., 15:1024–1049, 1966. Courtesy of The Williams & Wilkins Co.

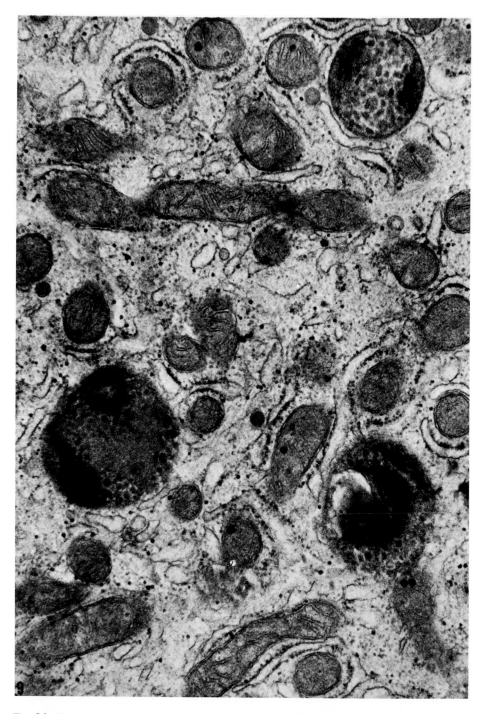

Fig. 34. Metaplastic intestinal epithelial cell of mucosa, human stomach. Details of endo-plasmic reticulum and mitochondria. From Rubin, Ross, Jeffries, and Sleisenger. Lab. Invest., 15:1024–1049, 1966. Courtesy of The Williams & Wilkins Co.

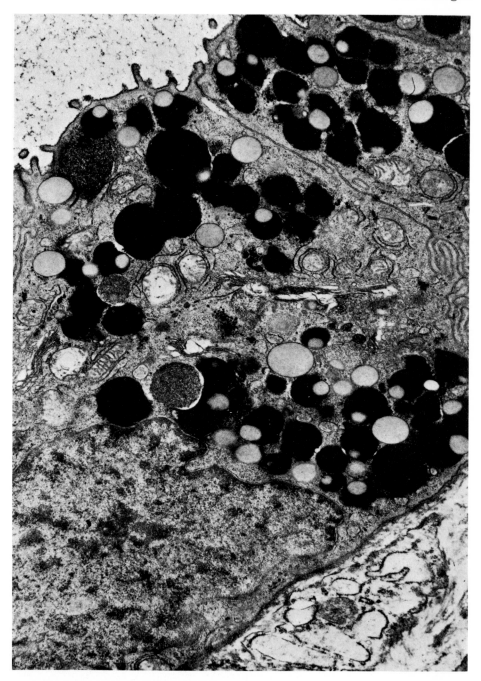

Fig. 35. Normal pyloric gland cell of mucosa, human stomach. Pyloric gland cells resemble mucous cells, but contain homogeneous granules like those of chief cells. Granules in basal cytoplasm. × 12,600. From Rubin, Ross, Jeffries, Sleisenger. Lab. Invest. 15: 1024–1049, 1966. Courtesy of The Williams & Wilkins Co.

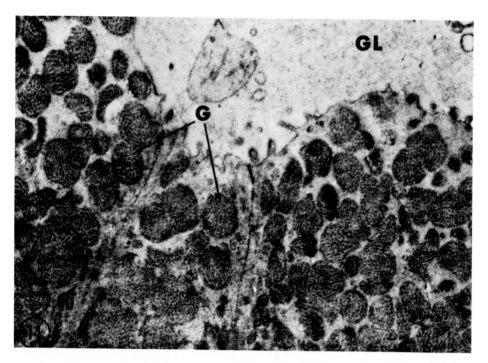

Fig. 36. Normal mucous epithelial cell of mucosa, human stomach. From Lillibridge. Gastroenterology, 47:269–290, 1964.

PRIOR OPERATION FOR "BENIGN" DISEASE. Six patients had prior gastric surgery for supposed benign disease as follows:

Case 141 (man 41)—antral mucous cell carcinoma widely metastatic to abdominal structures; gastrojejunostomy several months before admission for obstructive chronic duodenal ulcer.

Case 150 (woman 71)—antral mucous cell carcinoma widely metastatic to abdominal structures; gastrojejunostomy 2 years before admission for stenosing duodenal ulcer.

Case 161 (man 60)—diffuse mucous cell carcinoma widely metastatic to abdominal structures; gastrojejunostomy 5 years before admission for duodenal ulcer.

Case 186 (woman 69)—fundic mucous cell carcinoma metastatic to regional lymph nodes; partial gastrectomy and gastrojejunostomy 7 years 7 months before admission for lesion of undesignated type.

Case 247 (man 85)—antral intestinal cell carcinoma type 1; gastrojejunostomy several years before admission for chronic duodenal ulcer.

Case 263 (man 60)—two polypoid fundic intestinal cell carcinomas limited to the stomach; partial gastrectomy and gastrojejunostomy 22 years before admission for chronic duodenal ulcer; alive and free of recurrent carcinoma 19 months after esophagogastrectomy and esophagojejunostomy.

All but the last of these six patients died of recurrent gastric carcinoma.

Summary

The experience of the Colorado General Hospital with 268 cases of gastric carcinoma during the period 1927 through 1968 may be recapitulated as follows.

MUCOUS CELL CARCINOMA.

1. Male/female ratio: 2.18, about as expected for all gastric carcinoma.
2. Significant frequency before the age of 50 years; occurrence of about 60 percent past the age of 60 years.
3. Cancerization: directly by topical application of carcinogens or indirectly by localization of radioisotopes.

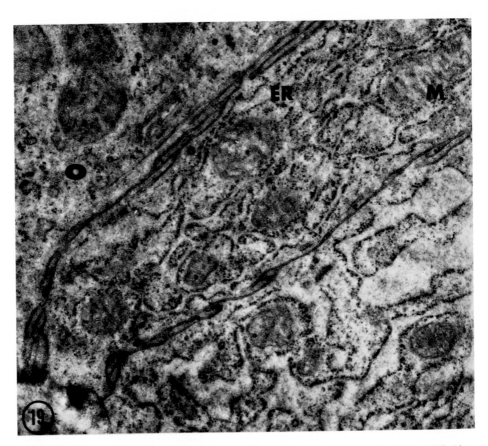

Fig. 37. Base of normal mucous epithelial cell of mucosa, human stomach. From Lillibridge. Gastroenterology, 47:269–290, 1964.

4. Origin in mucous neck and mucous epithelial cells.
5. Dominant localization in the antrum and a significant tendency to involve the entire stomach.
6. Less than 10 percent confined to the stomach.
7. Extension index (total number of extensions divided by the total number of carcinomas): 0.68.
8. Two times greater capacity to metastasize than pylorocardiac gland cell carcinoma and about three times greater than intestinal cell carcinoma.
9. Salvage: 5 percent.
10. Diffuse and subtle origin from gastric mucosa in nondelimited fashion.
11. Microscopic features of 121 carcinomas: undifferentiated 111, signet ring cells 106, mucin 101, incomplete small glands 70, rare mitoses, satellite foci of carcinoma in grossly normal mucosa.
12. Intense staining of many malignant mucous epithelial cells with periodic acid-fuchsin-sulfurous acid and mucicarmine methods.
13. Strong tendency to incite productive fibrosis in invaded tissues of host.

Pylorocardiac Gland Cell Carcinoma

1. Male/female ratio: 4.13, about twice that expected for all gastric carcinoma.
2. Occurrence: more than 75 percent in persons past the age of 60 years.
3. Protected position of pyloric and cardiac glands and high frequency in males compared to other two types of gastric carcinoma suggestive of genesis connected with steroid hormone imbalance.
4. Origin in pyloric and cardiac gland cells of stomach.
5. Dominant localization in the antrum and a significant tendency to originate in the cardia of the stomach.
6. More than 20 percent confined to the stomach.
7. Extension index: 0.64.
8. Tendency to metastasize: about half that of the mucous cell carcinoma.
9. Salvage: 15 percent.
10. Usual delimited growth fungated into lumen of stomach.
11. Microscopic features of 77 carcinomas: small glands 74, large glands 69, secretion 71, undifferentiated 14, frequent vacuolated cytoplasm in neoplastic cells, alternating stratification and single orientation of neoplastic epithelial cells, mitoses frequent when tumor cells stratified, satellite foci unusual in grossly normal mucosa.
12. Most brilliant staining of malignant pylorocardiac gland cells with periodic acid-fuchsin-sulfurous acid method.
13. Incitation of relatively little fibrous connective tissue reaction by the host to the invasive carcinoma.
14. Tendency to invade submucosal veins.

Intestinal Cell Carcinoma

1. Male/female ratio: 3.07, not significantly different from the average for all gastric carcinomas in this series.
2. Occurrence rate nearly 75 percent in persons past the age of 60 years.

3. Cancerization: possibility of anaplasia of metaplastic intestinal epithelial cells by absorption of fat-soluble carcinogens.
4. Origin in metaplastic intestinal epithelial cells of polypoid or flat mucosa.
5. Dominant localization in the antrum and notable tendency to arise in the fundus of the stomach.
6. More than 40 percent confined to the stomach.
7. Most predictable as the type of gastric carcinoma in pernicious anemia.
8. Only about 40 percent of the tendency of mucous cell and pylorocardiac gland cell carcinomas to extend beyond the stomach.
9. About one-third of the capacity of mucous cell carcinoma to metastasize.
10. Salvage: 38 percent.
11. Delimited, polypoid, fungated, or relatively flat nodular growth.
12. Notable frequency of two or more synchronous or metachronous, primary carcinomas.
13. Microscopic features of 68 carcinomas: IC-1 in 33: small glands 29, large glands 29, undifferentiated 9; IC-2 in 35: undifferentiated 32, small glands 30, focal large glands 7, prominent cytoplasmic basophilia; crossover between IC-1 and IC-2 patterns in same tumor or in two tumors in a single patient; frequent foci of carcinoma in situ adjacent to main carcinoma(s).
14. Weak or absent staining of neoplastic cells with periodic acid-fuchsin-sulfurous acid and mucicarmine methods.
15. Incitation of moderate to abundant lymphoid tissue of host; also relatively little connective tissue reaction by the host, unless peptic digestion of the carcinoma is severe.
16. Tendency to invade submucosal veins.

References

1. Mulligan, R. M., and Rember, R. R. Histogenesis and biologic behavior of gastric carcinoma: study of 138 cases. Arch. Path. (Chicago), 58:1–25, 1954.
2. Mulligan, R. M. Important aspects of the metabolism of the liver cell revealed in selected references. Exp. Med. Surg., 26:66–95, 1968.
3. Salenius, P. On the ontogenesis of the human gastric epithelial cells. Acta anat. (Basel), 50 (Suppl. 1):1–76, 1962.
4. Bélanger, L. F. Autoradiographic detection of sulphur-35 synthesis by the mucous neck cells of the rat's stomach. Nature (London), 172:1150, 1953.
5. Hunt, T. E., and Hunt, E. A. Radioautographic study of proliferation in the stomach of the rat using thymidine-H-3 and compound 48/80. Anat. Rec., 142:505–517, 1962.
6. MacDonald, W. C., Trier, J. S., and Everett, N. B. Cell proliferation and migration in the stomach, duodenum, and rectum of man: radioautographic studies. Gastroenterology, 46:405–417, 1964.
7. Teir, H., and Räsänen, T. A. A study of mitotic rate in renewal zones of nondiseased portions of gastric mucosa in cases of peptic ulcer and gastric cancer, with observations on differentiation and so-called "intestinalization" of gastric mucosa. J. Nat. Cancer Inst., 27:949–972, 1961.
8. Clark, R. H., and Baker, B. L. Effect of hypophysectomy on mitotic proliferation in gastric epithelium. Amer. J. Physiol., 204:1018–1022, 1963.

9. Lillibridge, C. B. The fine structure of normal human gastric mucosa. Gastroenterology, 47:269–290, 1964.
10. Helander, H., and Ekholm, R. Ultrastructure of epithelial cells in the fundus glands of the mouse gastric mucosa. J. Ultrastruct. Res., 3:74–83, 1959.
11. Loring, W. E., and Hartley, L. J. The destructive effects of DL-ethionine on the pancreas, stomach, and submaxillary glands. Amer. J. Path., 31:521–533, 1955.
12. Mulligan, R. M. Protein synthesis as a determining factor in carcinogenesis. Exp. Med. Surg., 24:288–302, 1966.
13. Baker, B. L., and Abrams, G. D. Effect of hypophysectomy on the cytology of the fundic glands of the stomach and the secretion of pepsin. Amer. J. Physiol., 177:409–412, 1954.
14. Debray, C., Laumonier, R., Hardouin, J. P., and Faye, C. M. Les lésions histologiques de la muqueuse gastrique au cours des altérations expérimentales des glandes endocrines chez la ratte. II. Action de la surréalectomie. C. R. Soc. Biol. (Paris), 154:283–284, 1960.
15. Lewinter, P., and Spiro, H. M. Gastric chief cell hyperplasia induced by hypercalcemia. Metabolism, 9:847–852, 1960.
16. Ballard, H. S., Frame, B., and Hartsock, R. J. Familial multiple adenoma—peptic ulcer complex. Medicine (Balt.), 43:481–516, 1964.
17. Nomura, Y. On the submicroscopic morphogenesis of parietal cell in the gastric gland of the human fetus. Z. Anat. Entwicklungsgesch., 125:316–356, 1966.
18. Ito, S. The endoplasmic reticulum of gastric parietal cells. J. Biophys. Biochem. Cytol., 11:333–347, 1961.
19. Gusek, W. Zur ultramikroskopischen Cytologie der Belegzellen in der Magenschleimhaut des Menschen. Z. Zellforsch., 55:790–809, 1961.
20. Lawn, A. M. Observations on the fine structure of the gastric parietal cell of the rat. J. Biophys. Biochem. Cytol., 7:161–166, 1960.
21. Sedar, A. W., and Friedman, M. H. F. Correlation of the fine structure of gastric parietal cell (dog) with functional activity in the stomach. J. Biophys. Biochem. Cytol., 11:349–363, 1961.
22. Carvalheira, A. F., Welsch, U., and Pearse, A. G. E. Cytological and ultrastructural observations on the argentaffin and argyrophil cells of the gastrointestinal tract in mammals and their place in the APUD series of polypeptide-secreting cells. Histochemie, 14:33–46, 1968.
23. Pearse, A. G. E. Common cytochemical and ultrastructural characteristics of cells producing polypeptide hormones (the APUD series) and their relevance to thyroid and ultimobranchial C cells and calcitonin. Proc. Roy. Soc. [Biol.[, 170:71–80, 1968.
24. Solcia, E., Vassallo, G., and Capella, C. Studies on the G cells of the pyloric mucosa, the probable site of gastrin secretion. Gut, 10:379–388, 1969.
25. Lattes, R., and Grossi, C. Carcinoid tumors of the stomach. Cancer, 9:698–711, 1956.
26. Laster, L., and Walsh, J. H. Enzymatic degradation of C-terminal tetrapeptide amide of gastrin by mammalian tissue extracts. Fed. Proc., 27:1328–1330, 1968.
27. Grossman, M. I. Physiological role of gastrin. Fed. Proc., 27:1312–1313, 1968.
28. Morley, J. S. Structure-activity relationships. Fed. Proc., 27:1314–1317, 1968.
29. Townsend, S. F. Regeneration of gastric mucosa in rats. Amer. J. Anat., 109:133–147, 1961.
30. Correia, J. P., Filipe, M. I., and Santos, J. C. Histochemistry of the gastric mucosa. Gut, 4:68–76, 1963.
31. Ragins, H., and Dittbrenner, M. Intracellular enzymatic histochemistry of the human stomach with special reference to atrophic gastritis. Gut, 6:357–363, 1965.
32. Villareal, R., and Burgos, M. H. A correlated biochemical and histochemical study of succinic dehydrogenase activity in the gastric mucosa of the rat and the frog. J. Cell. Comp. Physiol., 46:327–339, 1955.

33. Niemi, M., Siurala, M., and Sundberg, M. The distribution of cytochemically demonstrable diphosphopyridine nucleotide diaphorase and succinic and lactic dehydrogenases in the normal human gastric mucosa. Acta Path. Microbiol. Scand., 48:323–327, 1960.

34. Planteydt, H. T., and Willihagen, R. G. J. Enzyme histochemistry of gastric carcinoma. J. Path. Bact., 90:393:398, 1965.

35. Räsänen, T. Mucosal mast cells of rat stomach: influence of ACTH, cortisone, and growth hormone. Gastroenterology, 38:70–75, 1960.

36. Raskin, H. F., Palmer, W. L., and Kirsner, J. B. Benign and malignant exfoliated gastrointestinal mucosal cells. Arch. Intern. Med. (Chicago), 107:872–884, 1961.

37. Hoskins, L. C., and Zamcheck, N. Studies on the "mucous barrier:" evaluation of sialic acid as a protective factor against degradation of gastric mucus by pancreatic endopeptidases. Gastroenterology, 44:456–462, 1963.

38. Gottschalk, A. The basic structure of glycoproteins and problems of chemical and physiochemical analysis. Ann N.Y. Acad. Sci., 106:168–176, 1963.

39. Green, P., and Bergman, M. "Mucinemia:" report of a case of carcinomatosis with a unique serum protein. Canad. Med. Ass. J., 86:418–419, 1962.

40. Richmond, V., Caputto, R., and Wolf, S. Biochemical study of the large molecule constituents of gastric juice. Gastroenterology, 29:1017–1021, 1965.

41. Masamune, H., Kawasaki, H., Sinohara, H., Abe, S., and Abe, S. Molisch-positive mucopolysaccharides of gastric cancers as compared with corresponding components of normal mucosa. Tohoku J. Exp. Med., 72:328–337, 1960.

42. Schrager, J. Chromatographic studies of the carbohydrate components of gastric and salivary polysaccharides. Gut, 5:166–169, 1964.

43. Shimizu, F. Free amino acids in the gastric juice of patients with gastric cancer. Tohoku J. Exp. Med., 65:229–236, 1957.

44. Oh-Uti, K., and Awataguchi, J. Free amino acids in gastric juice of patients with gastric or duodenal ulcer and gastric carcinoma, with special reference to the change after operation. Tohoku J. Exp. Med., 67:123–130, 1958.

45. Abasov, I. T. Chromatographic analysis of free amino acids of gastric juice in patients with cancer and other stomach diseases. Neoplasma (Bratisl.), 14:429–434, 1967.

46. Hoedemaeker, P. J., Abels, J., Wachters, J. J., Arends, A., and Niewig, H. O. Investigations about the site of production of Castle's intrinsic factor. Lab. Invest., 13:1394–1399, 1965.

47. Hoedemaeker, P. J., Abels, J., Wachters, J. J., Arends, A., and Niewig, H. O. Further investigation about the site of production of Castle's gastric intrinsic factor. Lab. Invest., 15:1163–1173, 1966.

48. Solomon, S. P., and Spiro, H. M. The effects of glucagon and glucose on the human stomach. Amer. J. Dig. Dis., 4:775–786, 1959.

49. Dotevall, G. Gastric function in diabetes mellitus. Acta Med. Scand., 170 (Suppl. 368):1–36, 1961.

50. Hunt, J. N., and Knox, M. T. A. Relation between the chain length of fatty acids and the slowing of gastric emptying. J. Physiol., 194:327–336, 1968.

51. Hoar, C. S., Jr., and Browning, J. R. Plasma pepsinogen in peptic-ulcer disease and other gastric disorders. New Eng. J. Med., 255:153–158, 1956.

52. Bock, O. A. A., Arapakis, G., Witts, G. J., and Richards, W. C. D. The serum pepsinogen level with special reference to the histology of the gastric mucosa. Gut, 4:106–111, 1963.

53. Balfour, D. C., Jr. Increased uropepsin excretion during testosterone administration. Amer. J. Gastroent., 25:341–345, 1956.

54. Boles, R. S. Cancer of the stomach. Gastroenterology, 34:847–858, 1958.

55. Haenszel, W. Variation in incidence of and mortality from stomach cancer with particular reference to the United States. J. Nat. Cancer Inst., 21:213–262, 1958.

56. Sigurjonsson, J. Trends in mortality from cancer, with special reference to gastric cancer in Iceland. J. Nat. Cancer Inst., 36:899–907, 1966.
57. Dungal, N. The special problem of stomach cancer in Iceland. J.A.M.A., 178: 789–798, 1961.
58. Sigurjonsson, J. Occupational variations in mortality from gastric cancer in relation to dietary differences. Brit. J. Cancer, 21:651–656, 1967.
59. Videbaek, A., and Mosbech, J. ʾ ̖ ᴸe etiology of gastric carcinoma elucidated by a study of 302 pedigrees. Acta Med. Scand., 149:137–159, 1954.
60. Laurén, P. The two histological main types of gastric carcinoma: diffuse and so-called intestinal-type carcinoma. Acta Path. Microbiol. Scand., 64:31–49, 1965.
61. Kuru, M., and Ryozo, S. Histogenetical study of gastric carcinomas in the Japanese: analysis of 150 cases treated in relatively early stages. *In* Proceedings of the Ninth International Cancer Congress. UICC Monograph Series 10. Berlin, Springer-Verlag, 1967, pp. 1–30.
62. Munoz, N., Correa, P., Cuello, C., and Duque, E. Histologic types of gastric carcinoma in high- and low-risk areas. Int. J. Cancer, 3:809–818, 1968.
63. Mosbech, J., and Videbaek, A. Mortality from and risk of gastric carcinoma among patients with pernicious anemia. Brit. Med. J., 2:390–394, 1950.
64. Schell, R. F., Dockerty, M. B., and Comfort, M. W. Carcinoma of the stomach associated with pernicious anemia. Surg. Gynec. Obstet., 98:710–720, 1954.
65. Doehring, P. C. Carcinoma of the stomach associated with pernicious anemia. Western J. Surg., 62:391–394, 1954.
66. Rubin, C. E. The diagnosis of gastric malignancy in pernicious anemia. Gastroenterology, 29:563–584, 1955.
67. Siurala, M., Erämaa, E., and Tapiovaara, J. Pernicious anemia and gastric carcinoma. Acta Med. Scand., 164:431–436, 1959.
68. Siurala, M., and Seppala, K. Atrophic gastritis as a precursor of gastric carcinoma and pernicious anemia. Acta Med. Scand., 166:455–474, 1960.
69. Grable, E., Zamcheck, N., Jankelson, N., and Shipp, F. Nuclear size of cells in normal stomach, in gastric atrophy, and in gastric cancer. Gastroenterology, 32: 1104–1112, 1957.
70. Joske, R. A., Finckh, E. S., and Wood, I. J. Gastric biopsy: a study of 1000 consecutive successful gastric biopsies. Quart. J. Med., 24:269–294, 1955.
71. MacLean, L. D., and Sundberg, R. D. Incidence of megaloblastic anemia after total gastrectomy. New Eng. J. Med., 254:885–893, 1956.
72. Schmidt, A. Untersuchungen über das menschliche Magenepithel unter normalen und pathologischen Verhältnissen. Virchow. Arch. Path. Anat., 143:477–508, 1896.
73. Klein, N. C., Sleisenger, M. H., and Weiser, E. Disaccharidases, leucine aminopeptidase, and glucose uptake in intestinalized gastric mucosa and in gastric carcinoma. Gastroenterology, 55:61–67, 1968.
74. Rubin, W., Ross, L. L., Jeffries, G. H., and Sleisenger, M. H. Some physiologic properties of heterotopic intestinal epithelium: its role in transporting lipid into the gastric mucosa. Lab. Invest., 16:813–827, 1967.
75. Kimura, K., Hiramoto, T., and Buncher, C. R. Gastric xanthelasma. Arch. Path. (Chicago), 87:110–117, 1969.
76. Rubin, W., Ross, L. L., Jeffries, G. H., and Sleisenger, M. H. Intestinal heterotopia: a fine structural study. Lab. Invest., 15:1024–1049, 1966.
77. Geissendorfer, R. Untersuchungen über Vorkommen, Lokalisation und Ausbreitungsweise der Umbaugastritis in Carcinomägen. Arch. Klin. Chir., 153:235–252, 1928.
78. Järvi, O., and Laurén, P. On the role of heterotopias of the intestinal epithelium in the pathogenesis of gastric cancer. Acta Path. Microbiol. Scand., 29:26–44, 1951.

79. Morson, B. C. Intestinal metaplasia of the gastric mucosa. Brit. J. Cancer, 9:365–376, 1955a.

80. Gosset, A., and Masson, P. Cancer intestinal de l'estomac. Presse Med., 20:225–228, 1912.

81. Masson, P. Diagnostics de Laboratoire. II Tumeurs. Paris, A. Maloine et Fils, 1923, pp. 405–417.

82. Morson, B. C. Carcinoma arising from areas of intestinal metaplasia in the gastric mucosa. Brit. J. Cancer, 9:377–385, 1955b.

83. Nakamura, K., Sugano, H., and Tagaki, K. Carcinoma of the stomach in incipient phase: its histogenesis and histological appearances. Gann 59:251–258, 1968.

84. Morson, B. C. Gastric polyps composed of intestinal epithelium. Brit. J. Cancer, 9:550–557, 1955c.

85. Berg, J. W. Histological aspects of the relation between gastric adenomatous polyps and gastric cancer. Cancer, 11:1149–1155, 1958.

86. Monroe, L. S., Boughton, G. A., and Sommers, S. C. Epithelial hyperplasia and cancer. Gastroenterology, 46:267–272, 1964.

87. Mulligan, R. M. Comparative pathology of human and canine cancer. Ann. N.Y. Acad. Sci., 108:642–690, 1963.

88. McPeak, E., and Warren, S. Histologic features of carcinoma of the cardioesophageal junction and cardia. Amer. J. Path., 24:971–1001, 1948.

89. Steiner, P. E., Maimon, S. N., Palmer, W. L., and Kirsner, J. B. Gastric cancer: morphologic factors in five-year survival after gastrectomy. Amer. J. Path., 24:947–961, 1948.

90. Takeda, K. Cancer of the stomach in Japan from the viewpoint of pathological anatomy. Schweiz. Z. Path. Bakt., 18:538–550, 1955.

91. Katami, J. On the late results of ordinary gastric resection for cancer, with special reference between the results and the histopathologic findings. Tohoku J. Exp. Med., 62:117–127, 1955.

92. Ringertz, N. The pathology of gastric cancer and its relationship to gastritis, polyps and cancer. Acta Un. Int. Cancr., 17:289–295, 1961.

93. Kori, Y., Yamashita, S., Shimamoto, K., Ashikara, T., Takeoka, O., Fujita, K., Kawai, K., Kadotari, H., and Shinoda, M. Development of stomach cancer in the human body. Saishin Igaku, 24:471–481, 1969.

94. Kuru, M., ed. Atlas of Early Carcinoma of the Stomach. Tokyo, Nakayama Shorten Co. Ltd., 1967.

95. Mulligan, R. M. Geriatric cancer: analysis of 257 autopsied cancer patients 70 years of age and older. Cancer, 12:970–981, 1959.

96. Grant, R. N. Cancer Statistics. New York, American Cancer Society, 1969.

97. Alvarez, W. C., and McCarty, W. C. Sizes of resected gastric ulcers and gastric carcinomas. J.A.M.A., 91:226–231, 1928.

98. Lampert, E. G., Waugh, J. M., and Dockerty, M. B. The incidence of malignancy in gastric ulcers believed preoperatively to be benign. Surg. Gynec. Obstet., 91:673–679, 1950.

99. Marshall, S. F., and Welch, M. L. Results of surgical treatment for gastric ulcer. J.A.M.A., 136:748–752, 1948.

100. Sunderland, D. A., McNeer, G., Ortega, L. G., and Pearce, L. The lymphatic spread of gastric cancer. Cancer, 6:987–996, 1953.

101. Dochat, G. R., and Gray, H. G. Carcinoma of the stomach: prognosis based on a combination of Dukes and Broders methods of grading. Amer. J. Clin. Path., 13:441–449, 1943.

102. Dukes, C. The classification of cancer of the rectum. J. Path. Bact., 35:323–332, 1932.

103. Stout, A. P. Pathology of carcinoma of the stomach. Arch. Surg. (Chicago), 46:807–822, 1943.

104. Harding, W. G., Jr., and Harkins, F. D. Postmortem observations of 158 cases of carcinoma of the stomach. Amer. J. Cancer, 16:561–563, 1932.
105. Walther, H. E. Krebsmetastasen. Basel, Benno Schwabe and Co., 1948, p. 560.
106. Moore, G. E., State, D., Hebbel, R., and Treloar, A. E. Carcinoma of the stomach: the validity of basing prognosis upon Borrmann typing or the presence of metastases. Surg. Gynec. Obstet., 87:513–518, 1948.
107. Benedict, E. B. A clinicopathological study of carcinoma of the stomach using large microscopic sections and dissecting lymphatic spread. Edinburgh Med. J., 39:263–267, 1932.
108. Walters, W., Gray, H. K., and Priestley, J. T. Prognosis and end results in the treatment of cancer of the stomach. Arch. Surg. (Chicago), 46:939–943, 1943.
109. Borrmann, R. Geschwülste des Magens und Duodenums: III. Epitheliale Geschwülste; Karzinom. *In* Henke, F., and Lubarsch, O., eds. Handbuch der speziellen pathologischen Anatomie und Histologie. Berlin, Springer-Verlag, 1926, pp. 855–988.
110. Konjetzny, G. E. Der Magenkrebs. Stuttgart, Ferdinand Enke, 1938, p. 289.
111. Warwick, M. Analysis of 176 cases of carcinoma of the stomach submitted to autopsy. Ann. Surg., 88:216–226, 1928.

Addendum

In the review of literature not available or overlooked since publication of the foregoing paper in *Pathology Annual 1972,* the same sequence of headings is preserved insofar as practicable. Although the Laurén classification [1] has been adopted in several studies of gastric carcinoma, this has proved inadequate in the analysis of cases at the Colorado General Hospital. Either pylorocardiac gland cell carcinoma is not found elsewhere in the United States or in the world or it is not recognized by others. Dr. Peter B. Marcus of South Africa plans a project to follow in the footsteps of Dr. Pierre Masson [2] in classifying gastric carcinoma by the fundamental cell types so well described in 1923. Dr. Marcus has a unique opportunity to study the disease in several ethnic groups under different living and dietary conditions.

Pylorocardiac Gland Cell

In Figures 3 and 4 of their ultrastructural study of gastric carcinoma cells, Sasano et al [3] depicted normal pyloric gland cells containing prominent granules positive for methenamine silver in the cisternae of the endoplasmic reticulum.

Preliminary observations by light microscopy of normal pyloric gland cells of resected stomachs stained by azocarmine G and counterstained with metanil yellow have demonstrated numerous cytoplasmic granules interpreted as an almost insoluble spermine–azocarmine complex, which is the result of the combination of the two sulfonyl groups of two molecules of azocarmine with the four amino groups of spermine. In this laboratory, the evidence is mounting that spermine is abundant in cells containing zinc metalloenzymes, as other positive cells are observed with this stain. Erythrocytes staining intensely with azocarmine are rich in carbonic anhydrase. The epithelial cells of the small ducts of the pancreas contain numerous positive granules and could be the source of carboxypeptidase A, although this remains to be proved. The acinar cells of the normal prostate contain numerous positive granules when exposed to the dye and are well known for their high content of acid phosphatase, probably a zinc metalloenzyme. This is well established for the other two enzymes mentioned, carbonic anhydrase and carboxypeptidase A. By way of contrast, the cytoplasm of normal mucous epithelial cells of the mucosa of bronchus, stomach, and colon are negative for spermine–dye complex. Paneth cells remain to be investigated. The strong possibility exists that spermine stabilizes the internal structure of these enzymes.

Mucin

In a study of 24 specimens of gastric carcinoma, type unspecified, five resected stomachs with ulcer, and five normal stomachs obtained shortly after death, Schrager and Oates[4] found normal stomach:ulcer stomach approximate ratios of galactose, fucose, glucosamine, galactosamine on a molar basis at 4:3:3:1. Glycoprotein isolated from normal and neoplastic gastric mucosa revealed the following: (1) a protein core with a characteristic amino acid composition, (2) a comparable range of sugars forming characteristic side chains, and (3) absence of mannose. They also noted that the composition of glycoproteins of connective tissue and serum were significantly different; eg, protein–polysaccharide complex of connective tissue lacked galactose but was rich in uronic acid.

Comparative Pathology

Lingeman et al[5] studied spontaneous adenocarcinoma of the stomach of 22 dogs obtained from several sources. They pointed out that whereas this cancer is quite uncommon in the dog, in other domestic animals it is much rarer and suggests a close association with man with regard to possible etiologic factors.

Sugimura et al[6] were able to induce gastric carcinoma of variable extent by N-methyl-N'-nitro-N-nitrosoguanidine in drinking water, started in one male dog and three female dogs at four months of age and about 5 kg weight with dosage at 167 μg per ml for 30 days and then 83 μg per ml and with exposure for 518 to 1,045 days. In the photomicrographs, dog 1 revealed the suggestive small gland pattern of mucous cell carcinoma and dog 3 mucous cell carcinoma composed of signet ring cells with infiltration of the mucosa. Leiomyosarcoma developed in the small intestine of all four dogs.

Etiology

Haenszel et al[7] analyzed the diets of Japanese living in Hawaii, 220 afflicted with cancer of the stomach and 440 hospital patients as controls. They observed an elevated risk for gastric cancer proportional to the intake in both Issei and Nisei who ate pickled vegetables and dried-salted fish. Those patients who consumed raw fish and unprocessed fresh or cooked vegetables were *not* similarly at risk.

Intestinal Cell Metaplasia

Sugimura et al [8] developed a method for the gross detection of the intestinal cell metaplasia of the stomach so prevalent in Japan.[9, 10] Sucrase, an enzyme specific for intestinal mucosal epithelial cells, in the gastric mucosa was interpreted as indicating intestinal cell metaplasia. Two specimens of gastric cancer were depicted in stunning color. After gently cleansing the mucosa and spraying with 5 percent sucrose, incubation was continued for 5 minutes at 37 C. The Tes-tape strips set closely upon the mucosa around the tumor turned variable shades of green, but no reaction was noted in the tumor proper.

Pathology of Gastric Carcinoma

Sasano et al [3] also depicted by electron microscopy the cells of pattern 1 of intestinal cell carcinoma (IC-1) in their Figure 13 with the neoplastic cells marked by prominent microvilli, many mitochondria, and abundant endoplasmic reticulum. These features are compatible with the synthesis of a probable glycoprotein responsible for the incitation of the often observed rich lymphoid infiltration in the stroma around the carcinoma.

Take [11] extracted the deoxyribonucleic acid of the mitochondria of normal liver, of hepatoma, and of gastric cancer (number and types unspecified). The DNA content per mg of protein of the mitochondria was 10 times higher in normal liver than in hepatoma. The DNA of the three types of cells was in a circular form depicted in electron micrographs. The bibliography of his paper is replete with references to the deoxyribonucleic acid content of a wide variety of mitochondria.

Experience of Colorado General Hospital with Gastric Carcinoma, 1969–73

Table 1 summarizes the data for 22 new cases of gastric carcinoma seen during this period. The follow-up information is updated to August 1974. Such data have become available for two patients in the original series. A woman of 60 years had resection of a mucous cell carcinoma metastatic to lymph nodes in 1968. She died 17 months later with autopsy displaying no residual carcinoma, but a perforation of the jejunum, a subdiaphragmatic abscess, *P. vulgaris* and *E. coli* septicemia, and bronchopneumonia, complications likely related to chemotherapy. A man of 69 years had resection of a mucous cell carcinoma metastatic to lymph nodes in 1968. He was alive and free of clinical disease more than six years after operation. He stopped 5-fluorouracil on his own in December 1973.

TABLE 1. Cases of Gastric Carcinoma 1969–73, Colorado General Hospital

Sex	Age *	Type	Site	Size (cm)	Stage	Extension	Metastasis	Tissue	Prognosis
M	57	MC	Entire stomach	10+	IV	—	P,GB,App	A	DWD
M	71	MC	Antrum	4	IV	—	LN–abd,P	A	DWD (Gastric hemorrhage)
F	57	MC	Cardia	2	IV	P,vena cava	LN–abd, thor,cerv,Pl	A	DWD (Embolism, lungs)
F	22	MC	Fundus	2	IV	—	Li,Lu,Sp,Ov, LN–abd, thor,cerv, Bra,Ki,Ad	A	DWD (Septicemia)
F	47	MC	Entire stomach	10+	IV	—	P,Pa,Ad,Lu, Ov,LN– abd,thor, cerv	A	DWD (Embolism, lungs)
F	53	MC	Entire stomach	10+	IV	—	P,Int,Ov,Tu	A,S	DWD (4 mo po)
F	61	MC	Antrum	2	II	—	None–23 LN	S,G	AFOD (41 mo)
F	45	MC	Entire stomach	10+	IV	Je	LN–10 of 15	S,Gx2	DWD (11 mo)
M	38	MC	Antrum	1	II	—	BM–widespread	G,S	DWD (48 mo po)
F	47	MC	Cardia	3	IV	—	P,Ov,App	G,S	DWD (4 mo)
F	68	PGC	Cardia	8.5	IV	—	LN–1 of 10	G,S	DWD (22 mo)
M	65	PGC	Cardia	6	IV	—	LN–18 of 19,P,Li	G,S	DWD (1 mo)
M	62	PGC	Cardia	1	I	—	None–4 LN	G,S	AFOD (9 mo)
M	60	PGC	Cardia	3	IV	—	P,Om	Bx	DWD (1 mo)
M	67	PGC	Cardia	3	IV	—	Li	Bx	AWD (14 mo) ChRx
F	81	IC2	Fundus	6	III	—	None–13 LN	G,S	DFOD (cardiac infarction)
M	60	IC1	Fundus	7	IV	—	LN–26 of 26	G,S	DWD (19 mo)
M	65	IC2	Fundus	9	IV	—	LN–6 of 18	G,S	DWD (14 mo)
M	58	IC2	Fundus	8	IV	—	LN–8 of 43	G,S	AFOD (29 mo)
M	71	IC2	Antrum	8	IV	—	LN–10 of 13	G,S	DWD (5 mo)
F	56	IC1	Fundus	3.5	III	—	None–2 LN	G,S	AFOD (17 mo)
F	80	IC2	Fundus	6	IV	Li	None–1 LN	G,S	Alive (10 mo) ? disease

A: autopsy; abd: abdominal; Ad: adrenals; AFOD: alive and free of disease (carcinoma); App: appendix; AWD: alive with disease (carcinoma); BM: bone marrow; Bra: brain; Bx: biopsy; cerv: cervical; ChRx: chemotherapy; DFOD: dead and free of disease (carcinoma); DWD: dead with disease (carcinoma); G: gastrectomy; GB: gallbladder; IC: intestinal cell carcinoma, patterns 1 and 2; Int: intestines; Je: jejunum; Ki: kidneys; Li: liver; LN: lymph nodes; Lu: lungs; MC: mucous cell carcinoma; mo: months; Om: omentum; Ov: ovaries; P: peritoneum; Pa: pancreas; PGC: pylorocardiac gland cell carcinoma; Pl: pleura; po: postoperative; S: surgical specimen; Sp: spleen; thor: thoracic; Tu: tubes, uterine.
* At autopsy or first operation.

References

1. Laurén P: The two histological main types of gastric carcinoma: diffuse and so-called intestinal-type carcinoma. Acta Path Microbiol Scand 64:31, 1965
2. Masson P: Diagnostics de Laboratoire. II Tumeurs. Paris, A. Maloine et Fils, 1923, pp 405–417
3. Sasano N, Nakamura K, Arai M, Akazaki K: Ultrastructural cell patterns in human gastric carcinoma compared with non-neoplastic gastric mucosa: histogenetic analysis of carcinoma by mucin histochemistry. J Natl Cancer Inst 43:783, 1969
4. Schrager J, Oates MDG: A comparative study of the major glycoprotein isolated from normal and neoplastic gastric mucosa. Gut 14:324, 1973
5. Lingeman CH, Garner FM, Taylor DON: Spontaneous gastric adenocarcinoma of dogs: a review. J Natl Cancer Inst 47:137, 1971
6. Sugimura T, Tanaka N, Kawachi T, et al: Production of stomach cancer in dogs by N-methyl-N'-nitro-N-nitrosoguanidine. Gann 62:67, 1971
7. Haenszel W, Kurihara M, Segi M, Lee, RKC: Stomach cancer among Japanese in Hawaii. J Natl Cancer Inst 49:969, 1972
8. Sugimura T, Kawachi T, Kogure K, et al: A novel method for detecting intestinal metaplasia of the stomach with Tes-tape. Gann 62:237, 1971
9. Kuru M, Ryozo S: Histogenetical study of gastric carcinomas in the Japanese: analysis of 150 cases treated in relatively early stages. In Proceedings of the Ninth International Cancer Congress. UICC Monograph Series 10. Berlin, Springer-Verlag, 1967, pp 1–30
10. Nakamura K, Sugano H, Tagaki K: Carcinoma of the stomach in incipient phase: its histogenesis and histological appearances. Gann 59:251, 1968
11. Take S: DNAs from human hepatoma and gastric cancer mitochondria. Acta Med Okayama 23:465, 1969

TROPICAL SPRUE: SUBCLINICAL AND IDIOPATHIC ENTEROPATHY

PARVIZ HAGHIGHI AND
KHOSROW NASR

Tropical sprue is a well-recognized disease of unknown etiology occurring in the tropics.[7, 9, 10, 13, 19, 24, 28, 36, 50, 58, 62, 74, 77, 89, 93-95, 99, 109, 110, 116, 121, 125, 130] Its predominant features include diarrhea, malabsorption of at least two unrelated substances, megaloblastic anemia, glossitis, stomatitis, edema, and nutritional deficiencies.[12, 89, 99, 130] The major morphologic changes of the small intestine include decrease in villous height, increase in crypt length, and an increase in number of inflammatory cells of the lamina propria.[8, 50, 57, 93, 140, 147, 160] Although it occurs endemically in certain areas, there are also reports of epidemics of sprue, strengthening the hypothesis that the condition is infectious in etiology.[3, 10, 11, 111, 112] Further supports to the infectious theory are its occurrence in visitors to the tropics, improvement of the condition upon departure from the tropics (reversibility), and response to antibiotics.[9, 19, 20, 42, 50, 74, 81, 83, 90, 92, 94, 95, 98, 102, 120, 130, 147-149, 151, 157, 159, 160] Finally, the clinical manifestations may vary from those described above, depending on the duration and severity of the illness (for example, malabsorption) and the dietary reserve of the patient (for example, folate).[18, 19, 24, 28, 51, 78, 86, 91, 120, 126, 139, 184]

After recognition of tropical sprue, reports on the apparently normal population of the tropics appeared in the literature, and it was clear that these apparently normal individuals had more minor abnormalities of structure and function of the small intestine.[7, 8, 10, 11, 15, 19, 25-27, 31, 50, 51, 53, 67, 68, 79, 81, 89, 91-95, 98-100, 103, 111, 127, 129, 131, 135, 144, 148, 149, 155, 159, 165] Thus the interchangeable terms subclinical enteropathy,[100] subclinical malabsorption,[19] nonspecific jejunitis,[19] tropical enteropathy,[99] tropical jejunitis,[149] and tropical malabsorption syndrome [74] came into use. These emphasized the presence of small intestinal abnormality based on morphologic and/or absorptive abnormalities in the apparently normal segment of the population.

Subclinical enteropathy appeared to be *qualitatively* similar to tropical sprue, though *quantitatively* the abnormalities were of less severe proportions.[85, 91, 92] Since the etiology(ies) of subclinical enteropathy and tropical sprue is (are) unknown, it is not possible to consider both conditions definitively as varying presentations of the same disease.[99] On the other hand, the spectrum of both tropical sprue and subclinical enteropathy with their overlap, their similarities, and the presence of both conditions in the tropics is suggestive of some relationship between the conditions; and, at present, it is proper to assume that in the tropics there is (are) a factor(s) that leads to morphologic and/or absorptive abnormalities of varying severity and sequelae (for example, nutritional deficiencies).[84, 88]

It should be emphasized that the term "subclinical enteropathy" as we use it refers to the condition only in geographic areas with tropical sprue. Elsewhere, there have been references to an enteropathy characterized by morphologic and/or absorptive abnormalities of the small intestine in absence of tropical sprue.[15, 27, 67, 123, 127, 129, 165] We refer to this as "idiopathic enteropathy," and herewith report findings on this condition in Iran.

Idiopathic Enteropathy in Iran

Definition

As noted in the preceding discussion, idiopathic enteropathy is an entity by exclusion (absence of other recognized small intestinal disease) characterized by morphologic and/or absorptive abnormalities of the small intestine in regions with no tropical sprue. Of necessity, normality of morphology or absorptive tests (fat, xylose, and vitamin B_{12}) are comparisons with standards from northern Europe and the United States.

Study Population

In Iran we have studied a nearly random population of 100 villagers (Fars Province). The description of the area and details of the study are presented elsewhere.[123] Although patients with other diseases—whether gastrointestinal or others —were excluded, gastrointestinal symptoms were not selected against.

Absorptive Findings

The results of studies on fat, xylose, and vitamin B_{12} absorption are presented in Table 1. It is noteworthy that 3 percent had fecal fat of greater than 5 g/day, while 4 percent had xylose and 7 percent vitamin B_{12} (with intrinsic factor) malabsorption. Combined, one subject had all three abnormalities; one other, two; and nine, only one abnormality.

**TABLE 1. Absorptive Findings in 100 Apparently Normal
Villagers Selected at Random**[*]

Test[†]	Percent Abnormal
Fat	3
Xylose	4
Vitamin B_{12} (with intrinsic factor)	7

[*]In all, 11 percent had one or more abnormalities of absorption as defined by the three tests.

[†]Normals: fat, less than 5 g/day; xylose, greater than 20 percent excretion within 5 hours after a 25-g intake; vitamin B_{12} (Schilling) with intrinsic factor, greater than 7 percent excretion in 24 hours.

Morphologic Abnormalities

Evaluation by light microscopy included (1) the appearance of the villous epithelium; (2) the villous core; and (3) the crypts and the lamina propria lying between the crypts.

1. Villous epithelium—abnormalities included
    Loss of clarity of the interepithelial cell membrane (Fig. 1)
    Frayed basement membrane, usually under the villous tips (Fig. 2)
    Loss of polarity of absorptive cell nuclei with occasional tendency of same to pseudostratification (Fig. 3)
    Enlargement of the nuclei usually associated with pallor of same
    Transepithelial lymphocytic migration (Fig. 4)
    Occasional loss of clear brush border (Fig. 5)
2. Villous core—abnormalities included
    Hypercellularity, predominantly that of plasma cells (Fig. 6)
    Lymphangiectasia, usually near the tip of villous (Fig. 7)
    Gruenhagen spaces
3. Crypts—abnormalities included
    Pallor and enlargement of crypt nuclei (Fig. 8)
    Apparent increase in the cells of the lamina propria lying between crypts (Fig. 9)
    Occasional instances of transepithelial lymphocytic migration (Fig. 10)

Grading of these abnormalities ranged from normal to slightly, moderately, and severely abnormal (Figs. 11 and 12). The predominant criteria for grading were villous epithelial abnormalities, transepithelial lymphocytic migration in the villous epithelium, and the villous core hypercellularity. The findings are presented in Table 2. No case with flat mucosa was encountered. Using strict criteria, significant morphologic changes were defined as presence of moderate (17 cases) or

TABLE 2. Morphologic Evaluation of Peroral Biopsies
of 100 Apparently Normal Villagers
Selected at Random

Findings	Percent
Normal	9
Slightly abnormal	42
Moderately abnormal	17
Severely abnormal	3
Subtotal	71
Inadequate biopsy	26
Not performed	3
Total	100

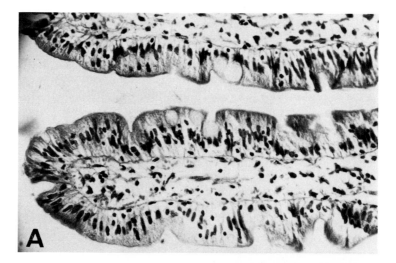

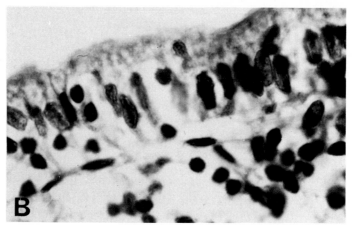

Fig. 1. Peroral biopsy showing loss of clarity of the interepithelial cell membrane of the villus. A. H&E × 100. B. H&E × 400.

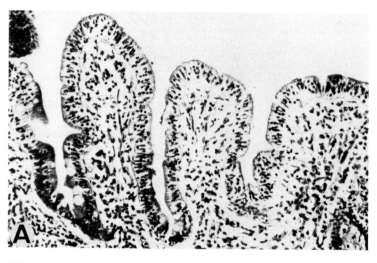

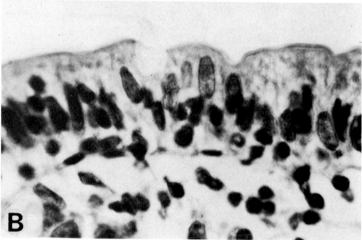

Fig. 2. Peroral biopsy. Frayed basement membrane under villous tip. A. H&E × 63. B. H&E × 400.

severe (3 cases) abnormalities (Fig. 12). Of 71 specimens (belonging to 71 cases) that were adequate for evaluation, 20 specimens (29 percent) were abnormal. Of the 20 abnormal small intestinal biopsies, four also had one or more abnormalities of absorption. Combining morphologic and absorptive abnormalities, one had all four; one had three; two had two; and twenty-three had one abnormality. In all, 27 percent had one or more abnormalities of function and/or morphology of small intestine as defined above. Except for those few with severe morphologic abnormalities, there was no correlation between structural and functional (absorptive) abnormalities.

Of the 27 subjects who had one or more abnormalities of small intestinal

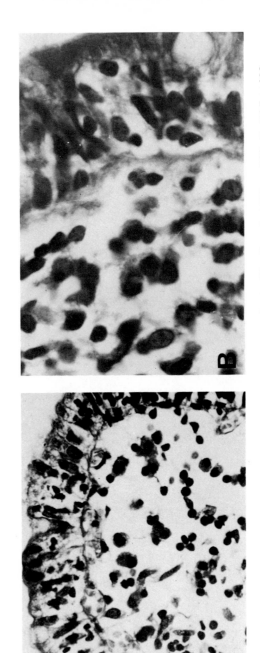

Fig. 3. Peroral biopsy. Loss of polarity of absorptive cell nuclei with pseudo-stratification. A. H&E × 200. B. H&E ×400.

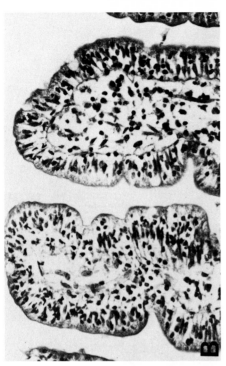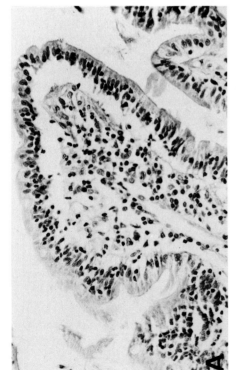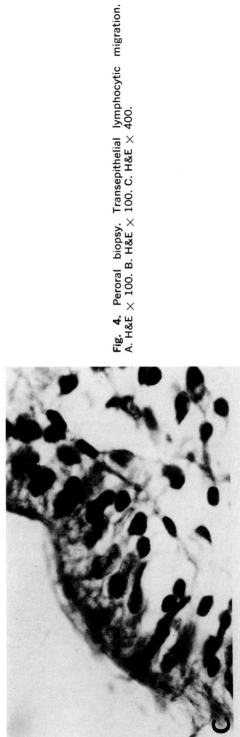

Fig. 4. Peroral biopsy. Transepithelial lymphocytic migration.
A. H&E × 100. B. H&E × 100. C. H&E × 400.

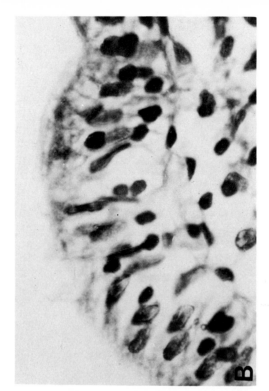
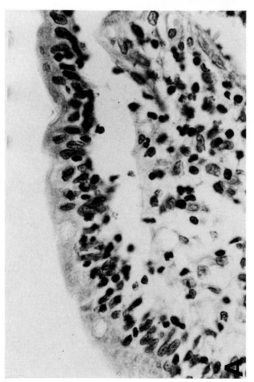

Fig. 5. Peroral biopsy. Loss of clear brush border. A. H&E × 200. B. H&E × 400.

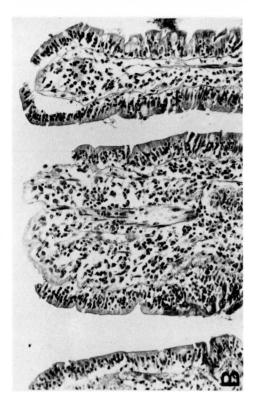

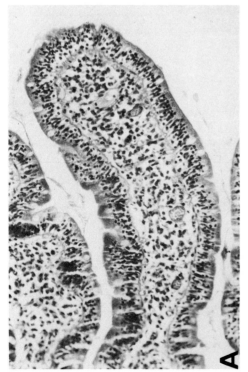

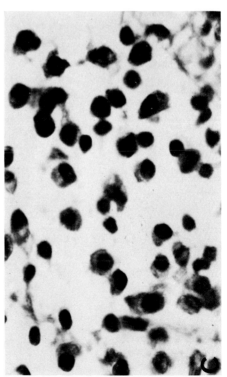

Fig. 6. Peroral biopsy. Hypercellularity, predominantly of plasma cells, of the villous core. A. H&E × 63. B. H&E × 63. C. H&E × 400.

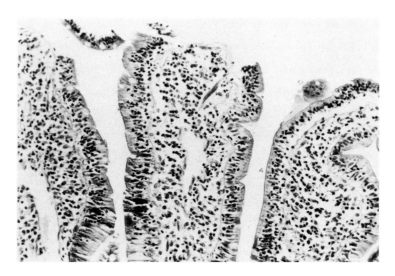

Fig. 7. Peroral biopsy. Lymphangiectasia of the villous core near the tip of the villous. H&E × 63.

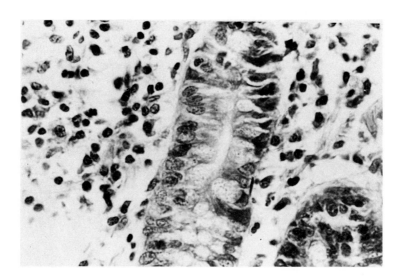

Fig. 8. Peroral biopsy. Pallor of crypt nuclei. H&E × 200.

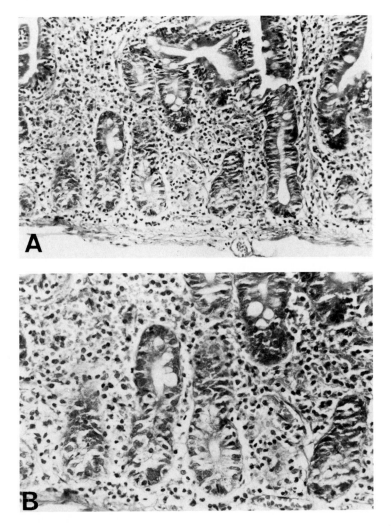

Fig. 9. Peroral biopsy. Increase in cells of lamina propria lying between crypts. A. H&E × 63. B. H&E × 100.

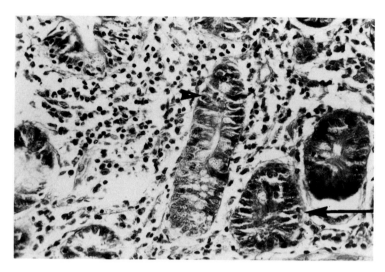

Fig. 10. Peroral biopsy. Crypt transepithelial lymphocytic migration (arrow). H&E × 100.

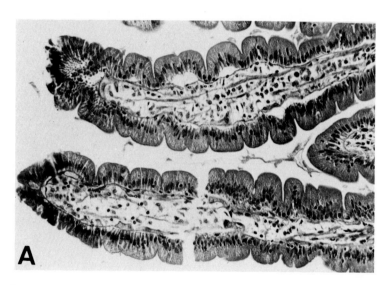

Fig. 11. Peroral biopsy. Normal western pattern. A. Normal villous architecture. Note serrated lateral villous border, delicate basement membrane, tall columnar epithelium, rare lymphocytes in the epithelial layer, and sparse cell population of the villous core. H&E × 63.

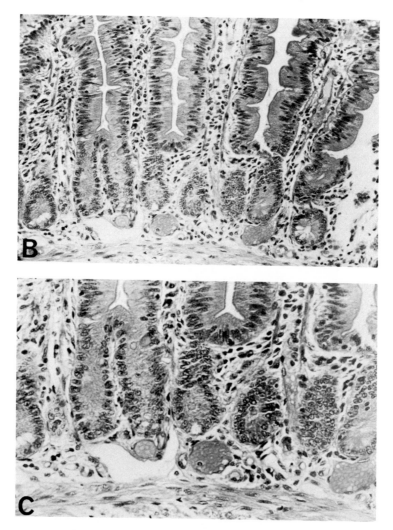

Fig. 11. (cont.) B. Villous base and the crypts. H&E $\times$ 63. C. Detail of crypt area with sparse intercrypt cell population. H&E $\times$ 100. (Courtesy of Dr. John H. Yardley, Johns Hopkins University School of Medicine)

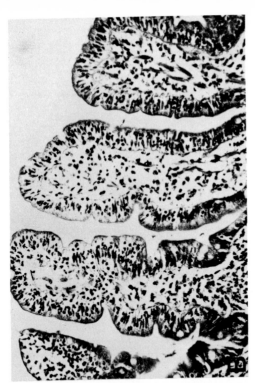

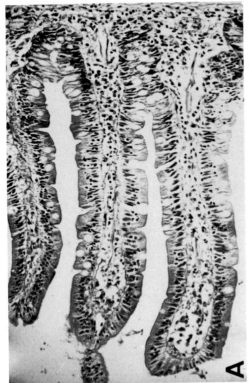

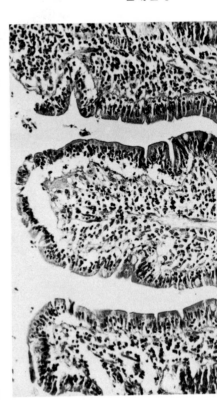

Fig. 12. Peroral biopsy. Histologic abnormalities. H&E $\times$ 63. A. Slightly abnormal. B. Moderately abnormal. C. Severely abnormal. Note villous width, degree of loss of serration, epithelial damage, transepithelial lymphocytic migration, and villous core hypercellularity.

function and/or morphology, only one had an increase in number of bowel movements per day; and that particular subject had 5.7 g fat in stool, Schilling test (with intrinsic factor) of 1.5 percent excretion and severe abnormalities of the small intestine on peroral biopsy.

In summary, of 100 randomly selected apparently normal villagers, there were no cases of severe malabsorption, only one case had symptoms suggestive of malabsorption, but nearly one-third had one or more abnormalities of jejunal morphology or absorption (fat, xylose, or vitamin B_{12}). The etiology of this enteropathy remains unknown; none of our subjects had parasites, infections, or consumption of drugs known to be associated with malabsorption.[22]

Geographic Pattern

Tropical sprue, because of malabsorption, is an identifiable entity and its geographic pattern can thus be clarified. But, lacking an etiologic agent, perhaps it should not be concluded that malabsorption states with similar clinical presentations from Central and South America, Africa, and Asia are actually the same disease.[7, 9-11, 13, 19, 24, 28, 36, 50, 58, 62, 74, 89, 94, 95, 99, 109, 110, 116, 121, 130] In almost every country where tropical sprue has been recognized, subclinical enteropathy has also been found.[7, 8, 10, 11, 15, 19, 24-27, 50, 51, 67, 68, 79, 81, 89, 91-93, 95, 98-101, 103, 111, 127, 129, 131, 135, 144, 148, 149, 155, 159, 165]

There have been far fewer studies on idiopathic enteropathy than on subclinical enteropathy; at present limited studies are available from Liberia, Egypt, Israel, and Uganda. These studies suggest the presence of an enteropathy of more minor proportion in the absence of tropical sprue.[15, 27, 67, 127, 129] Iran can now be added to this list. Studies from Nigeria and Thailand are not clear, and firm conclusions cannot be made without more extensive studies.[17, 53, 165] This list is far from complete, but it does suggest that an enteropathy of unknown etiology does exist in the nontropical regions, at least in populations that continue to have a low socioeconomic, nutritional, and hygienic status.

Comparison of Idiopathic Enteropathy with Subclinical Enteropathy—Tropical Sprue Complex

Except for geographic location in which each entity is found, the major difference between these entities may be quantitative in that although tropical sprue may be associated with severe malabsorption, idiopathic enteropathy is milder in degree and more similar to subclinical enteropathy.

Absorption of fat, xylose, and vitamin B_{12} is less abnormal in subclinical enteropathy and idiopathic enteropathy when compared to tropical sprue.[24, 74, 91, 92, 99, 120] The same is also true of morphologic changes.[7, 24] Furthermore, in tropical sprue there is a greater possibility of involvement of the ileum.[7] Tropical sprue and subclinical enteropathy are acquired, in that the newborn's small intestine appears normal.[6, 8, 50] Furthermore, the abnormalities in these conditions are reversible, treatable (with folate or tetracycline), and found in visitors to the region. [9, 19, 20, 50, 74, 81, 83, 92, 94, 95, 98, 102, 120, 130, 147-149, 151, 157, 160] Similar studies in idiopathic enteropathy are not available. Finally, tropical sprue and, to a lesser degree, subclinical enteropathy lead to nutritional deficiencies.[99, 130] Sequelae of idiopathic enteropathy are less clear.

Leaving out what is unknown about idiopathic enteropathy and considering only the morphologic and absorptive abnormalities, this entity is similar to sub-clinical enteropathy with changes that are quantitatively milder than those noted in tropical sprue.[15, 27, 67, 123, 127, 129, 165]

The problem is further complicated because of recognition of protein mal-nutrition leading to abnormalities of morphology and absorption. These intestinal changes have been shown in protein-deficient animals,[43, 161] as well as in humans with kwashiorkor[25, 27, 156] and adult protein malnutrition.[25, 62, 93, 115, 175] The rever-sibility of intestinal changes after correction of the protein malnutrition suggests further that protein malnutrition enteropathy may be a real entity.[64, 114, 156] But certainly in cases of tropical sprue and subclinical enteropathy, well-nourished individuals moving into the tropics can, within a very brief period, develop the morphologic or absorptive abnormalities, suggesting that protein malnutrition is not the major cause of the illness in the tropics.[12, 98, 102, 103, 147-149, 151, 157] Little information is available in idiopathic enteropathy.

These and other findings in various gastrointestinal infections suggest that the highlight is the similarity of end results (absorptive and morphologic changes) that differ only in degree of abnormality rather than in any qualitative difference. With this background, perhaps it is best to consider tropical sprue, subclinical entero-pathy, and idiopathic enteropathy as separate entities with perhaps different etiolo-gies in which the small intestine responds in a basically similar manner.

Morphology: Normal Appearance

The detailed morphologic comparisons of necessity must include descriptions of the normal small intestine as seen in the United States or in northern Europe. This seems justified since normal Western type of small bowel mucosa has been observed in asymptomatic subjects of the tropics.[75, 139]

Comparisons can be made from aspects found by dissecting and light micro-scopy. In general, findings of dissecting and light microscopy correlate both in health and disease and may thus be regarded as complementary.[19, 132, 159]

DISSECTING MICROSCOPY. Normally, the villi of the jejunum are finger-shaped; leaf-shaped villi have been described in the duodenum, occasionally in the upper jejunum, and rarely in the ileum.[8, 21, 133]

LIGHT MICROSCOPY. Normally, the mucosal height of the small intestine as measured from the crypt base to the villous tip has been estimated to be 0.78 to 0.91 mm (average 0.85 mm).[28, 93, 159] Villous height seems to vary with the degree of villous smooth muscle contraction, bowel distension, and plane of section.[142] It has been given variously as 300 to 1,000 μ,[21, 142, 147] with a mean of 450 μ.[147] Normal villous width has been estimated at 90 to 145 μ (mean 120 μ).[147] Consider-able variation in size and shape of villi, according to age and bowel segment, may normally be expected.[21, 22, 73, 87, 133, 142] Normal crypt depth has been stated to be 0.12 to 0.26 mm.[142]

The mucosal epithelium may be divided into crypt and villous epithelium. The villous epithelial cells originate by differentiation and migration of crypt cells along the villous length where they desquamate at the villous tip.[73, 134] The cell life of normal villous epithelium is estimated to be one to seven days.[73, 134] The villous epithelium includes goblet cells, pigmented cells (also referred to as Astaldi-Strosseli cells), and absorptive cells. The absorptive cells are of tall columnar type, 22 to 31 μ in height with gradual decrease of same as the villous tip is reached.[155] Nuclei are round to oval and usually lie at or near the base of each cell. Mitoses are rarely present.[142, 173] A limited number of lymphocytes and histiocytes may normally be seen between the villous epithelial cells.[2, 25, 118] The well-defined brush border corresponding electron microscopically to microvilli gradually becomes less distinct near the villous base. The villous-crypt junction has been regarded as the crucial region in regard to cell maturation.[23, 134]

Within the crypt epithelium are found Paneth cells, argentaffin cells, undifferentiated cells, immature cells, and goblet cells.[134, 150] Normal crypt depth is given as 0.12 to 0.26 mm.[142] Mitotic figures are usually seen in the middle third of the crypt.[57, 73] The normal mitotic index of the crypt epithelium, as defined by the number of cells in mitosis per 100 cells of the crypt epithelium, is around 1.1.[138, 142] The nuclei of the crypt epithelium are usually moderately dense and round to oval in shape. Normally, the crypt lumen does not contain cellular elements. The goblet cells are found mostly at the upper third of the crypt and lower third of villus. Their number decreases markedly as the villous tip is reached.[28] Goblet cell differentiation from crypt cells occurs near the crypt base.[142]

The villous epithelial cells rest over a thin membrane that, under normal circumstances, stains like reticulin and is PAS positive. This basement membrane becomes less distinct as one approaches the crypts.[142] The villous core contains few lymphocytes, histiocytes, plasma cells, eosinophils, mast cells, and the so-called globular leukocytes.[2, 142] There is a centrally located lacteal surrounded by smooth muscle cells that are apparently extensions of the muscularis mucosae (Bruecke's muscle). The vascular network in the villous core appears delicate. The cell population of the lamina propria between the crypts is essentially similar to that in the villous core with perhaps more eosinophils. With lipid stains, fat is usually distributed throughout the villous core and can be demonstrated in lacteals and occasionally in some histiocytes.[96, 142, 159]

Tropical Sprue

For brevity, changes as seen in autopsy,[1, 4, 105, 108, 158] open biopsy,[28] and peroral biopsy specimens[8, 10, 50, 140, 159] will be described together. These changes appear to be identical in epidemic and endemic forms, in both adults and children.[111, 113] There is a considerable range in the severity of alterations.[8, 75, 85, 159]

DISSECTING MICROSCOPY. Leaf-shaped villi or ridges may be found in the jejunum[8, 159] and convoluted mucosa is occasionally seen.[9, 20, 50, 159] The ileum may be involved; when so, it is less severely involved[8, 50, 126] or at the most equally involved[19, 171] as compared with the jejunum.

LIGHT MICROSCOPY.   The villous epithelium shows one or more of the following changes:

Indistinct or fragmented brush border.[10, 147]

Decrease in cell height, so that the normal columnar epithelium may be replaced by cuboidal epithelium.[50, 57, 138, 139, 147]

Pseudostratification and loss of polarity and regularity of epithelial cell nuclei.[93, 142, 147]

Possible increase in the number of goblet cells in the villous epithelium so that these cells may be observed at the villus tip.[28] Alternately, a decrease in goblet cell number in villi with an increase of same in crypts may occur.[93, 142, 159] However, quantitative data on the normal and abnormal number of goblet cells are not sufficient and great variation may occur under normal conditions.[138, 142]

Various degrees of transepithelial lymphocytic migration.[10, 57, 85, 111, 139] This may be the predominant abnormality in early or mild cases.[50, 142, 147]

An increase [10, 50, 142, 159] or, rarely, a decrease (in advanced cases) [147, 159] in mitotic index of the crypt epithelium.

Pallor and enlargement of the nuclei of the crypt epithelial cells.[10, 19, 28, 143, 150, 159, 162] This is referred to as megalocytosis; it appears related to folate deficiency, may revert to normal upon folate repletion,[162] and may represent part of a more widespread change in the epithelial nuclei observed outside the small intestine, such as the stomach.[9, 10, 28, 113, 167]

Nuclear enlargement and rounding of villous epithelial cells with altered position of cell nuclei.[57]

Subnuclear vacuolization.[10, 28, 57]

Subepithelial edema, at times to the point of vesicle formation (Gruenhagen spaces).[28, 92, 147, 153]

Change in tinctorial characteristics, usually basophilia, of the villous epithelial cytoplasm.[57, 93]

Occasionally, an increase in mitotic figures in villous epithelium.[57]

Villous core edema.[28, 50, 159]

Villous core lymphangiectasis.[28]

Perivascular eosinophilic infiltrate in muscle wall of the small bowel and submucosal edema are less constant features.[28]

Loss of delicate ruffling of the villi.[28]

Thickening of the basement membrane with change in tinctorial characteristics from those of reticulin to collagen fibers have been noted, particularly at the villous tip,[78, 86, 138-140, 170] although a basically similar phenomenon has been recently described in a variant of celiac disease called collagenous sprue.[170] Lipid stains reveal collection of lipids essentially in or under the lamina densa of basement membrane. This again has been regarded as a helpful morphologic criterion in the diagnosis of tropical sprue.[85, 93, 96, 139, 140, 159]

Lymphocytic transepithelial migration through the crypt epithelium; this is less constant than the same phenomenon in regard to the villous epithelium. Nuclear debris may be observed within the crypt lumen (necrocytosis).[57, 155]

In terms of the overall villous architecture, shortening of villi may be associated with lengthening or tortuosity of crypts leading to a decreased or at times to a relatively normal mucosal thickness as well as reduction of the total absorptive surface.[28, 85, 93, 139, 140] Shortened, blunted, clubbed, and broadened villi may be seen creating leaves, ridges, or convolutions, in that order, depending on the severity of change.[8, 10, 21, 50, 56, 85, 93, 102, 139, 157] This villous shortening has been referred to, perhaps incorrectly, as partial villous atrophy.[46] Flat mucosa is a rare feature of tropical sprue.[10, 21, 50, 51, 85, 92, 93, 147] Synechiae formation and coalescence of adjacent villi, as well as pseudocrypt formation, have also been described, accounting for at least some of the abnormal appearance by dissecting microscopy.[28, 57, 85, 139, 141]

The preceding changes are severer in the proximal small intestine, and, although the ileum may be less, equally, or more severely involved, a normal ileum is not a rarity.[85, 171] Ileal involvement was emphasized in the early autopsy series.[11, 108, 171] Jejunal changes are said to antedate the ileal abnormalities.[87, 99] Duodenal changes are similar to those described in the jejunum.[169] In terms of the length of bowel involved, the alterations are thought to be patchy or diffuse.[139] Some workers have developed their own grading system of dissecting and light microscopic abnormalities, depending on the severity of changes.[15, 48, 121, 149, 159] The described histologic changes can be seen within two weeks of development of clinical symptoms.[147] In experimental situations spruelike changes have been noted in as little as 24 hours after intestinal injury.[153]

In general, there seems to be a good correlation between the degree of histologic, absorptive, and radiologic abnormalities.[18, 55, 171] Also, the histologic abnormalities tend to revert to normal with considerable individual variation after folate, vitamin B_{12}, and antibiotic therapy.[85, 146, 171] With occasional exceptions,[8] the severity of histologic abnormalities appears to correlate with the duration of the illness.[28, 51, 78] For descriptions of the electron microscopy, enzyme histochemistry, and immunology of the small intestine under normal conditions and in tropical sprue-subclinical enteropathy, the reader is referred to several articles that have appeared in recent literature.[24, 37, 38, 41, 70, 85, 104, 107, 122, 134, 142, 152, 164]

Subclinical and Idiopathic Enteropathies

The dissecting and light microscopy findings of the small intestine in subclinical enteropathy are, in general, similar to those described for tropical sprue.

The scanty literature available does not permit singling out any abnormality that might be considered specific for idiopathic enteropathy. Thus far, the reported alterations seem indistinguishable from those noted in subclinical enteropathy.[15, 67, 123, 127, 165]

Specificity of the Intestinal Changes

As described previously, changes in the villous architecture, as well as the epithelial and villous core alterations, are generally regarded as nonspecific and may represent a characteristic response of the bowel mucosa to a large variety of noxious agents.[22-24, 66, 83, 85, 98, 99, 139, 149, 153, 155, 163, 174, 184] More than fifty conditions, including animal experiments, cited in review of the literature have been associated with these changes,[24, 72, 122] including various bacterial,[26, 54, 65, 71, 78, 82, 97, 98, 145, 153, 154] viral, and parasitic infections,[22, 27, 99] as well as drugs [45, 80, 117] and deficiency states.[25-27, 43, 44, 58, 62, 93, 94, 114-116, 128, 156, 175]

Despite the general impression that the described lesions are nonspecific, several observers feel that certain features are characteristic of the tropical sprue-subclinical enteropathy entities.[24, 139, 140] These so-called specific features include a combination of thickening of the basement membrane under the villous epithelium, lipid deposits in the thickened basement membrane, the possible predominance of the IgA-containing plasma cells in the lamina propria,[139] and changes in the enzyme histochemistry of the small bowel mucosa.

Mention should be made of celiac disease as compared to tropical sprue. Celiac disease predominantly involves the upper small intestine and is associated with flat mucosa with plasmacytic rather than lymphocytic infiltration of the lamina propria.[110, 133]

Relation to Lymphoma

Discussion of idiopathic enteropathy cannot be complete without reference to its possible relation to primary upper small intestinal lymphoma.[5, 166, 99] Similar to the celiac disease-lymphoma relationship, it has been postulated that, in Iran, this idiopathic enteropathy may be predisposing to lymphoma formation.[48, 66] This is strengthened by morphologic changes in the nontumor tissue adjacent to the intestinal lymphoma.

Summary and Conclusions

Presented is a study of an enteropathy of unknown etiology in Iran characterized by minor morphologic and absorptive abnormalities noted in nearly one-third of randomly selected villagers. Similar studies have been available for very few nontropical regions, although this entity (called idiopathic enteropathy) is similar to a subclinical enteropathy noted in tropical sprue regions. Rather than lumping together all such entities, we have attempted to differentiate between tropical sprue and subclinical enteropathy and idiopathic enteropathy. The reasons have been the lack of etiologic agent(s) and the probability that the small intestine responds in a limited way to varying injuries. This implies that many etiologic agents may produce qualitatively similar changes, although quantitatively there may be differences. Further proof for this hypothesis are changes noted with protein malnutrition and postcholera and other gastrointestinal infections. Obviously, there is much need for research in etiologies of tropical sprue, subclinical enteropathy, and idiopathic enteropathy.

Acknowledgments

The authors wish to thank Dr. John H. Yardley, Johns Hopkins University, Baltimore, Maryland, for providing normal small intestinal peroral biopsies; Dr. E. A. Mohallatee, Nemazee Hospital, Shiraz, Iran, for his permission to use the

Nemazee Hospital material; Mrs. Afsar Mansoorzadeh, for providing locally unavailable references; Mrs. Parvin Ghazi for valuable secretarial assistance; Miss Nasrin Ghazi for photomicrographs; and Mr. Hassan Shoorangiz for technical assistance.

References

1. Adlersberg D, Schein J: Clinical and pathologic studies in sprue. JAMA 134: 1459, 1947
2. Astaldi G, Strosselli E: Biopsy of the normal intestine. Am J Dig Dis 5:175, 1960
3. Avery F: Outbreaks of sprue during the Burma campaign. Trans R Soc Trop Med Hyg 41:377, 1948
4. Bahr PH: A Report on Researches on Sprue in Ceylon, 1912–1914. London, Cambridge Univ Press, 1915
5. Baker SJ: Tropical sprue. Br Med Bull 28:87, 1972
6. Baker SJ: Discussion, workshop on malabsorption and malnutrition, Am J Clin Nutr 25:107, 1972
7. Baker SJ, Mathan VI: Tropical enteropathy and tropical sprue. Am J Clin Nutr 25:1047, 1972
8. Baker SJ, Ignatius M, Mathan VI, Vaish SK, Chacko CC: Intestinal biopsy in tropical sprue. In Wolstenholme GEW, Cameron MP (eds): Intestinal Biopsy, Ciba Foundation Study Group No. 14. Boston, Little, Brown, 1962, pp 84–99
9. Baker SJ, Mathan VI: Syndrome of tropical sprue in south India. Am J Clin Nutr 21:984, 1968
10. Baker SJ, Mathan VI: Tropical sprue. In Card WI, Creamer B (eds): Modern Trends in Gastroenterology. London, Butterworth, 1970, pp. 198–228
11. Baker SJ, Mathan VI: The epidemiology of tropical sprue. In Tropical Sprue and Megaloblastic Anemia. Wellcome Trust Collaborative Study. Edinburgh and London, Churchill, 1971, pp 159–88
12. Baker SJ, Mathan VI: Tropical sprue in southern India. In Tropical Sprue and Megaloblastic Anemia. Wellcome Trust Collaborative Study. Edinburgh and London, Churchill, 1971, pp 189–260
13. Banwell JG, Gorbach SD, Mitra R: Tropical sprue and malnutrition in west Bengal. II. Fluid and electrolyte transport in the small intestine. Am J Clin Nutr 23:1559, 1970
14. Banwell JG, Hutt MSR, Marsden PD, Blackman V: Malabsorption syndromes amongst African people in Uganda. East Afr Med J 41:188, 1964
15. Banwell JG, Hutt MSR, Tunnicliffe R: Observations on jejunal biopsy in Ugandan Africans. East Afr Med J 41:46, 1964
16. Bayless TM: Tropical sprue: a comparison with celiac disease. Am J Dig Dis 9:779, 1964
17. Bayless TM: Discussion, workshop on malabsorption and malnutrition. Am J Clin Nutr 25:1074, 1972
18. Bayless TM, Swanson VL, Wheby MS: Jejunal histology and clinical status in tropical sprue and other chronic diarrheal disorders. Am J Clin Nutr 24:112, 1971
19. Bayless TM, Wheby MS, Swanson VL: Tropical sprue in Puerto Rico. Am J Clin Nutr 21:1030, 1968
20. Booth CC, Mollin DL: Chronic tropical sprue in London. Am J Dig Dis 9:770, 1964
21. Booth CC, Stewart JS, Holmes R, Brackenbury W: Dissecting microscope appearances of intestinal mucosa. In Wolstenholme GEW, Cameron MP (eds): Intestinal Biopsy. Ciba Foundation Study Group No. 14. Boston, Little, Brown, 1962, pp 2–19
22. Brandborg LL: Structure and function of the small intestine in some parasite diseases. Am J Clin Nutr 24:124, 1971

23. Br Med J: Intestinal villi. 21:1330, 1965
24. Brunser O, Eidelman S, Klipstein FA: Intestinal morphology of rural Haitians: a comparison between overt tropical sprue and asymptomatic subjects. Gastroenterology 58:655, 1970
25. Brunser O, Reid A, Monckeberg F, Maccioni A, Contreras I: Jejunal biopsies in infants with malnutrition with special reference to mitotic index. Pediatrics 38:605, 1966
26. Brunser O, Reid A, Monckeberg F, Maccioni A, Contreras I: Jejunal mucosa in infant malnutrition. Am J Clin Nutr 21:976, 1968
27. Burman D: The jejunal mucosa in kwashiorkor. Arch Dis Child 40:526, 1965
28. Butterworth CE Jr, Perez-Santiago E: Jejunal biopsies in sprue. Ann Int Med 48:8, 1958
29. Cameron GR, Khanna SD: Regeneration of the intestinal villi after extensive mucosal infarction. J Pathol Bacteriol 77:505, 1959
30. Cocco AF, Dohrmann MJ, Hendrix TR: Reconstruction of normal jejunal biopsies: three-dimensional histology. Gastroenterology 51:305, 1966
31. Collins JR: Small intestinal mucosal damage with villous atrophy. Am J Clin Pathol 44:36, 1965
32. Colwell EJ, Welsh JE, Letgers LJ, Proctor RR: Jejunal morphological characteristics in South Vietnamese residents. JAMA 206:2273, 1968
33. Conrad ME, Schwartz FD, Young AA: Infectious hepatitis—a generalized disease. Am J Med 37:789, 1964
34. Cook GC, Kajubi SK, Lee FD: Jejunal morphology of the African in Uganda. J Pathol 98:157, 1969
35. Cooke WT, Cox EV, Fone DJ, Meynell MJ, Gaddie R: The clinical and metabolic significance of jejunal diverticula. Gut 4:115, 1963
36. Cowan D, Satja VK, Malvea BP: Steatorrhea in the Punjab: the results of a village survey. J Trop Med 74:137, 1971
37. Crabbe PA, Carbonarei AO, Heremans JF: The normal human intestinal mucosa as a major source of plasma cells containing gamma-a-immunoglobulin. Lab Invest 14:235, 1965
38. Crabbe PA, Heremans JF: The distribution of immunoglobulin-containing cells along the human gastrointestinal tract. Gastroenterology 51:305, 1966
39. Creamer B: Variations in small-intestinal villous shape and mucosal dynamics. Br Med J 2:1371, 1964
40. Creamer B, Dutz WF, Post C: Small intestinal lesion of chronic diarrhea and marasmus in Iran. Lancet 1:18, 1970
41. Curran RC, Creamer B: Ultrastructural changes in some disorders of the small intestine associated with malabsorption. J Pathol Bacteriol 86:1, 1963
42. Dean AF, Jones TC: Seasonal gastroenteritis and malabsorption at an American military base in the Philippines. I. Clinical and epidemiological investigations of the acute illness. Am J Epidemiol 95:111, 1972
43. Deo MG, Ramalingaswami V: Absorption of Co[58]-labeled cyanocobalamin in protein deficiency. An experimental study in the rhesus monkey. Gastroenterology 45:167, 1964
44. Desai HG, Merchant PC, Antia FP: Tropical sprue versus protein malnutrition. Indian J Med Sci 26:356, 1972
45. Dixon JMS, Paulley JW: Bacteriological and histological studies of the small intestine of rats treated with mecamylamine. Gut 4:169, 1963
46. Doniach I, Shiner M: Duodenal and jejunal biopsies. II. Histology. Gastroenterology 33:71, 1957
47. Douglas AP, Crabbe PA, Hobbs JR: Immunochemical studies of the serum, intestinal secretions and intestinal mucosa in patients with adult celiac disease and other forms of the celiac syndrome. Gastroentrology 59:414, 1970
48. Dutz W, Asvadi S, Sadri S, Kohout E: Intestinal lymphoma and sprue: a systematic approach. Gut 12:804, 1971

49. Einstein LP, Mackay DM, Rosenberg IH: Pediatric xylose malabsorption in East Pakistan: correlation with age, growth retardation, and weanling diarrhea. Am J Clin Nutr 25:1230, 1972
50. England NWJ: Intestinal pathology of tropical sprue. Am J Clin Nutr 21:961, 1968
51. England NWJ, O'Brien W: Appearances of the jejunal mucosa in acute tropical sprue in Singapore. Gut 7:128, 1966
52. Falaiye JM: Tropical sprue in Nigeria. J Trop Med Hyg 73:119, 1970
53. Falaiye JM: Present status of subclinical intestinal malabsorption in the tropics. Br Med J 4:454, 1971
54. Fischer W: In Henke F, Lubarsch O (eds): Handbuch v. der Spez. Path. Anat. u. Hist. Berlin, Springer, 1929, Vol 14, No 3, p 425
55. Floch MH, Caldwell WL, Sheehy TW: A histopathological basis for the interpretation of small bowel roentgenography in tropical sprue. Am J Roentgenol Radium Ther Nucl Med 87:709, 1962
56. Fone DJ, Meynell MJ, Harris EL, et al: Jejunal biopsy in adult celiac disease and allied disorders. Lancet 1:933, 1960
57. Frazer AC: On the significance of mucosal damage. In Wolstenholme GEW, Cameron MP (eds): Intestinal Biopsy. Ciba Foundation Study Group No. 14. Boston, Little, Brown, 1962, pp 59–66
58. Garcia S: Malabsorption and malnutrition in Mexico. Am J Clin Nutr 21:1066, 1968
59. Gardner FH: Malabsorption syndrome in military personnel in Puerto Rico. Arch Int Med 98:44, 1955
60. Gardner FH: Tropical sprue. N Engl J Med 258:791, 835, 1958
61. Gerson CD, Kent TH, Saha JR, Siddiqi N, Lindenbaum J: Recovery of small-intestinal structure and function after residence in the tropics. II. Studies in Indians and Pakistanis living in New York City. Ann Int Med 75:41, 1971
62. Ghitis J, Tripathy K, Mayoral G: Malabsorption in the tropics. 2. Tropical sprue versus primary protein malnutrition: vitamin B_{12} and folic acid studies. Am J Clin Nutr 20:1206, 1967
63. Goldstein F, Dammin GJ, Mandle RJ, Wirts CW: Clinical syndrome resembling tropical sprue in lifelong residents of temperate zone. Am J Dig Dis 17:407, 1972
64. Gorbach SL, Banwell JG, Jacobs B, et al: Tropical sprue and malnutrition in West Bengal. I. Intestinal microflora and absorption. Am J Clin Nutr 23:1545, 1970
65. Gottlieb S, Brandborg LL: Reversible flat mucosal changes of the small bowel occurring with an acute diarrheal disease. Gasteroenterology 51:1037, 1966
66. Haghighi P, Nasr K: Primary upper small intestinal lymphoma, so-called "Mediterranean lymphoma." Pathol Ann 8:231–255, 1973
67. Halstead CH, Sheir S, Sourial N, Patwardhan VN: Small intestinal structure and absorption in Egypt. Am J Clin Nutr 22:744, 1969
68. Harper GP: Xylose malabsorption and growth retardation in East Pakistani children. Am J Clin Nutr 25:1227, 1972
69. Harries JR: Tropical sprue in the African. East Afr Med J 41:180, 1964
70. Hartman RS, Butterworth CE Jr, Hartman RE, Crosby WH, Shizai A: An electron microscopic investigation of the jejunal epithelium in sprue. Gastroenterology 38:506, 1960
71. Herskovic TJ, Katz J, Floch MH, Spencer RP, Spiro HM: Small intestinal absorption and morphology in germ-free, monocontaminated and conventional mice. Gastroenterology 52:1136, 1967
72. Hindle W, Creamer B: Significance of a flat intestinal mucosa. Br Med J 3:455, 1965
73. Hourihane DO'B: The pathology of malabsorption states. In Harrison CV (ed): Recent Advances in Pathology. London, Churchill, 1966, pp 320–347

74. Jeejeebhoy KN, Desai HG, Borkar AV, Deshpande V, Pathare SM: Tropical malabsorption syndrome in West India. Am J Clin Nutr 21:994, 1968
75. Jeejeebhoy KN, Desai HG, Noronha M, Anita FP, Parekh DV: Idiopathic tropical diarrhea with or without steatorrhea (tropical malabsorption syndrome). Gastroenterology 51:333, 1966
76. Kean BH, Hoskins DW, Kammerer WH: Tropical medicine in New York City. Bull NY Acad Med 40:43, 1964
77. Keele KD, Bound JP: Sprue in India: clinical survey of 600 cases. Br Med J 1:77, 1946
78. Kent TH, Lindenbaum J: Correlation of jejunal function and morphology in patients with acute and chronic diarrhea in East Pakistan. Gastroenterology 52:966, 1967
79. Keusch GT: Subclinical malabsorption in Thailand. I. Intestinal absorption in Thai children. Am J Clin Nutr 25:1062, 1972
80. Keusch GT, Buchanan RD, Bahmarapravathi N, Troncale FJ: Neomycin enteropathy in man. Clin Res 15:237, 1967
81. Keusch GT, Plaut AG, Troncale FJ: Subclinical malabsorption in Thailand. II. Intestinal absorption in American military and Peace Corps personnel. Ann J Clin Nutr 25:1067, 1972
82. King MJ, Joske RA: Acute enteritis with temporary intestinal malabsorption. Br Med J 1:1324, 1960
83. Klipstein FA: Tropical sprue in New York City. Gastroenterology 47:457, 1964
84. Klipstein FA: Tropical sprue—an iceberg disease? Ann Int Med 66:622, 1967
85. Klipstein FA: Progress in gastroenterology: tropical sprue. Gastroenterology 54:275, 1968
86. Klipstein FA: Intestinal morphology in tropical malabsorption. Proc Western Hemisphere Nutrition Congr II. Chicago, AMA, 1968
87. Klipstein FA: Foreword: symposium on malabsorption and malnutrition in the tropics. Am J Clin Nutr 21:939, 1968
88. Klipstein FA: Regarding the definition of tropical sprue. Gastroenterology 58:717, 1970
89. Klipstein FA: Recent advances in tropical malabsorption. Scand J Gastroenterol (suppl 6), 93:114, 1970
90. Klipstein FA: Tropical sprue in the Western Hemisphere. In Tropical Sprue and Megaloblastic Anemia. Wellcome Trust Collaborative Study. Edinburgh and London, Churchill, 1971, pp 129–158
91. Klipstein FA, Baker SJ: Regarding the definition of tropical sprue. Gastroenterology, 58:717, 1970
92. Klipstein FA: Falaiye JM: Tropical sprue in expatriates from the tropics living in the continental United States. Medicine 48:475, 1969
93. Klipstein FA, Samloff IM, Schenk EA: Tropical sprue in Haiti. Ann Int Med 64:575, 1966
94. Klipstein FA, Samloff IM, Smarth G, Schenk EA: Malabsorption and malnutrition in rural Haiti. Am J Clin Nutr 21:1042, 1968
95. Klipstein FA, Samloff IM, Smarth G, Schenk EA: Treatment of overt and subclinical malabsorption in Haiti. Gut 10:315, 1969
96. Klipstein FA, Schenk EA, Samloff IM: Folate repletion associated with oral tetracycline therapy in tropical sprue. Gastroenterology 51:317, 1966
97. Lindenbaum J: Malabsorption during and after recovery from acute intestinal infection. Br Med J 11:326, 1965
98. Lindenbaum J: Small intestine dysfunction in Pakistanis and Americans resident in Pakistan. Am J Clin Nutr 21:1023, 1968
99. Lindenbaum J: Tropical enteropathy. Gastroenterology 64:637, 1973
100. Lindenbaum J, Alam AKMJ, Kent TH: Subclinical small intestinal disease in East Pakistan. Br Med J 2:1616, 1966

101. Lindenbaum J, Gerson CD, Kent TH: Recovery of small intestinal structure and function after residence in the tropics. 1. Studies in Peace Corps volunteers. Ann Int Med 74:218, 1971
102. Lindenbaum J, Harmon JW, Gerson CD: Subclinical malabsorption in developing countries. Ann J Clin Nutr 25:1056, 1972
103. Lindenbaum J, Kent TH, Sprinz H: Malabsorption and jejunitis in American Peace Corps volunteers in Pakistan. Ann Int Med 65:1201, 1966
104. Lojda Z, Fric PL, Jodl J, Chmelik V: Cytochemistry of the human jejunal mucosa in the norm and in malabsorption syndrome. Curr Top Pathol 52:1, 1970
105. Mackie FP, Fairley NH: The morbid anatomy of sprue. Indian J Med Res 16:797, 1929
106. Madanagopalan N, Shiner M, Rowe B: Measurements of small intestinal mucosa obtained by peroral biopsy. Am J Med 38:42, 1965
107. Maldonado N, Sanchez NJ: Immunologic studies in tropical sprue. Am J Gastroenterol 52:141, 1969
108. Manson-Bahr PH: The riddle of tropical sprue. J Trop Med Hyg 63:49, 1960
109. Manson-Bahr PH: Tropical Diseases. Baltimore, Williams & Wilkins, 1966, pp 464–476
110. Mathan VI: Tropical sprue. In Sleisenger MH, Fordtran JS (eds): Gastrointestinal Disease: Pathophysiology, Diagnosis, Management. Philadelphia, Saunders, 1973, pp 978–988
111. Mathan VI, Baker SJ: Epidemic tropical sprue and other epidemics of diarrhea in features. Ann Trop Med Parasitol 64:439, 1970
112. Mathan VI, Baker SJ: An epidemic of tropical sprue in southern India. I. Clinical south Indian villages. A comparative study. Am J Clin Nutr 21:1077, 1968
113. Mathan VI, Joseph S, Baker SJ: Tropical sprue in children. A syndrome of idiopathic malabsorption. Gastroenterology 56:556, 1969
114. Mayoral LG, Tripathy K, Bolanos O, et al: Intestinal functional and morphologic abnormalities in severely protein-malnourished adults. Am J Clin Nutr 25:1084, 1972
115. Mayoral LG, Tripathy K, Garcia FT, et al: Malabsorption in the tropics: a second look. I. The role of protein malnutrition. Am J Clin Nutr 20:866, 1967
116. Mayoral LG, Tripathy K, Garcia FT, Bolanos O, Ghitis J: Protein malnutrition-induced malabsorption and other enteropathies in Colombia. Am J Clin Nutr 21:1053, 1968
117. McPherson JR, Summerskill WHJ: An acute malabsorption syndrome with reversible mucosal atrophy. Gastroenterology 44:900, 1963
118. Meader RD, Landers DF: Electron and light microscopic observations on relationship between lymphocytes and intestinal epithelium. Am J Anat 121:763, 1965
119. Misra RC, Kasthuri D, Chuttani HK: Adult coeliac disease in the tropics. Br Med J 2:1230, 1966
120. Misra RC, Kasthuri D, Chuttani HK: Correlation of biochemical, clinical, radiological and histological findings in tropical sprue. J Trop Med 70:6, 1967
121. Misra RC, Krishnan N, Ramalingaswami V, Chuttani HK: Tropical sprue in northern India. Scand J Gastroenterol 2:192, 1967
122. Montgomery RD, Beale DJ, Sammons HG, Schneider R: Postinfection malabsorption: a sprue syndrome. Br Med J 2:265, 1973
123. Nasr K, Haghighi P, Abadi P, Hedayati H, Reinhold JG: Idiopathic enteropathy in Iran. Submitted for publication.
124. O'Brien W: Acute military tropical sprue in South-East Asia. Am J Clin Nutr 21:1007, 1968
125. O'Brien W: Historical survey of tropical sprue affecting Europeans in South-East Asia. In Tropical Sprue and Megaloblastic Anemia. Wellcome Trust Collaborative Study. Churchill, Edinburgh and London, 1971, pp 13–24

126. O'Brien, England NWJ: Military tropical sprue from South-East Asia. Br Med J 2:1157, 1966

127. Parkins RA, Eidelman S, Perrin EB, Rubin CE: A preliminary study of factors affecting blood lipid levels in three groups of Yeminite Jews. Am J Clin Nutr 18:134, 1966

128. Platt BS, Heard CRC, Stewart RJC: The effects of protein-calorie deficiency on the gastrointestinal tract. In The Role of the Gastrointestinal tract in Protein Metabolism. Philadelphia, Davis, 1964, p 227

129. Rhodes AR, Shea N, Lindenbaum J: Malabsorption in asymptomatic Liberian children. Am J Clin Nutr 24:574, 1971

130. Rivera JV, DeLaobra FR, Maldonado MM: Anemia due to vitamin B_{12} deficiency after treatment with folic acid in tropical sprue. J Clin Nutr 18:110, 1966

131. Robins SJ, Garcia-Palmieri M, Rubio C: Low serum cholesterol levels and subclinical malabsorption. Ann Int Med 66:556, 1967

132. Roy-Choudhury D, Cooke WT, Tan DT, Banwell JG, Smits BJ: Jejunal biopsy: criteria and significance. Scand J Gastroenterol 1:57, 1966

133. Rubin CE, Dobbins WO III: Peroral biopsy of the small intestine: a review of its diagnostic usefulness. Gastroenterology 49:676, 1965

134. Rubin W: The epithelial "membrane" of the small intestine. Am J Clin Nutr 24:45, 1971

135. Russel PK, Aziz MA, Ahmad N, Kent TH, Gangarosa EJ: Enteritis and gastritis in young asymptomatic Pakistani men. Am J Dig Dis 11:296, 1966

136. Santiago-Borrero PJ, Maldonado N, Horta E: Tropical sprue in children. J Pediatr 76:470, 1970

137. Schenk EA: Summation, session II, part I, workshop on malabsorption and malnutrition. Am J Clin Nutr 25:1107, 1972

138. Schenk EA, Klipstein FA: A protocol for the evaluation of small bowel biopsies. Appendix to session II, part I, workshop on malabsorption and malnutrition. Am J Clin Nutr 25:1108, 1972

139. Schenk EA, Klipstein FA, Tomasini JT: Morphologic characteristics of jejunal biopsies from asymptomatic Haitians and Puerto Ricans. Am J Clin Nutr 25:1080, 1972

140. Schenk EA, Samloff IM, Klipstein FA: Morphologic characteristics of jejunal biopsies in celiac disease and in tropical sprue. Am J Pathol 47:765, 1965

141. Schenk EA, Samloff IM, Klipstein FA: Pathogenesis of jejunal mocosal alterations: synechia formation. Am J Pathol 50:523, 1967

142. Schenk EA, Samloff IM, Klipstein FA: Morphology of small bowel biopsies. Am J Clin Nutr 21:944, 1968

143. Sheehy TW: Megalocytic changes in tropical sprue. Am J Gastroentrol 42:30, 1964

144. Sheehy TW: Enteric disease among U.S. troops in Vietnam. Gastroenterology 55:105, 1968

145. Sheehy TW, Artenstein MS, Green RW: Small intestinal mucosa in certain viral diseases. JAMA 120:1023, 1964

146. Sheehy TW, Baggs B, Perez-Santiago E, Floch MH: Prognosis of tropical sprue. Ann Int Med 57:892, 1962

147. Sheehy TW, Cohen WH, Brodsky JP: The intestinal lesion in the initial phase of tropical (military) sprue. Am J Dig Dis 8:826, 1963

148. Sheehy TW, Cohen WH, Wallace DK, Legters LJ: Tropical sprue in North Americans. JAMA 194:1069, 1965

149. Sheehy TW, Letgers LJ, Wallace DK: Tropical jejunitis in Americans serving in Vietnam. Am J Clin Nutr 21:1013, 1968

150. Shiner M: The histology of the small intestine: In Girdwood RH, Smith AN (eds): Malabsorption. Edinburgh, Edinburgh Univ Press, 1969, pp 134–148

151. Sparberg M, Knudson KB, Frank S: Tropical sprue from the Philippines: report

of three cases. Milit Med 132:809, 1967

152. Spiro HM, Filipe MI, Stewart JS, Booth CC, Pearse AGE: Functional histochemistry of the small bowel mucosa in malabsorptive syndromes. Gut 5:145, 1964

153. Sprinz H: Morphologic response of intestinal mucosa to enteric bacteria and its implications for sprue and Asiatic cholera. Fed Proc 21:57, 1962

154. Sprinz H, Kundel DW, Dammin GJ, et al: The response of the germ-free guinea-pig to oral bacterial challenge with Escherischia coli and Shigella flexneri. Am J Pathol 39:681, 1961

155. Sprinz H, Sribhibhadh R, Gangarosa EJ, et al: Biopsy of small bowel of Thai people: with special reference to recovery from Asiatic cholera and to an intestinal malabsorption syndrome. Am J Clin Pathol 38:43, 1962

156. Stanfield JP, Hutt MSR, Tunnicliffe R: Intestinal biopsy in kwashiorkor. Lancet 2:519, 1965

157. Stefanini M: Clinical features and pathogenesis of tropical sprue: observations on a series of cases among Italian prisoners of war in India. Medicine 27:379, 1948

158. Suarez RM, Spies TD, Suarez RM Jr: Use of folic acid in sprue. Ann Int Med 26:543, 1947

159. Swanson VL, Thomassen RW: Pathology of the jejunal mucosa in tropical sprue. Am J Pathol 46:511, 1965

160. Swanson VL, Wheby MS, Bayless TM: Morphologic effects of folic acid and vitamin B_{12} on the jejunal lesion of tropical sprue. Am J Pathol 49:167, 1966

161. Takano J: Intestinal changes in protein-deficient rats. Exp Mol Pathol 3:224, 1964

162. Ten Thije OJ, Veeger W, Braams WG, Nieweg HO: Sprue associated with folic acid deficiency. Am J Dig Dis 9:774, 1964

163. Townley RRW, Cass MH, Anderson CM: Small intestinal mucosal patterns of celiac disease and idiopathic steatorrhea seen in other situations. Gut 5:51, 1964

164. Trier JS, Rubin CE: Electron microscopy of the small intestine: a review. Gastroenterology 49:574, 1965

165. Troncale FJ, Keusch GT, Miller LH, Olsson RA, Buchanan RD: Normal absorption in Thai subjects with non-specific jejunal abnormalities. Br Med J 4:578, 1967

166. Tropical Sprue and Megaloblastic Anemia. Wellcome Trust Collaborative Study. Edinburgh and London, Churchill, 1971, pp 269–291

167. Vaish SK, Sampathkumar J, Jacob R, Baker SJ: The stomach in tropical sprue. Gut 6:458, 1965

168. Walia BNS, Sidhy JR, Tandon BN, Ghai OP, Bhargava S: Celiac disease in North Indian children. Br Med J 2:1233, 1966

169. Webb JF, Simpson B: Tropical sprue in Hong Kong. Br Med J 2:1162, 1966

170. Weinstein WM, Saunders DR, Tytgat BGN, Rubin CE: Collagenous sprue—an unrecognized type of malabsorption. N Engl J Med 283:1297, 1970

171. Wheby MS, Swanson VL, Bayless TM: Comparison of ileal and jejunal biopsies in tropical sprue. Am J Clin Nutr 24:117, 1971

172. Wheby MS, Swanson VL, Bayless TM: Jejunal crypt cell and marrow morphology in tropical sprue. Ann Int Med 1969

173. Whitehead R: Interpretation of mucosal biopsies from the gastrointestinal tract. In Dyke VSC (ed): Recent Advances in Pathology and Clinical Pathology. Series V. Boston, Little, Brown, 1968 pp 375–400

174. Winawer SJ, Sullivan LW, Herbert V, Zamchek N: The jejunal mucosa in patients with nutritional folate deficiency and megaloblastic anemia. N Engl J Med 272:892, 1965

175. Zubiran S: Nutritional aspects of gastrointestinal disease. Am J Dig Dis 6:336, 1961

PRIMARY UPPER SMALL INTESTINAL LYMPHOMA (SO-CALLED MEDITERRANEAN LYMPHOMA)

PARVIZ HAGHIGHI and KHOSROW NASR

Primary small intestinal lymphoma has recently attracted attention, mainly due to the identification of a geographically distinct primary upper small intestinal lymphoma (also referred to as Mediterranean lymphoma) with its noteworthy features including steatorrhea and an associated heavy chain protein abnormality.[1, 10, 28, 31, 50, 53, 69, 71, 72, 77, 78, 92] However, primary small intestinal lymphoma has been recognized as far back as 1838 when Priquet (cited by Skrimshire [97]) described enlarged gastric rugae due to lymphoid growth together with granulomatous tumors throughout the intestine accompanied by a generalized glandular enlargement. Since then, numerous other reports describing lymphoma solely in the intestine have appeared in the literature.[6, 13, 15, 26, 33, 34, 37, 51, 52, 60, 63, 65, 68, 93]

In 1961 Dawson et al.[26] reviewed the literature and established the criteria for classification of primary small intestinal lymphoma. Meanwhile studies from Israel and Iran emphasized the special features and the geographic distribution of primary upper small intestinal lymphoma (heretofore referred to as PUSIL).[31, 69, 71, 78] All this has led to a certain degree of confusion especially in terminology, so that the terms *abdominal lymphoma, intestinal lymphoma, primary intestinal lymphoma,* and *primary upper small intestinal lymphoma* are usually used interchangeably and often incorrectly. To clarify this matter, the following needs to be emphasized:

1. *Abdominal lymphoma* is a clinical term and refers to lymphoma involving the intraabdominal organs. However, in the literature this term usually refers to lymphoma involving mesenteric or paraaortic lymph nodes, or both, with or without small bowel involvement.[31, 50, 72, 77]

2. *Intestinal lymphoma* refers to lymphoma involving the intestinal tract, either primarily or in association with lymphoma elsewhere.[30, 110]

3. *Primary gastrointestinal lymphoma* refers to lymphoma originating in the gastrointestinal tract. This means that at the earliest point of the disease, the lymphoma is found solely in the gastrointestinal tract. Of special note in this

category is *primary upper small intestinal lymphoma* (PUSIL) where, in terms of origin, the lymphoma must be found solely in the upper small intestine (duodenum-jejunum) before this terminology can be properly applied. This present report reviews our understanding of primary small intestinal lymphoma with a particular attention to PUSIL.

Primary Small Intestinal Lymphoma

Lymphoma reports from Europe and the United States have included cases of primary small intestinal lymphoma though they emphasize its relatively rare occurrence. In fact, 2 or possibly 3 cases in a review of 618 cases of lymphoma by Gall and Mallory [35] as well as reports of only a few cases from other large medical centers over a prolonged period, exemplify this rarity.[26, 34, 63, 82, 105] Small intestinal tumors in general are also relatively rare, and these lymphomas comprise one-third to one-half of all such tumors [13] or 16 percent of all primary malignant neoplasms of the small bowel.[113] One out of four primary gastrointestinal tract lymphomas occurs in the small intestine,[31, 68, 113] and the frequency of segmental involvement increases from duodenum to ileum.[14, 33, 63, 93, 100] The more frequent involvement of the terminal ileum has been related to its rich lymphoid tissue.[22, 106]

This type of lymphoma primarily affects the older age group in the fifth and sixth decades and males.[26, 33, 34, 60, 63, 68, 113] The symptoms and findings usually suggest an intraabdominal disease.[34] The lymphomatous lesions tend to be patchy, probably accounting for the low diagnostic value of the peroral intestinal biopsy. Their gross appearance in the approximate order of frequency may be described as ulcerative, aneurysmal, polypoid, and constricting.[75, 113] Within this basic framework some reporters have recognized infiltrative, submucosal, and nodular variants. The ulcerative type is more common in the jejunum and the proximal ileum, having a high rate of perforation [108] and fistula formation, while the polypoid type frequently occurs in the distal ileum where it predisposes to intussusception.[33, 113] Multiple sites of involvement occur in 20 to 40 percent of the cases,[61, 93] and mesenteric node involvement may be an associated finding. Histologically, all types of malignant lymphoma have been described in primary small intestinal lymphoma. The difficulty has been the differences in criteria for classification among various series.[26, 108] With this qualification in mind, reticulum cell sarcoma appears the most frequent while Hodgkin's disease and giant follicle lymphoma are rare.[6, 26, 75, 97, 108, 113] There does not appear to be a significant correlation between the cell type and the gross findings. On the other hand, well-differentiated lymphosarcoma and giant follicle lymphoma carry the best prognoses.[61, 63, 93, 100, 108]

The previous description of primary small intestinal lymphoma was from reports from the Western countries. Small intestinal lymphomas fitting this description probably do exist in other areas of the world with slight differences, including the age of onset and possibly the frequency.[71] The major geographic difference appears to be the segment involved. In the West this is usually the ileum, while in the Middle East, for example, there is a preponderance of upper small intestinal involvement.[77, 78, 85]

Primary Upper Small Intestinal Lymphoma (PUSIL)

This is only one category in the already referred to primary small intestinal lymphoma. Reasons for its separation include its distinct geographic distribution and clinical presentation.

Our criterion for diagnosis of this entity is pathologically proved lymphoma originating in the upper small intestine. To remove any question regarding the intestinal origin, our studies have been based on cases that on extensive evaluation were found to have this lymphoma solely in the upper small intestine.[69]

Clinical Presentation

Our patients are Moslems from Southern Iran, primarily from the rural and low socioeconomic bracket. The majority are men under 30 years of age. The complaints and findings suggest an intraabdominal disease. The main complaints include abdominal pain and diarrhea, singly or in combination. Weight loss, nausea, and vomiting seem to be common, while fever is rarely observed. Perforation and obstruction are occasional findings. The physical examination abnormalities include abdominal tenderness, distention, or a mass. Edema and ascites are found in about 20 percent of the cases. Of special note is the high frequency of associated clubbing and osteoarthropathy.[70] In fact, in our area the triad of chronic abdominal pain, diarrhea, and clubbing, especially in a young patient, is regarded as PUSIL until proved otherwise.[3, 66]

Reports from Israel [31, 77] and South Africa [72] present a very similar clinical picture save for the differences in religion and ethnic backgrounds. Cases from India,[62, 103] Iraq,[2] and Mexico [53] are insufficient for generalizations. In fact, it is not certain whether or not the cases from India and Iraq indeed represent PUSIL.

The usual laboratory tests are not of help in diagnosis of this disease. On the other hand, the barium meal shows an abnormal upper small intestine described as a "malabsorption-like" pattern.[24, 36, 69] More specifically, this includes areas of dilatation, segmentation, and puddling with abnormalities of the mucosal pattern.[71] With the suggestive clinical presentation and the abnormal barium meal our next step has been the histopathologic proof of the diagnosis. This is initially attempted with a peroral small intestinal suction biopsy.[16, 83] Failing this or needing further clarification, laparotomy may be the procedure of choice.

Gross Pathologic Findings

Pathologic findings may be described under gross and microscopic observations. As in the Israeli series [78] various gross presentations were noted in our cases. These include diffusely infiltrative, ulcerative, and nodular forms (Figs. 1–4).[17] Perforation was occasionally present associated with the ulcerative type. The relative frequencies of these various forms are not available at present.[28] More than one gross feature may be present in the same specimen. In one case, for ex-

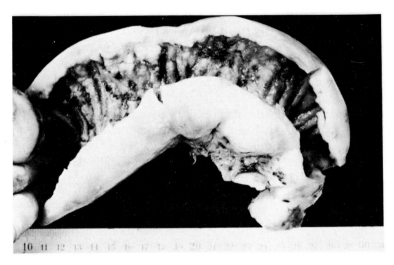

Fig. 1. Small bowel. Lymphosarcoma, infiltrative type. Note the diffusely thickened wall of the small bowel.

ample, ulceration was seen in association with annular constriction (Fig. 3). In the infiltrative form the diffuse infiltration of the bowel wall by tumor may be associated with a rigid bowel segment not unlike the leather-bottle effect seen in linitis plastica of the stomach (Figs. 1, 2).

Laparotomy with full-thickness small intestinal and mesenteric node biopsy has been helpful in arriving at the diagnosis. In three of our cases, laparotomy

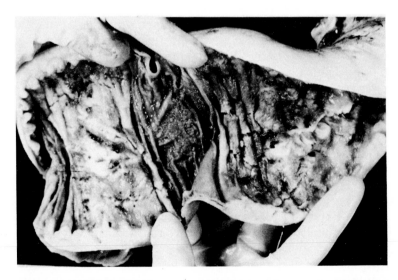

Fig. 2. Small bowel (same patient as in Figure 1). Lymphosarcoma. Note the mucosa uniformly destroyed by tumor.

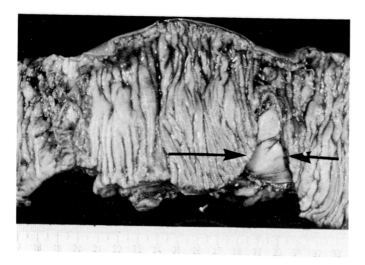

Fig. 3. Small bowel. Reticulum cell sarcoma, ulcerative type. Two separate circumferential tumor ulcers are seen, one (*right*) producing marked luminal constriction at the same time. Adjacent to and below the latter (*arrows*), involved mesenteric lymph nodes are present.

showed a perfectly normal serosal surface of the bowel with no apparent enlargement of the mesenteric lymph nodes. The surgeon did not perform a full-thickness intestinal biopsy, considering the clinical impression an error. These three cases were reexplored within 1 month of the initial exploration, again the finding being one of normal appearance of the bowel. However, this time a full-thickness biopsy was obtained and the lymphoma diagnosis established histologically. Thus, the

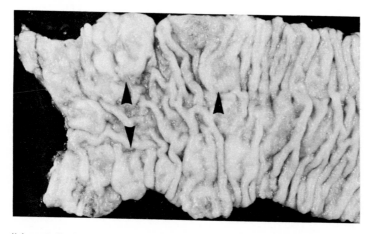

Fig. 4. Small bowel. Reticulum cell sarcoma. In this case the lymphoma infiltrate presents as discrete, nonulcerated tumor plaques and nodules on the mucosal surface (*arrowheads*).

gross serosal appearance of an intestine with this type of lymphoma may be perfectly normal. It should be stressed that the usual appearance is that of patchy abnormalities of the serosa with intestinal segmentation.

Mesenteric nodes are often involved and frequently display a fish-flesh appearance on cut surfaces.[32]

Microscopic Findings

For discussion purposes findings as seen in peroral biopsies and in open biopsy-resection specimens will be described separately.

Peroral Biopsy Findings

Except for the infrequent failures where the biopsy specimens were quantitatively insufficient for evaluation, and save for the occasional biopsy in the "minimal change" group (Fig. 5, see next paragraph), all other biopsy specimens were either positive for lymphoma (70 percent of the quantitatively sufficient biopsies) or definitely abnormal (30 percent) (Figs. 6–11). Sometimes several biopsies had to be performed (as many as five in one case) before the lymphoma diagnosis was reached. In these cases the "prefinal" biopsies were invariably abnormal.

"MINIMAL CHANGE" BIOPSIES. At this moment it is not exactly clear what constitutes a "normal" peroral small bowel biopsy in the Iranian population. Studies are currently underway to answer this question. Preliminary work by Dutz

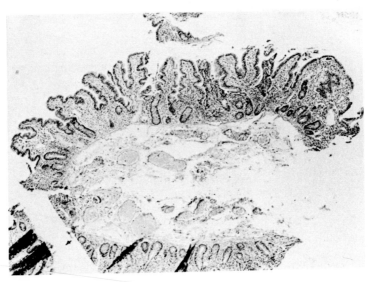

Fig. 5. Peroral biopsy. "Minimal change." Allowing for the slightly tangential section, the villi have almost normal configuration. The lamina propria is, at the most, minimally hypercellular. (H&E × 10.)

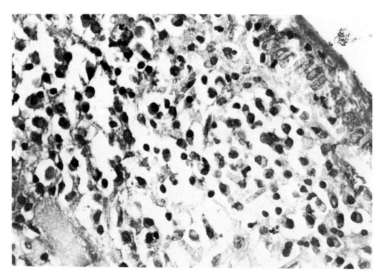

Fig. 6. Peroral small bowel biopsy. Mature plasma cells and not tumor cells lie directly beneath the surface epithelium. Note loss of demarcation between the surface epithelium and the villous core. (H&E × 160.)

et al.[28] on necropsy bowel specimens of children more than 1 year of age as well as adults indicates a 15 percent incidence of flat mucosa. However, necropsy material may not necessarily reflect the true situation in life.[31] The single case in this category (Fig. 5) merely showed "de-ruffled" villous epithelium and possibly a mild increase in plasma cells in villous core and the lamina propria.

"ABNORMAL" BIOPSIES. The degree of "abnormality" was variable but never so mild as to permit one to disregard them as possible regional normal variation. These abnormalities consisted of the following:

Abnormal Villous Shapes. Blunting, branching, and flattening of the villi were noted in those cases in which the orientation of the biopsy sections permitted evaluation of the villi from this standpoint. It must be remembered that unless the sections are perpendicular to the long axis of the bowel, such evaluation is fraught with danger of misinterpretation.

Disturbed Villous Height-to-Crypt Ratio. Usually it was in the "diminished" direction. This again requires properly oriented specimens.

Surface Epithelial Abnormalities. At times this finding was rather striking (Figs. 6, 7). The surface epithelial cells lose their sharply demarcated contours, including their brush borders as well as their normally sharp delineation from the underlying lamina propria. They may not be quite perpendicular to the basement membrane. The epithelial cell nuclei may be disproportionately large and vesicular or small and dense. (Figs. 6, 8, 9).

Crypt Cell Abnormalities. The crypt epithelium may also display nuclear enlargement or hyperchromasia. Mitoses were frequent. Paneth cells could not be critically evaluated owing to the quality of sections with regard to preservation of the cell granules.

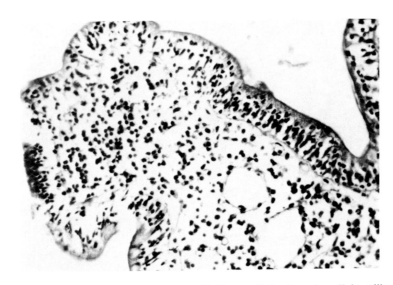

Fig. 7. Peroral small bowel biopsy. "Abnormal" biopsy. Note densely cellular villous core. (Most of these are plasma cells at higher magnifications not shown here). Also note lymphangiectasis of the villous core and intense lymphocytic transmigration through the surface epithelium. Mesenteric lymph node and another peroral biopsy (not illustrated) showed reticulum cell sarcoma. (H&E × 100.)

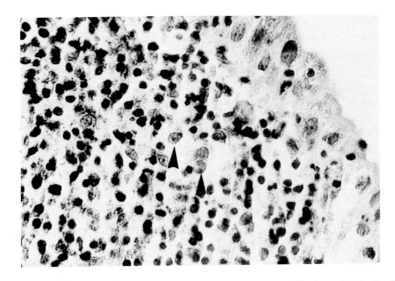

Fig. 8. Peroral small bowel biopsy (same case as in Figure 12). Lymphoblastic lymphosarcoma. Higher magnification of the villous tip. Note lack of sharp distinction between the surface epithelium and the villous core on one hand and between the individual epithelial cells on the other. The epithelial cell nuclei have lost their polarity and are large and vesicular. Large, bare vesicular nuclei probably belonging to tumor cells are present in the villous core (*arrowhead*). This field by itself, though abnormal, is not regarded as diagnostic of lymphoma. (H&E × 200.)

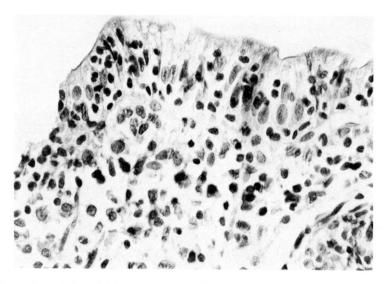

Fig. 9. Peroral small bowel biopsy (same biopsy as in Figure 10). "Abnormal" biopsy. Higher magnification of the superficial portion of the specimen. Note marked alterations in the surface epithelium with essentially the same changes as in Figure 7 plus lymphocytic transmigration. Large, bare nuclei of reticulum cells are noted in the villous core. (H&E × 100.)

Lymphocytic Epithelial Transmigration. In mild forms this appears to be a normally occuring event.[107] However, in our biopsies this frequently constituted a striking finding (Figs. 7, 10, 11). Transmigration occurred through the surface as well as the crypt epithelium.

Lymphangiectasis. This was noted both within the villous lacteals and deeper in the submucosa (Fig. 7). It was sometimes associated with a similar phenomenon in the mesenteric lymph nodes. It probably represents the effect of obstruction to the lymph flow.

Hypercellularity of the Lamina Propria. In mild forms this is rather subjective and open to debate.[31] The cells responsible for this finding are usually the mature plasma cells and abound immediately under the surface epithelium (Figs. 6, 7). A variable number of lymphocytes and reticulum cells may be found in association with these plasma cells. The reticulum cells are usually found deeper in the villous core and particularly in the lamina propria, although they may occasionally reach the villous tips (Figs. 8, 9). Finding these cells, especially in atypical forms and in large numbers, should alert one to the presence of lymphoma (Figs. 8, 9). Eosinophils were not a feature in our cases. Polymorphonuclear neutrophils were occasionally noted within the villi and the lamina propria. According to Eidelman et al.[31] these cells are almost never found outside the blood vessels in normal lamina propria.

Lymphoid follicles as normally occurring structures were occasionally noted in the peroral biopsies. The germinal centers were variably developed in these follicles. Care must be exercised in differentiating these "benign" follicles from the

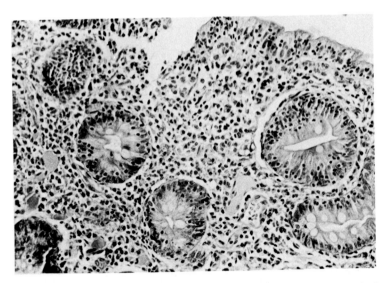

Fig. 10. Peroral small bowel biopsy. "Abnormal" biopsy. Intense hypercellularity of the lamina propria and lymphocytic migration through the surface and crypt epithelium are seen. (H&E × 63.)

"malignant" follicles that occur in some forms of lymphosarcoma, reticulum cell sarcoma, and the giant follicle lymphoma.[45-47, 54, 64, 109]

"LYMPHOMA" BIOPSIES. The criteria for diagnosis of malignant lymphoma on peroral small bowel biopsies do not differ basically from those employed to diagnose lymphoma in other locations. In other words, recognizable tumor cells must be present in the specimen. In this context we concur with Eidelman et al.[31] that the single most important criterion for diagnosis of lymphoma in these biopsies is cytology of the cells (Figs. 12–16).

In 28 percent of the lymphoma biopsies a subsequent laparotomy was performed, and the peroral biopsy–rendered diagnosis was confirmed by open biopsy of the small bowel. In another 43 percent the bowel was not biopsied at laparotomy, but biopsy of the mesenteric lymph nodes revealed lymphoma; and in at least a third of these there was a grossly visible abnormality of the small bowel at laparotomy.

Most of the biopsies were lymphosarcoma (usually lymphoblastic). Others were reticulum cell sarcoma, and one was an unclassified lymphoma. No case of Hodgkin's disease was present in the peroral biopsy series. A partly follicular feature was present in two of the lymphosarcomas, and one lymphosarcoma had a plasmacytoid feature. Unfortunately no immunoglobulin work-up is available in any of our plasmacytoid lymphomas. Besides the lymphoma infiltrate which displayed its invasive nature in some biopsies, various degrees of abnormalities in the villous architecture and relative number of crypts were noted. The latter feature

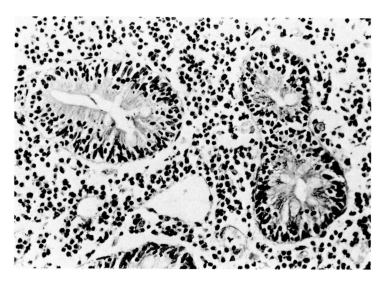

Fig. 11. Peroral small bowel biopsy (same biopsy as in Figure 7 but deeper in the lamina propria). "Abnormal" biopsy. Marked hypercellularity, lymphangiectasis, and transmigration through the crypt epithelium. (H&E × 100.)

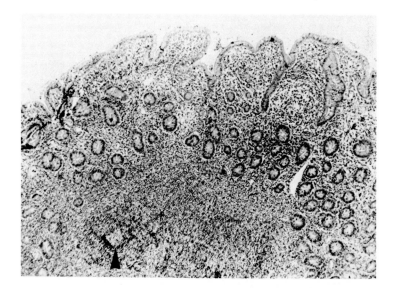

Fig. 12. Peroral small bowel biopsy. Lymphoblastic lymphosarcoma, focally follicular. At this magnification, severe hypercellularity of the villous core, lamina propria, and submucosa with total destruction of the muscularis mucosae are seen. One area (*arrowhead*) suggests a follicular arrangement. No comment can be made regarding villous configuration owing to the tangential section. (H&E × 16.)

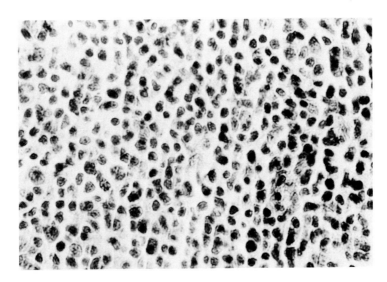

Fig. 13. Peroral small bowel biopsy (same biopsy as in Figures 8 and 12). Lymphoblastic lymphosarcoma. Tumor infiltrate in the lamina propria. (H&E × 200.)

is emphasized by some workers [31] as a helpful clue to the presence of lymphoma since it does not take place in celiac sprue, a condition which can pose problems in differential diagnosis. [7, 48, 56, 58, 80, 84, 95, 96, 101, 102]

In many cases, though present in considerable number in the deeper portion of the villous core and elsewhere in the lamina propria, the tumor cells did not

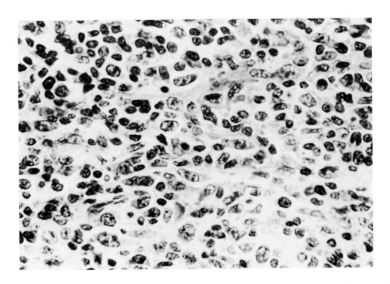

Fig. 14. Open biopsy of the small bowel (same case as in Figures 9 and 10). Reticulum cell sarcoma. Note the large, vesicular, bare nuclei essentially similar to the few seen in the peroral biopsy of Figure 10. (H&E × 200.)

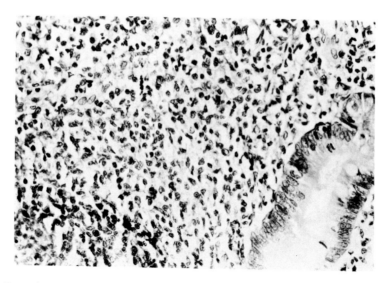

Fig. 15. Peroral small bowel biopsy (small biopsy as in Figure 6). Reticulum cell sarcoma. Note many tumor cells with vesicular nuclei lying between crypts. (H&E × 100.)

reach the villous tips. Instead, a rather dense aggregate of mature plasma cells separated the tumor cells from the surface epithelium (Fig. 6). Presence of plasma cells in large numbers, a phenomenon referred to by Novis et al.[72] as "plasma cell transformation," although not diagnostic by itself, appears to be associated with PUSIL frequently.

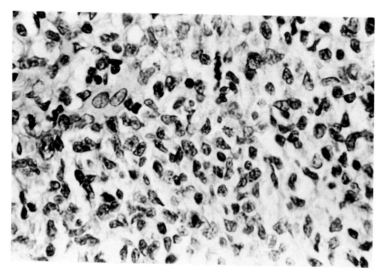

Fig. 16. Peroral biopsy (same biopsy as in Figure 15). Reticulum cell sarcoma. Higher magnification of tumor cells. (H&E ×200.)

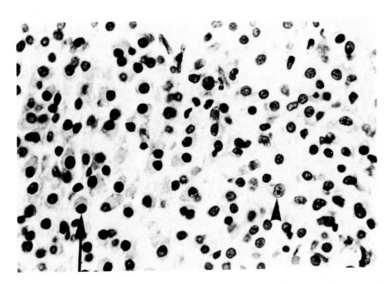

Fig. 17. Open biopsy of the small bowel. "Plasmacytoid" lymphoma. This figure illustrates the tumor infiltrate deep in the lamina propria. Two morphologically distinct types of cells are present: reticulum or lymphoblast-like cells (*arrowhead*) and plasmacytoid cells (*arrow*). (H&E × 200.)

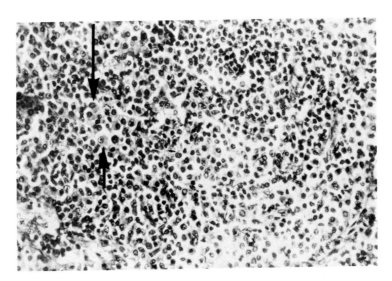

Fig. 18. Mesenteric lymph node biopsy (same case as in Figure 17). "Plasmacytoid" lymphoma. Note the diffuse tumor infiltrate with plasmacytoid cells (*arrows*). (H&E × 200.)

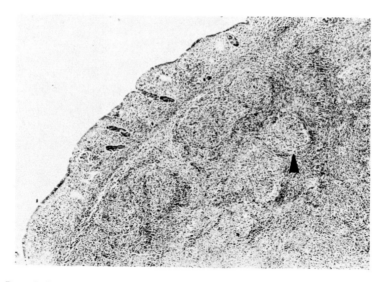

Fig. 19. Resected small bowel. Reticulum cell sarcoma, focally follicular. Near-total destruction of the bowel mucosa by lymphoma. Note the follicular arrangement of tumor (*arrowhead*). (H&E × 10.)

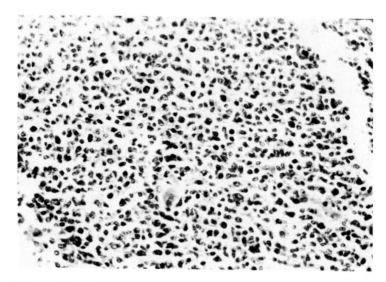

Fig. 20. Resected small bowel (same specimen as in Figure 19). Reticulum cell sarcoma, focally follicular. Detail of tumor cells within follicles. Note the nearly homogeneous cell population and absence of phagocytosis in contradistinction to reactive follicles. (H&E × 100.)

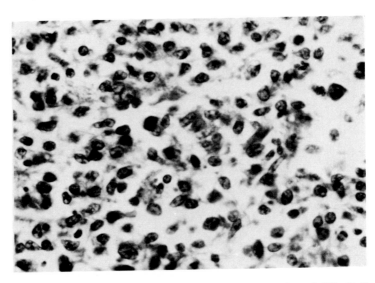

Fig. 21. Resected small bowel (same specimen as in Figures 19 and 20). Reticulum cell sarcoma, focally follicular. Higher magnification of tumor cells in the bowel wall. (H&E × 200.)

Findings in Open Bowel Biopsy-Resection Specimens

There was complete agreement as regards the histologic type of lymphoma between the positive peroral biopsies and the subsequent laparotomy. However, in the open biopsy-resection specimens (Figs. 17–21) some variation in the histology of the neoplasm was at times observed in different portions of the same specimen. In this series reticulum cell sarcoma outnumbered lymphosarcoma. Plasmacytoid differentiation was again seen on occasion. Two of the lymphosarcomas and one reticulum cell sarcoma displayed focal areas of follicular arrangement of the tumor cells. In the entire series of PUSIL under study, Hodgkin's disease was diagnosed only once and this was on a mesenteric lymph node only (Fig. 22).

In this group the lymphoma diagnosis was obvious on histologic examination. Tumor infiltration was often transmural. The changes described under "abnormal peroral biopsies" were almost invariably present in the areas of the gut immediately adjacent to the tumor. Sections of the small bowel distant from the tumor area were not available in most instances. Dutz et al.[28] have described flat mucosa as a very frequent finding in the necropsy material of the cases they considered primary small intestinal lymphoma.

Findings in the Mesenteric Lymph Nodes

In a majority of instances the resected mesenteric lymph nodes revealed lymphoma of the same variety as in the small bowel (Figs. 22–24). Other mesen-

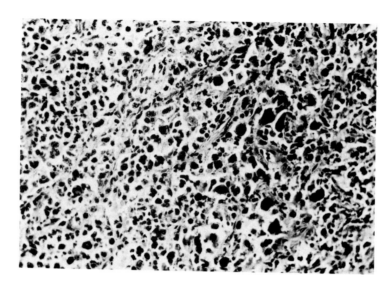

Fig. 22. Mesenteric lymph node biopsy. Hodgkin's disease. No histology is available from the bowel wall. However, multiple constrictive lesions of the small bowel were present at laparotomy. (H&E × 63.)

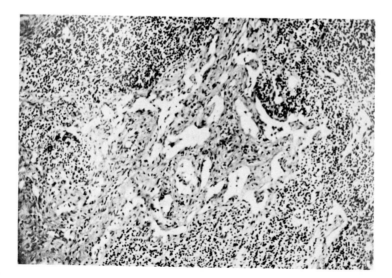

Fig. 23. Mesenteric lymph node biopsy. Marked vascular proliferation, probably a response to long-standing mechanical obstruction produced by tumor. (H&E × 40.)

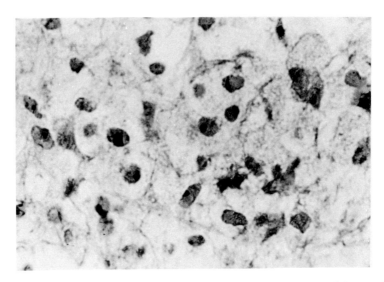

Fig. 24. Mesenteric lymph node biopsy (same biopsy as in Figure 23). High magnification of the lipophages accumulated in the same lymph node. (H&E × 320.)

teric lymph nodes showed varying degrees of follicular or sinus histiocytic hyperplasia. The hyperplasia was at times atypical, the lymph nodes containing variable number of large cells morphologically resembling "transformed lymphocytes" such as those found in lymph nodes responding to antigenic challenge. Thus far, however, we have not been able to find cases described by Robb-Smith [81] as "fibrillary histiocytic medullary reticulosis" and by Whitehead [112] as "steatorrhea lymphadenopathy."

In occasional cases, there was a remarkable vascular proliferation in the mesenteric lymph nodes quite similar to that described in lymph nodes in other locations as a response to obstruction. In certain instances (Fig. 24) many lipid-laden macrophages were seen within such lymph nodes.[39, 84]

In summary, then, we accept only the findings diagnostic of lymphoma as proof for same. The "minimal changes" may be a reflection of similar changes in the general rural population, in the same manner as reported in the peroral small bowel biopsies of volunteers in some developing countries.[31, 40, 55, 57, 59] On the other hand, changes more than "minimal" are considered definitely abnormal but not diagnostic with our present criteria.

Staging of the PUSIL has been difficult from our study since it includes only the early cases involving solely the small intestine and possibly mesenteric nodes. We have encountered cases with lymphoma elsewhere but otherwise having this same upper small intestinal involvement, suggesting the possibility of progression of disease initially originating in the small intestine. Others have suggested a staging system from I to IV according to the extent of primary tumor, presence of regional or distant nodes, invasion of adjacent abdominal viscera, and distant metastases.[28, 68] Considering the clinical difficulties of definitely delineating the extent of the small intestinal disease and mesenteric node involvement, we prefer a simple and clinically practical staging which, with our presently available therapeutic regimens, is clinically helpful:

Stage I. Lymphoma solely involving the small intestine and possibly the mesenteric nodes.

Stage II. Lymphoma also involving other intraabdominal organs.

Stage III. Lymphoma present distally and outside the abdomen.

Special Features

Malabsorption

Diarrhea and steatorrhea have been recorded as frequently associated with PUSIL.[31, 42, 77, 86] The steatorrhea is at least partially antibiotic responsive suggesting bacterial overgrowth or an abnormal bacterial population.[42] An associated xylose and vitamin B_{12} malabsorption may also be explained by these intestinal bacterial changes though the villous atrophy noted in the biopsies may be an important contributing facor. The most reasonable explanation for these intestinal bacterial changes remains alteration in the upper small intestinal motility leading to a stasis syndrome phenomenon. An alternate explanation may be an abnormal immunologic milieu of the upper small intestine promoting an altered bacterial population.[4, 12, 18-20, 27, 49, 74] This malabsorption is a rare finding in other small intestinal lymphomas, i.e., those not involving the upper small intestine.[25, 31, 98, 99] An exception to this may be the small intestinal lymphoma complicating gluten enteropathy.[5, 9, 29, 31, 38, 41, 98, 111]

Heavy Chain Disease

Normally the plasma cells in the lamina propria of the small intestine are engaged in the synthesis of IgA (80 percent), IgM (15 percent), IgG (less than 5 percent), IgD, and IgE.[19, 21, 43, 44, 93, 104] In 1968 Seligmann et al.[87] described a young Syrian woman with primary small intestinal lymphoma whose intestinal tumor infiltrate was of the "plasmacytoid" variety associated with an abnormal protein in the patient's serum, urine, and saliva. This protein was further characterized as an alpha-1 heavy chain, related to the Fc fragment.[76, 87] Subsequent reports have confirmed this finding and shown it also to be present in the jejunal fluid.[88-90] Reports from geographic areas with PUSIL have confirmed the coexistence of this heavy chain disease in some of the patients.[1, 10, 72, 78, 79, 90, 91]

Etiology

The etiology of this lymphoma remains to be determined. The two noteworthy features appear to be its geographic distribution and the susceptible population. By far, most of the PUSIL cases have been reported from the Middle East,[31, 69, 77] some from South Africa,[72] and more recently, a few from Italy.[10] This geographic distribution was initially emphasized by the term "Mediterranean" lymphoma [76, 86] which, considering the reports from other areas, does not appear to be presently fitting.

Still, this geographic distribution probably represents environmental factors. It also defines the susceptible population. But, this susceptibility is not simply that of moving from a no-PUSIL area to a PUSIL one. The same applies to immigration of genetically similar populations.[31, 77] All of this has suggested an exposure very early in life to environmental factors promoting PUSIL formation. Our few cases of familial lymphoma can be confirmatory to this hypothesis though genetic susceptibility cannot be excluded definitely.[8] Confirming the predisposition hypothesis are reports relating to patients with celiac disease eventually developing an intestinal lymphoma.[11, 38, 41]

Perhaps the flat villi noted in PUSIL cases adjacent to lymphomatous tissue are an indication of an earlier intestinal injury.[28] Biopsies in apparently normal villagers from our area [40] and necropsies on dying infants with diarrhea and marasmus from the same population [23] do show structural abnormalities by Western standards. Reasons for these structural abnormalities and their predisposition to lymphoma later in life are, of course, speculative. This structural abnormality, even if etiologically significant, does not exclude the possible importance of other factors that may occur later in life. In our population the low intake of protein, especially animal protein, and a marginal malnutrition may also promote cancer formation in presence of other "carcinogens." [59, 94]

Therapy

Reported cases, including our own, have been too few to comment definitely on the proper therapeutic program.[67] Surgical resection does not appear possible, especially since the extent of the intestinal involvement is presently impossible to define. Still, if there is clear-cut segmental disease or a complication such as perforation or obstruction, resection may be ameliorating or even "curative." X-ray therapy,[67] chemotherapy including use of cyclophosphamide, corticosteroids, antimicrobial therapy, and vitamin B_{12} or K, as need be, have been employed according to the individual case requirements.[73]

Conclusion

Primary small intestinal lymphoma, though relatively uncommon, has a worldwide prevalence which geographically differs primarily in its segment of involvement. Thus primary upper small intestinal lymphoma (PUSIL), involving the duodenum and upper jejunum, is becoming a clearly recognizable disease with a distinct geographic distribution. It is common in the Middle East and very rare in Northern Europe and the United States. Its clinical features are nonspecific though they suggest an intraabdominal disease. Clubbing and osteoarthropathy are frequent. Special features of this lymphoma are steatorrhea, which is at least partly antibiotic responsive, and an abnormal protein best described as an alpha heavy chain. The importance of peroral biopsy in the diagnosis of this entity is emphasized. The etiology of PUSIL is not clear, though being in the PUSIL area at a susceptible time (early life) seems to be a prerequisite.

Acknowledgements

We wish to acknowledge the assistance of Mr. John T. Flannery, Tumor Registry Supervisor, State of Connecticut, State Department of Health, for making the unpublished data on small bowel lymphomas in the Connecticut Tumor Registry available to us; Mr. H. Shurangiz and Mrs. E. Rafailzadeh for technical assistance; Miss N. Ghazi and Z. Naziri for photographs; Mrs. L. Banisadre, Miss P. Ghazi, and H. Kohanim for secretarial assistance; and Dr. Mohallatee, Associate Professor of Pathology, for permission to use the material of Nemazee Hospital.

References

1. Aia, F. A., and Khodadoust, J. Alpha chain disease in Iran. Third Pahlavi Medical Congress, Shiraz, Iran, April 1972.
2. Al-Khateeb, A. K. Primary malignant lymphoma of the small intestine. Int Surg 54:295, 1970.
3. Armine, K. Frequence, images histologiques et formes atypiques de la lympho-granulomatose maligne en Iran. (Extract) Rev Med Moyen Orient 24(2):97, 1967.
4. Asquith, P., Thompson, R. A., and Cooke, W. T. Serum immunoglobulins in adult celiac disease. Lancet 2:129, 1961.
5. Austad, W. I., Cornes, J. S., Gough, K. R., McCarthy, C. F., and Read, A. E. Steatorrhea and malignant lymphoma. The relationship of malignant tumors of lymphoid tissue and celiac disease. Am J Dig Dis 12:475, 1967.
6. Azzopardi, J. G., and Menzies, T. Primary malignant lymphoma of the alimentary tract. Br J Surg 47:358, 1960.
7. Baker, S. J. Tropical sprue. Br Med Bull 28:87, 1972.
8. Banihashemi, A., and Nasr, K. Familial lymphoma. In press.
9. Benson, G. D., Kowlessar, O. D., and Sleisenger, M. H. Adult celiac disease with emphasis upon response to the gluten-free diet. Medicine (Baltimore) 43:1, 1964.
10. Bonomo, L., Dammacco, F., Marano, R., and Bonomo, G. M. Abdominal lymphoma and alpha chain disease. Report of three cases. Am J Med 52:73, 1972.
11. Brunt, P. W., Sircus, W., and Maclean, N. Neoplasia and the celiac syndrome in adults. Lancet 1:180, 1969.
12. Bull, D. M., and Tomasi, T. Deficiency of immunoglobulin A in intestinal disease. Gastroenterology 54:313, 1968.
13. Burman, S. O., and VanWyk, F. A. K. Lymphoma of the small intestine and cecum. Ann Surg 143:349, 1955.
14. Bush, R. S., and Ash, C. L. Primary lymphoma of the grastrointestinal tract. Radiology 92:1349, 1969.
15. Charache, H. Lymphosarcoma in infancy and childhood including a case of twenty-two years' duration. Am J Roentgenol Radium Ther Nucl Med 76:594, 1956.
16. Ciba Foundation Monograph Series. Intestinal Biopsy. Wolstenholme, G. E. W., and Cameron, M. D., eds. London, Churchill, 1962.
17. Cornes, J. S. Multiple lymphomatous polyposis of the gastrointestinal tract. Cancer 14:249, 1961.
18. Crabbe, P. A., and Heremans, J. F. Lack of gamma-A immunoglobulin in serum of patients with steatorrhoea. Gut 7:119, 1966.
19. Crabbe, P. A. Significance du Tissue Lymphoide des Muqueuses Digestives. Brussels, Arscia & Paris, Maloine, 1967.

20. Crabbe, P. A., and Heremans, J. F. Selective IgA deficiency with steatorrhea. Am J Med 42:319, 1967.
21. Crabbe, P. A., and Heremans, J. F. Normal and defective production of immunoglobulins in the intestinal tract. In Modern Problems in Pediatrics. Basel and New York, Karger, 1968, Vol. 11, pp. 161–181.
22. Crabbe. P. A. The lymphoid tissue of the gastrointestinal mucosa and its possible clinical significance. In Glass, G. B. J., ed. Progress in Gastroenterology. New York, Grune and Stratton, 1970, Vol. 2, pp. 1–12.
23. Creamer, B., Dutz, W., and Post, C. Small intestinal lesion of chronic diarrhea and marasmus in Iran. Lancet 1:18, 1970.
24. Cupps, R. E., Hodgson, J., Dockerty, M. B., and Adson, M. Primary lymphoma in the small intestine: Problems of roentgenologic diagnosis. Radiology 92:1355, 1969.
25. Cutler, G. D., Stark, R. B., and Scott, H. W. Lymphosarcoma of the bowel in childhood. N Engl J Med 232:665, 1945.
26. Dawson, I. M. P., Cornes, J. S., and Morson, B. C. Primary malignant lymphoid tumors of the intestinal tract. Report of 37 cases with a study of factors influencing prognosis. Br J Surg 49:80, 1961.
27. Douglas, A., Crabbe, P. A., and Hobbs, J. R. Immunocytochemical studies of the serum, intestinal secretions and intestinal mucosa in patients with adult celiac disease and other forms of the sprue syndrome. Gastroenterology 59:414, 1970.
28. Dutz, W., Asvadi, S., Sadri, S. and Kohout, E. Intestinal lymphoma and sprue: A systematic approach. Gut 12:804, 1971.
29. Eakins, D., Fulton, T. and Hadden, D. R. Reticulum cell sarcoma of the small bowel and steatorrhoea. Gut 5:315, 1964.
30. Ehrlich, A. N., Stalder, G., Geller, W., and Sherlock, P. Gastrointestinal manifestations of malignant lymphoma. Gastroenterology 54:1115, 1968.
31. Eidelman, S., Parkins, R. A., and Rubin, C. E. Abdominal lymphoma presenting as malabsorption: A clinico-pathologic study of nine cases in Israel and a review of the literature. Medicine (Baltimore) 45:111, 1966.
32. Fairley, N. H., and Mackie, F. P. The clinical and biochemical syndrome in lymphadenoma and allied diseases involving the mesenteric lymph glands. Br Med J, 1:375, 1937.
33. Faulkner, J. W., and Dockerty, M. B. Lymphosarcoma of the small intestine. Surg Gynecol Obstet 95:76, 1952.
34. Fu, Y., and Perzin, K. H. Lymphosarcoma of the small intestine: A clinico-pathologic study. Cancer 29:645, 1972.
35. Gall, E. A., and Mallory, T. B. Malignant lymphoma: A clinico-pathologic survey of 618 cases. Am J Pathol 18:381, 1942.
36. Golden, R. Small intestine and diarrhea. Am J Roentgenol Radium Ther Nucl Med 36:892, 1936.
37. Good, A. Tumors of the small intestine. Am J Roentgenol Radium Ther Nucl Med 89:685, 1963.
38. Gough, K. R., Read, A. E., and Naish, J. M. Intestinal reticulosis as a complication of idiopathic steatorrhoea. Gut 3:232, 1962.
39. Gull, W. Fatty stools from disease of the mesenteric glands. Guys Hosp Rep 1:369, 1855.
40. Haghighi, P., and Nasr, K. Histology of peroral small intestinal biopsies in apparently normal villagers of Southern Iran. In press.
41. Harris, O. D., Cooke, W. T., Thompson, H., and Waterhouse, J. A. H. Malignancy in adult celiac disease and idiopathic steatorrhea. Am J. Med 42:899, 1967.
42. Hedayati, H., Lahimgarzadeh, A., Bakhshandeh, K., Dehghan, R., Reinhold, J. G., and Nasr, K. Steatorrhea in primary upper small intestinal lymphoma. Abstr. Third Pahlavi Medical Congress, Shiraz, Iran, 1972, p. 125.

43. Heremans, J. F., and Crabbe, P. A. IgA deficiency: General considerations and relation to human disease. In Bergsma, D., ed. Immunologic Deficiency Diseases in Man. Birth Defects, Original Article Series. New York, National Foundation-March of Dimes, 1968, Vol. 4, pp. 298–310.

44. Heremans, J. F. Immunoglobulin formation and function in different tissues. Curr Top Microbiol Immunol 45:131, 1968.

45. Hermans, P. E., Huizenga, K. A., Hoffman, H. N., Brown, A. L., and Markowitz, H. Dysgammaglobulinemia associated with nodular lymphoid hyperplasia of the small intestine. Am J Med 40:78, 1966.

46. Hermans, P. E. Nodular lymphoid hyperplasia of the small intestine and hypogammaglobulinemia: Theoretical and practical considerations. Fed Proc 26:1606, 1967.

47. Hourihane, D. O'B. The histology of intestinal biopsies. Proc R Soc Med 56:1073, 1963.

48. Hourihane, D. O'B. The pathology of malabsorption states. In Harrison, C. V., ed. Recent Advances in Pathology, 8th ed. London, Churchill, 1966, pp. 320–345.

49. Huizenga, K., Wollaeger, E. E., Green, P. A., and McKenzie, B. F. Serum globulin deficiencies in nontropical sprue with report of two cases of acquired agammaglobulinemia. Am J Med 31:572, 1961.

50. Hulu, N., Ramot, B., and Sheehan, W. Childhood abdominal lymphoma in Israel. Isr J Med Sci 6:246, 1970.

51. Irvine, W. T., and Johnstone, J. M. Lymphosarcoma of the small intestine with special reference to perforating tumours. Br J Surg 42:611, 1955.

52. Jenkin, R. D. T., Sonley, M. J., Stephens, C. A., Darte, J. M. M., and Peters, M. V. Primary gastrointestinal lymphoma in childhood. Radiology 92:763, 1969.

53. Jinich, H., Rojas, E., Webb, J., and Kelsey, J. R. Lymphoma presenting as malabsorption. Gastroenterology 54:421, 1968.

54. Kent, T. H. Malabsorption syndrome with malignant lymphoma. Arch Pathol 78:97, 1964.

55. Kent, T. H., and Lindenbaum, J. Correlation of jejunal function and morphology in patients with acute and chronic diarrhea in East Pakistan. Gastroenterology 52:972, 1967.

56. Lasch, E. E., Ramot, B., and Neumann, G. Childhood celiac disease in Israel. Isr J Med Sci 4:1260, 1968.

57. Lindenbaum, J., Alam, A. K. J., and Kent, T. H. Subclinical small intestinal disease in East Pakistan. Br Med J 2:1616, 1966.

58. Lindenbaum, J., Kent, T. H., and Sprinz, H. Malabsorption and jejunitis in American Peace Corps volunteers in Pakistan. Ann Intern Med 65:1201, 1966.

59. Lindenbaum, J. Small intestine dysfunction in Pakistanis and Americans resident in Pakistan. Am J Clin Nutr, 21:1023, 1968.

60. Loehr, W. J., Mujahed, Z., Zahn, F. D., Gray, G. F., and Thorbjarnarson, B. Primary lymphoma of the gastrointestinal tract: A review of 100 cases. Ann Surg 170:232, 1969.

61. Maclean, N. The pathology of malignant lymphomas of the alimentary tract. In Goslings, W. R. O., ed. Diseases of the Gastrointestinal Tract. Leiden, Leiden Univ. Press, 1970, pp. 82–90.

62. Madhavan, M., Chandra, K., and Balassoubramaniane, R. Lymphomas of gastrointestinal tract (a study of 18 cases). Indian J Cancer 00:115, 1971.

63. Marcuse, P. M., and Stout, A. P. Primary lymphosarcoma of the small intestine. Analysis of thirteen cases and review of the literature. Cancer 3:459, 1950.

64. McCarthy, C. F., Fraser, I. D., Evans, K. T., and Read, A. E. Lymphoreticular dysfunction in idiopathic steatorrhoea. Gut 7:140, 1966.

65. Mestel, A. L. Lymphosarcoma of the small intestine in infancy and childhood. Ann Surg 149:87, 1959.

66. Modan, B., Goldman, B., Shani, M., Meytes, D., Mitchell, B. Epidemiological aspects of neoplastic disease in Israeli migrant population. V. The lymphomas. J. Natl. Cancer Inst., 42:375, 1969.
67. Mortazavi, S. H., Dehghan, R., Haghighi, P., and Sepehri, B. Primary small intestinal lymphoma in Southern Iran. In press.
68. Naqvi, M. S., Burrows, L., and Kark, A. E. Lymphomas of the gastrointestinal tract. Prognostic guides based on 162 cases. Ann Surg 170:221, 1969.
69. Nasr, K., Haghighi, P., Bakhshandeh, K., and Haghshenas, M. Primary lymphoma of the upper small intestine. Gut 11:673, 1970.
70. Nasr, K., Bakhshandeh, K., Haghighi, P., and Haghshenas, M. Clubbing and osteoarthropathy associated with primary upper small intestinal lymphoma. J Trop Med Hyg 74:117, 1971.
71. Nasr, K. Personal communication.
72. Novis, B. H., Bank, S., Marks, I. N., Selzer, G., Kahn, L., and Sealy, R. Abdominal lymphoma presenting with malabsorption. Q J Med 40:521, 1971.
73. Pack, G. T., and Ariel, I. M., eds. Treatment of Cancer and Allied Diseases. IX. Lymphomas and Related Diseases, 2nd ed. New York, Hoeber Medical Division, Harper & Row, 1964, Vol. 9, pp. 155–156.
74. Pellkonen, R., Siurala, M., and Vuopio, P. Inherited agammaglobulinemia with malabsorption and marked alterations in the gastrointestinal mucosa. Acta Med Scand 173:549, 1963.
75. Perzin, K. H. Personal communication.
76. Rambaud, J. C., Bognel, C., Prost, A., Bernier, J. J., Quintrec, Y., Lambling, A., Danon, F., Hurez, D., and Seligmann, M. Clinicopathological study of a patient with "Mediterranean" type of abdominal lymphoma and a new type of IgA abnormality (alpha chain disease). Digestion 1:321, 1968.
77. Ramot, B., Shahin, N., and Bubis, J. J. Malabsorption syndrome in lymphoma of small intestine. A study of 13 cases. Isr J Med Sci 1:221, 1965.
78. Ramot, B. Malabsorption due to lymphomatous disease. Ann Rev Med 22:19, 1971.
79. Ramot, B. The relationship between intestinal lymphoma and heavy chain of IgA. Abstr. Third Pahlavi Medical Congress, Shiraz, Iran, 1972, p. 100.
80. Read, A. E. Malignancy and Steatorrhea. In Modern Problems in Pediatrics. Basel and New York, Karger, 1968, vol. 11, pp. 182–190.
81. Robb-Smith, A. H. T. The classification and natural history of lymphadenopathies. In Pack, G. T., and Ariel, I. M., eds. Treatment of Cancer and Allied Diseases. IX. Lymphomas and Related Diseases, 2nd ed. New York, Hoeber Medical Division, Harper & Row, 1964, Vol. 9.
82. Rosenberg, S. A., Diamond, H. D., Jaslowitz, B., and Craver, L. F. Lymphosarcoma: A review of 1269 cases. Medicine (Baltimore) 40:31, 1961.
83. Rubin, C. E., and Dobbins, W. O. Peroral biopsy of the small intestine. Gastroenterology 49:676, 1965.
84. Rubin, C. E., Eidelman, S., and Weinstein, W. M. Sprue by any other name. Gastroenterology 58:409, 1970.
85. Sacks, M. I., and Seijffers, M. J. Clinico-pathological conference. Isr J Med Sci 4:164, 1968.
86. Seijffers, M. J., Levy, M., and Hermann, G. Intractable watery diarrhea, hypokalemia and malabsorption in a patient with Mediterranean type of abdominal lymphoma. Gastroenterology 55:118, 1968.
87. Seligmann, M., Danon, F., Jurez, D., Mihaesco, E., and Preud'homme, J. L. Alpha chain disease: A new immunoglobulin abnormality. Science 162:1396, 1968.
88. Seligmann, M., Mihaesco, E., Hurez, D., Mihaesco, C., Preud'homme, J. L., and Rambaud, J. C. Immunochemical studies in four cases of alpha chain disease. J. Clin Invest 48:2374, 1969.

89. Seligmann, M., and Rambaud, J. C. IgA abnormalities in abdominal lymphoma (alpha-chain disease). Isr J Med Sci 5:151, 1969.
90. Seligmann, M., Mihaesco, E., and Frangione, B. Studies on alpha chain disease. Ann NY Acad Sci 190:487, 1971.
91. Seligmann, M. Personal communication.
92. Shani, M., Modan, B., Goldman, B., Branstaeter, S., and Ramot, B. Primary gastrointestinal lymphoma. Isr J Med Sci 5:1173, 1969.
93. Sherlock, P., Winawer, S., Goldstein, M., and Bragg, D. G. Malignant lymphoma of the gastro-intestinal tract. In Progress in Gastroenterology. New York, Grune and Stratton, 1970, Vol. 2, pp. 367–391.
94. Shiner, M. The dynamic morphology of the normal and abnormal small intestinal mucosa of man. In Modern Problems in Pediatrics. Basel and New York, Karger, 1968, Vol. 11, pp. 5–21.
95. Shiner, M. The histology of the small intestine: The relation of crypts to villi in the normal jejunal mucosa and in the abnormal histological appearances of steatorrhoea. In Girdwood, R. H., and Smith, A. N., eds. Malabsorption. Edinburgh, Edinburgh University Press, 1969, pp. 134–147.
96. Sircus, W., Brunt, P. W., Maclean, N. Neoplasia of the small intestine: Villous structure and malabsorption. In Girdwood, R. H., and Smith, A. N., eds. Malabsorption. Edinburgh, Edinburgh University Press, 1969, pp. 260–268.
97. Skrimshire, J. F. P. Lymphoma of the stomach and intestine. Q J Med 24:203, 1955.
98. Sleisenger, M. H., Almy, T. P., and Barr, D. P. The sprue syndrome secondary to lymphoma of the small bowel. Am J Med 15:666, 1953.
99. Spence, J. E., and Ritchie, S. Lymphomas of small bowel and their relationship to idiopathic steatorrhea. S Can J Surg 12:207, 1969.
100. Sperling, L. Malignant lymphoma of the gastrointestinal tract. Prog Clin Cancer 2:338, 1966.
101. Sprinz, H., Scribhibhadh, R., Gargarosa, E. J., Benyajati, C., Kundel, D., and Halstead, S. Biopsy of small bowel of Thai people with special reference to recovery from Asiatic cholera and to an intestinal malabsorption syndrome. Am J Clin Pathol 38:43, 1962.
102. Swanson, V. L., and Thomassen, R. W. Pathology of the jejunal mucosa in tropical sprue. Am J Pathol 46:511, 1965.
103. Talvalkar, G. V. Primary malignant lymphoma of the small and large intestines. Indian J Cancer 5:238, 1968.
104. Tomasi, T. B., and Czervinski, D. S. The secretory IgA system. In Bergsma, D., ed. Birth Defects, Original Article Series. New York, National Foundation— March of Dimes, 1968, Vol. 4, pp. 270–282.
105. Ulmann, A., and Abeshouse, B. S. Lymphosarcoma of the small and large intestines. Ann Surg 95:878, 1932.
106. Valdes-Dapena, A. M., and Stein, G. N., eds. Morphologic Pathology of the Alimentary Canal. Philadelphia, Saunders, 1970.
107. Watson, D. W. Immune responses and the gut. Gastroenterology 56:944, 1969.
108. Weaver, D. K., and Batsakis, J. G. Primary lymphomas of the small intestine. Am J Gastroenterology 42:620, 1964.
109. Weaver, D. K., and Batsakis, J. G. Pseudolymphomas of small intestine. Am J Gastroenterology 44:374, 1965.
110. Welborn, K., Rebuck, J. W., and Ponka, J. Intestinal lymphosarcoma. Arch Surg 94:717, 1967.
111. Weser, E., and Sleisenger, M. H. Pathophysiology of sprue syndromes. Adv Intern Med 15:253, 1969.
112. Whitehead, R. Primary lymphadenopathy complicating idiopathic steatorrhoea. Gut 9:569, 1968.
113. Wood, D. A. Tumors of the Intestines. Armed Forces Institute of Pathology. 1967, Series VI, Fascicle 22, pp. 96–100.

Addendum

Little has been added to our understanding of primary upper small intestinal lymphoma (PUSIL) since our 1973 review of the subject. We continue not to know much about its etiology or proper management. Advancement in our knowledge relating to this disease over the past few years has predominantly included its pathology, geographic distribution, and the associated immunologic abnormalities.[1-12]

Pathologically, it is becoming apparent that the plasma cell infiltrate, usually with a benign cytologic character, is a prominent accompaniment of PUSIL (Fig. 1).[6, 9-11] It has even been postulated that the plasmacytosis and alpha-chain disease may be precursors to the later development of PUSIL.[6, 10, 13, 14] This hypothesis is attractive in that it suggests an early-in-life antigenic stimulation of the small intestinal mucosa followed by a benign plasmacytic infiltration that later becomes malignant and, in so doing, either retains the plasma cell appearance[7, 14] or transforms into other type of lymphoma (histiocytic type in particular) through a monoclonal[10, 15] or a biclonal[7, 11, 13] evolution of neoplasia (Fig. 2). However, the antigenic stimulus thus far has not been clearly defined, although protozoal,[16] helminthic, bacterial, and viral[14] antigens have been suggested.

The geographic distribution of PUSIL with or without alpha-chain disease includes cases from areas characterized by poor hygienic conditions and a high frequency of intestinal infections.[1-4, 6-8, 10-12] The presence of PUSIL/alpha-chain disease in the Middle East and the Mediterranean region now appears well established.[8, 9] Reports of the disease occurring in patients of North African,[7, 8, 13, 17] South African,[5, 6] South American,[11] and Southeast Asian origin are becoming more numerous but not sufficiently so for the making of a disease map.[18, 19] We are not aware of reports from Europe (except for some regions of the Mediterranean basin such as Southern Italy, Southern Spain, and Greece)[3] or North America at this time save for two cases of alpha-chain disease, apparently of the respiratory tract, from the Netherlands[20] and New England.[12]

Remissions, at times prolonged, have been recorded in patients with alpha-chain disease treated with antibiotics alone[21, 22] or in combination with steroids and cytotoxic agents.[3, 6, 19, 23] No controlled study, however, is available to determine the optimal therapy.

The immunoglobulin in alpha-chain disease is now identified as an electrophoretically heterogeneous,[11] carbohydrate-rich,[24, 25] monoclonal (ie, alpha-1 subclass)[11, 12, 24] portion of the alpha-heavy chain, approximately two-thirds to three-quarters the length of the normal alpha chain,[25-27] containing the Fc and a portion of the Fd fragment[26, 28] with the missing part of the latter involving the V and the C1 regions.[11, 13] It is further characterized by the variable length of the polypeptide chain from patient to patient and the high affinity for polymerization.[11] It is synthesized by the plasma cell infiltrate within the small bowel wall and the mesenteric lymph nodes,[3, 26, 28] and may be detected by immunofluorescence in the plasma cell infiltrate within and outside the small bowel–mesenteric

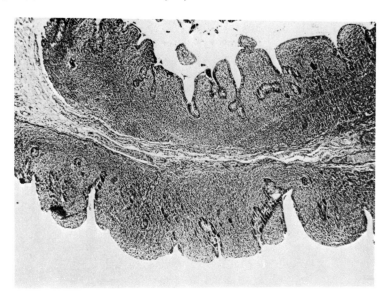

Fig. 1. Alpha-chain disease: low-power photomicrograph of open biopsy of the small intestine. Diffuse infiltrate involving the lamina propria. H&E. × 10.

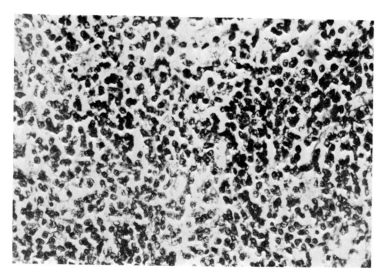

Fig. 2. Alpha-chain disease. Higher magnification of the infiltrate in the lamina propria of the small intestine. This might be classified as histiocytic lymphoma. H&E. × 100.

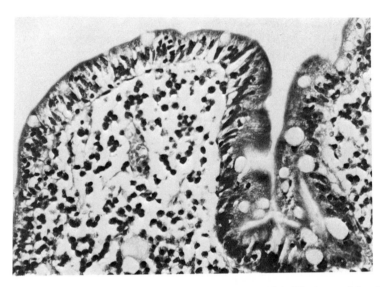

Fig. 3. Alpha-chain disease. Rather dense mature plasma cell infiltrate overlying the tumor infiltrate depicted in Figures 1 and 2 and not shown here. The surface epithelium is abnormal and shows loss of nuclear polarity of the epithelial cells plus transepithelial lymphocytic migration. H&E. × 100.

node complex.[18] An internal deletion within the heavy chain molecule followed by a limited intracellular postribosomal proteolysis of same has been proposed.[11, 27, 28] Morphologic criteria of the malignant nature of the plasma cell infiltrate at the cell level have not always been fulfilled (Fig. 3).[3, 6, 7, 29, 30]

Extraintestinal spread of the plasma cell infiltrate in cases of alpha-chain disease has now been documented. This includes spread to the rectum,[13, 23] stomach,[14] portal spaces,[14] bone marrow, and blood.[3]

Alpha-chain disease has been the most frequently reported of the heavy chain diseases to date.[26] One case of a young Polish man of Middle Eastern descent with diffuse nodular "early" lymphoma of the gastrointestinal tract associated with an IgG3 kappa type monoclonal gammapathy has recently been described.[31] The exact place of this single case within the PUSIL group is at present not clear.

Finally, alterations in the level of the serum IgA among relatives of alpha-chain disease patients and those with PUSIL,[5, 7, 10] raised serum levels of the intestinal alkaline phosphatase isoenzymes in patients with PUSIL/alpha-chain disease and in the relatives of PUSIL cases [3, 14] and a subnormal delayed hypersensitivity in a case of alpha-chain disease [13] are among the intriguing recent findings in this disease complex and are in need of further study.[32, 33]

References

1. Al-Bahrani ZR, Bakir F: Primary intestinal lymphoma: a challenging problem in abdominal pain. Ann R Coll Surg Engl 49:103, 1971

2. Al-Saleem T, Al-Bahrani Z: Malignant lymphoma of the small intestine in Iraq (Middle East lymphoma). Cancer 31:291, 1973
3. Doe WF, Henry K, Hobbs JR et al: Five cases of alpha-chain disease. Gut 13:947, 1972
4. Nasr K, Abadi P, Haghighi P, Rezai HR: Primary upper small intestinal lymphoma: two special features. Part II: Heavy chain disease. Abstracts Fifth Pahlavi Medical Congress April 1974, p 48
5. Novis BH, Bank S, Young G: Alpha-chain disease. Lancet II:498, 1973
6. Novis BH, Kahn LB, Bank S: Alpha-chain disease in Subsaharan Africa. Am J Dig Dis 18:679, 1973
7. Rambaud JC, Matuchansky C, Bognel JC, et al: Nouveau cas de maladie des chaines alpha chez un Eurasien. Ann Med Interne 121:135, 1970
8. Ramot B: Intestinal lymphoma with malabsorption in Mediterranean populations. Isr J Med Sci 7:1488, 1971
9. Ramot B, Many A: Primary intestinal lymphoma: clinical manifestations and possible effects of environmental factors. In Rentchnick P (ed): Recent Results in Cancer Research: Current Problems in the Epidemiology of Cancer and Lymphomas. Berlin, Springer-Verlag, 1972, pp 193–99
10. Rappaport H, Ramot B, Hulu N, Park JK: The pathology of so-called Mediterranean abdominal lymphoma with malabsorption. Cancer 29:1502, 1972
11. Seligmann M: Heavy chain diseases. Rev Eur Etudes Clin Biol 17:349, 1972
12. Seligmann M: Alpha-chain disease. Gastroenterology 63:914, 1972
13. Bognel JC, Rambaud JC, Modigliani R, et al: Etude clinique, anatomo-pathologique, et immunochimique d'un nouveau cas de maladie des chaines alpha suivi pendant cinq ans. Rev Eur Etudes Clin Biol 17:362, 1972
14. Rambaud JC, Matuchansky C: Alpha-chain disease: pathogenesis and relation to Mediterranean lymphoma. Lancet I:1430, 1973
15. Stein H, Lennert K, Parwaresch MR: Malignant lymphoma of the B-cell type. Lancet II:855, 1971
16. Henry K, Bird RG, Doe WF: Intestinal coccidiosis in a patient with alpha-chain disease. Br Med J 1:542, 1974
17. Irunberry J, Banllegue A, Illoul G, et al: Trois cas de maladie des chaines alpha observé en Algerie. Nouv Rev Fr Hematol 10:609, 1970
18. Bernadou A, Segond P, Bilski-Pasquier G, et al: La maladie des chaines lourdes alpha: à propos d'une observation. Nouv Rev Fr Hematol 12:333, 1972
19. Zlotnick A, Levy M: Alpha heavy chain disease: a variant of Mediterranean lymphoma. Arch Intern Med 128:432, 1971
20. Stoop JW, Ballieux RE, Hijmans W, Zegers BJM: Alpha-chain disease with involvement of the respiratory tract in a Dutch child. Clin Exp Immunol 9:625, 1971
21. Roge J, Druet P, Marche C: Lymphome mediterranéeen avec maladie des chaines alpha: triple remission clinique, anatomique et immunologique. Pathol Biol 18:851, 1970
22. Roge J: Lymphome mediterranéen avec maladie des chaines alpha. Effet d'une antibiotherapie continué pendant un an. Ann Med Interne 122:55, 1971
23. Laroche C, Seligmann M, Merillon H, et al: Nouvelle observation d'une maladie des chaines lourdes alpha. Presse Med 78:55, 1970
24. Dorrington KJ, Mihaesco E, Seligmann M: The molecular size of three alpha-chain disease proteins. Biochim Biophys Acta 221:647, 1970
25. Seligmann M: La maladie des chaines alpha. Acta Gastroentol Belg 33:841, 1970
26. Seligmann M: La maladie des chaines alpha. Presse Med 78:51, 1970
27. Wolfenstein-Todel C, Mihaesco E, Frangione B: Alpha-chain disease protein DEF: internal deletion of a human immunoglobulin A1 heavy chain. Proc Natl Acad Sc USA 71:974, 1974
28. Buxbaum J, Preud'homme JL: Alpha and gamma heavy chain diseases in man: intracellular origin of the aberrant polypeptides. J Immunol 109:1131, 1972

29. Pittman FE, Pittman JC: Ultrastructure of intestinal mucosa in alpha heavy chain disease. Gastroenterology 60:794, 1971
30. Scotto J, Stralin H, Caroli J: Ultrastructural study of two cases of alpha-chain disease. Gut 11:782, 1970
31. Kopec M, Swierczynska Z, Pazdur J, et al: Diffuse lymphoma of the intestine with a monoclonal gammaopathy of IgG3 kappa type. Am J Med 56:381, 1974
32. Lageron A, Theodoropoulos, Caroli J: La maladie des chaines lourdes alpha; étude histoenzymologique d'un cas. Nouv Presse Med 1:945, 1972
33. Laroche C, Merillon H, Turpin G: Le lymphome mediterranéeen. Presse Med 78:53, 1970

SCHISTOSOMIASIS:

A CLINICOPATHOLOGIC EVALUATION

VICTOR M. AREÁN

Schistosomiasis is a parasitic infection caused by the blood flukes, *Schistosoma mansoni, S. japonicum,* and *S. haematobium.* Although certain basic ecologic factors are necessary for the establishment of endemic foci, increased travel and migration of individuals have resulted in growing numbers of affected persons in areas where the disease was previously unknown. The large majority of infected individuals have mild or no symptoms related to this parasitosis; yet there is increasing evidence that it may play a major role in the lag of both physical and mental development of persons living in endemic areas.[27,60] In others, clinical syndromes of varying severity may appear which endanger life or cause death. The pathologic lesions responsible for the disease are chiefly related to the eggs released by the parasites in various tissues and organs. However, it is also apparent that ancillary factors, such as repeated exposures, poor diet and undernourishment, multiple parasitosis, and concomitant bacterial infections, are influential in the development of the disease.[3]

HISTORICAL. The first description of schistosomiasis is found in an Egyptian papyrus of about 1500 BC, as well as in Babylonian inscriptions. Proof that the disease existed at that time was given by Ruffer,[138] who identified schistosome eggs in tissues of mummies from the Twentieth Dynasty (1250–1000 BC). Later cases of the infection were observed among the French Army of occupation in Egypt (1799–1801). In Japan, the first description of Katayama disease or Oriental schistosomiasis was made by Fujii in 1847.[41]

The first identification of a schistosome parasitic for man was made by Bilharz,[20] who in 1851 recovered adult worms from the mesenteric veins of an Egyptian peasant and established its causal relationship with a chronic intestinal and urinary ailment, widespread among fellaheen since time immemorial and characterized by persistent hematuria and the passage with urine and feces of large quantities of eggs with a terminal spine (*S. haematobium*). Bilharz also observed in a female worm eggs with a lateral rather than terminal spine, but he failed to recognize the significance of this finding. Manson, in 1903, while examining fecal material of a patient from the West Indies who had never been to Africa, noted eggs with a lateral spine.[95] He stressed absence of eggs in the urine and suggested the existence of another species of schistosome that deposited eggs exclusively in the intestine, whereas *S. haematobium* deposited eggs both in the intestine and bladder. In 1904, Letulle [78] verified the existence of the infection in Martinique, and Gonzalez Martinez [49] found the parasite in Puerto Ricans. Soto, in 1906, observed it in Venezuelans.[145] Sambon [140] proposed for the new organism the name of *S. mansoni,* although at that time (1907) there were doubts regarding the existence of two different species. Pirajá da Silva,[24,120,121] who in 1904 had found eggs with lateral spines in the feces of patients from Bahia, Brazil, reported his observations on the morphologic characteristics of the adults and established their difference from those of *S. haematobium* (1909).

Fujinami, in 1904, observed adult worms in the portal vein of a patient from Japan and found eggs in the tissues to which he attributed the etiology of the lesions.[41] Katsurada (1904) encountered the parasite in man, dogs, and cats and named it *S. japonicum.*[41]

Cobbold,[29] in 1864, surmised from his field observations that the larvae of the parasite would be found in molluscs, a hypothesis confirmed in 1913 by Miyairi [41] (1913) for *S. japonicum* and in 1915 by Leiper [77] for *S. mansoni* and *S. haematobium.* Allen [2] was the first to call attention to the close relationship between bathing in polluted waters and the incidence of the disease. Fujinami and Nakamura,[41] in 1909, demonstrated the penetration of the cercaria through the skin of mammals and, in 1911, transmitted the disease to guinea pigs, white mice, and monkeys. Lutz [89] in a series of experiments (1915–1917) observed the complete cycle of the parasite by infecting snails (*Australorbis olivaceus*) and produced the disease in guinea pigs and rabbits.

GEOGRAPHIC DISTRIBUTION AND EPIDEMIOLOGY (FIG. 1). It is estimated that over 200 million people throughout the world are infected by schistosomes. The infection is spreading at an alarming pace because of the development of irrigation projects and the migration of infected populations into areas where ecologic conditions favorable for the completion of the parasite's life cycle prevail.[3,64,75] In Southern Rhodesia [156] a 10 million dollar irrigation project had to be abandoned within 10 years of its initiation for this reason. Deficient planning, substandard economies, and poor education contribute greatly to the persistence and dissemination of the disease. In certain areas of Africa the infection rate reaches 100 per cent of the population over 2 years of age.[3]

Schistosomiasis was introduced into the Americas by the African slaves.[119] It is prevalent in northeastern Brazil and other isolated foci, in the coastal region of Dutch Guiana and Venezuela, and in several Caribbean Islands. In Puerto Rico where there are numerous well-entrenched foci, the incidence of infection in the general population is 14 per cent. Koppisch [73] found this incidence in his autopsy cases, and the figure has not changed in recent years.[46] As the number of Puerto Ricans who have migrated to the United States is estimated to be over one million, it follows that at the present time there are over 140,000 individuals with schistosomiasis within the continental United States. The problem is of major importance

Figure I.　WORLD　DISTRIBUTION　OF　BILHARZIASIS

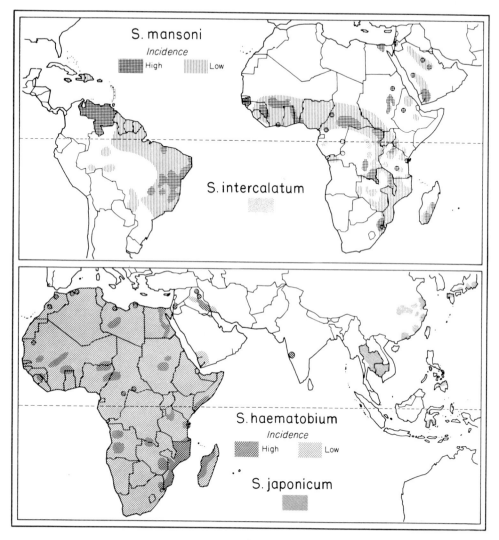

Fig. 1. World distribution of bilharziasis. (Courtesy of Dr. John Weir.)

in large cities (New York, Philadelphia, Chicago, Los Angeles) where most of the Puerto Ricans have established residence; however, with the trend to movement to smaller cities there is an increasing need for awareness of this infection. A considerable number of infections were acquired by American soldiers in the Philippines during World War II,[21] as well as among other persons working in endemic areas.[130]

Isolated cases of the disease, acquired while visiting endemic areas, have been reported.[101]

The infection is initiated in nonendemic areas and maintained in endemic ones when fecal matter or urine from infected subjects reaches bodies of fresh water where a suitable intermediary host lives. For *S. mansoni* the main reservoir of infection is man, although in highly endemic areas monkeys and wild rodents have been incriminated also. In Asia, the extensive use of night soil as fertilizer and the high rate of infection among domestic and wild animals as well as man perpetuate the infection and account for its spreading to areas where the host snails live.

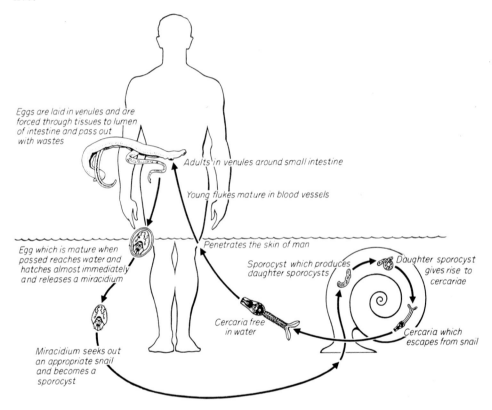

Fig. 2. Schistosoma life cycle. (Courtesy of Dr. John Weir.)

The disease is acquired while swimming, bathing, wading, working, or washing clothes and more rarely by drinking infected waters. The high temperature and humidity prevalent in endemic areas invite the population to seek relief from the oppressive climatic conditions in the waters of infested rivers. Children's common habit of urinating while swimming contributes to the perpetuation of *S. haematobium* infections. The disease is usually acquired in childhood and is more prevalent among males.

LIFE CYCLE AND MODE OF PENETRATION (FIG. 2). The fully mature eggs hatch

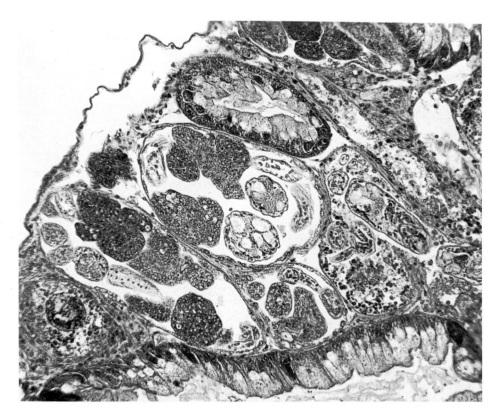

Fig. 3. Developing cercariae in tissues of a snail. H&E. × 325. (Section courtesy of Dr. G. W. Hunter, III.)

on reaching a body of water, and the embryo (miracidium) swims about freely until it dies or encounters a suitable snail intermediary host, varying with the species of schistosome and also with the geographic locations. For *S. japonicum* the snail host is *Oncomelania* sp.; for *S. mansoni,* either *Australorbis* sp. or *Tropicorbis* sp. in the Western Hemisphere or *Biomphalaria* sp. in Africa. *S. haematobium* parasitizes snails of the genus *Bulinus* (*Physopsis*). The miracidium upon entering the snail develops into a mother sporocyst which produces daughter sporocysts that migrate to the gonads and digestive glands of the mollusc and give rise to hundreds or thousands of cercariae (Fig. 3). The completion of the molluscan cycle requires from four to eight weeks. Once the cercariae have attained the infective stage they abandon the intermediary host and swim freely until they encounter a suitable definitive host. The fork-tailed cercariae (Fig. 4) measure from 100 to 250 microns in length and usually leave the snail when it is at or just below the water level.

Cercariae possess two pairs of large, anterior glands with coarsely granular acidophilic cytoplasm that stains with alizarine and is periodic acid-Schiff-negative (preacetabular glands) and three to four pairs of posteriorly located smaller glands with finely granular basophilic cytoplasm that stain intensely positive with PAS

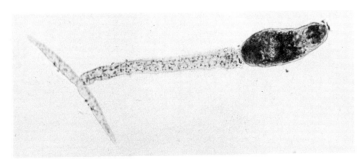

Fig. 4. Infective fork-tailed cercaria. × 325.

(postacetabular glands).[147,148] Two sets of ducts carry the glandular secretions into
the lumen of the oral sucker after they have pierced its musculature through hollow
spicules. Cercariae are phototropic so that infections are more likely to occur when
immersion of the host takes place during bright sunlight hours of the day. As the
cercaria contacts the skin of the vertebrate host it makes a number of contractile
movements causing it to bend ventrally and facilitating the application of the oral
sucker onto the skin surface. Muscular contractions squeeze out secretions from the
postacetabular glands. These appear at the site of the oral sucker and in the
adjacent epidermis as masses of intensely PAS-positive material (a lipomuco-
protein).[147] Apparently these secretions enhance the adherence of the parasite to the
epidermis and possibly limit the site of action of other lytic enzymes (Figs. 5 and
6). The parasites lose their tails and enter readily through the horny and malpighian
layers, destroying the squamous cells as they advance. They are called thenceforth
metacercariae or schistosomules. Before entering the dermis the parasite is temporarily detained by the basement membrane, which shortly thereafter disintegrates
focally allowing the cercariae to enter the papillary dermis. Lewert [79-81] has shown
this tissue alteration to be due to a collagenase-like substance secreted by the
parasite that causes depolymerization of the dermal ground substance with increase
in its water content and facilitates migration of the schistosomule. In man, the time
of penetration has been determined to be about one minute.[146]

Penetration of the parasite is felt by the patient within minutes or hours after
exposure as an intense itching, similar to pin pricks, which may last a few minutes
or several days. Occasionally there is an erythematous papular (urticariform) rash
with or without vesiculation.[152] The local inflammatory response is minimal or
absent and in most instances is caused by scratching rather than by direct action of
the parasite. Monkeys may show local pinpoint lesions and even pronounced edema;
guinea pigs given water containing cercariae will refuse more than the initial
drops.[94]

Once the cercaria has reached the papillary dermis it enters the venules and
lymphatics and disappears from the site, although in experimental animals schistosomules have been found at the site of inoculation four days after exposure. Some
may go to the regional lymph nodes, but most are carried by the blood stream to
the lungs. The pulmonary stage of the parasite is critical, for it appears that here

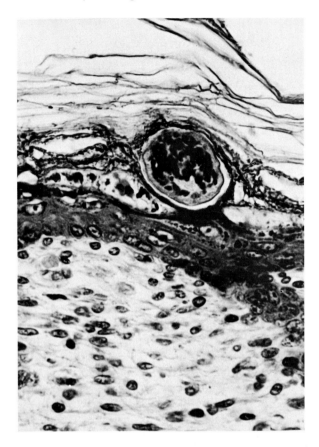

Fig. 5. Cercaria entering skin of mouse; note edema and degeneration of adjacent squamous cells. H&E. × 440.

the largest numbers are destroyed. Those which survive make their way into the left side of the heart, whence they are carried by the systemic circulation and may reach the mesenteric arteries and the intrahepatic radicles of the portal vein. Only about 20 per cent of the parasites reach maturity.

The symptomatology from the time of skin invasion to the time the parasites reach the portal system is minimal or absent despite the fact that focal hemorrhages and inflammatory foci at sites of destroyed schistosomules have been found in experimental animals. Krakower et al.[74] have described vascular lesions and necrosis in experimental animals which they attributed to toxic products released by the worms.

The parasites mature in the intrahepatic radicles of the portal vein, whence, with the help of the two suckers, they move against the venous blood stream to lodge in the mesenteric veins.[30,99] The adult schistosomes range from 0.6 to 2.5 cm in length, the females being longer and thinner than the males. The males have a midventral infolding (gynecophoric canal) occupied by the female during copulation as well as during the migration along the mesenteric vessels (Fig. 7). Oviposi-

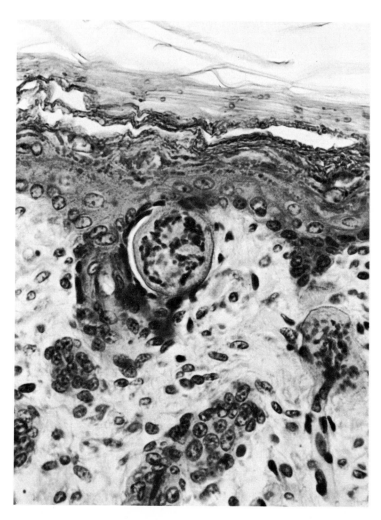

Fig. 6. Schistosomule located in upper dermis; another (right) is in a lymphatic. H&E. × 440.

tion occurs in the finer venous radicles of the intestinal or bladder mucosa and submucosa in rows or singly. By mechanisms to be discussed later, the eggs break through the vascular wall, enter the interstitial space, and are either retained causing a granulomatous reaction or discharged into the lumen of the hollow viscus (intestine or bladder) to be passed with the feces or urine. In some instances adults of *S. mansoni* and even more often those of *S. japonicum* may reach the inferior vena cava by anastomotic venous channels, whence they travel to ectopic sites (lungs, genitourinary tract, vertebral venous plexuses, brain). *S. haematobium* migrates from the mesenteric veins by way of the inferior hemorrhoidal and pudendal veins to the vesical and pelvic plexuses. The incubation period varies from species to species and ranges from 21 days to 12 weeks.[154] Worms may live 26 years or longer.[153]

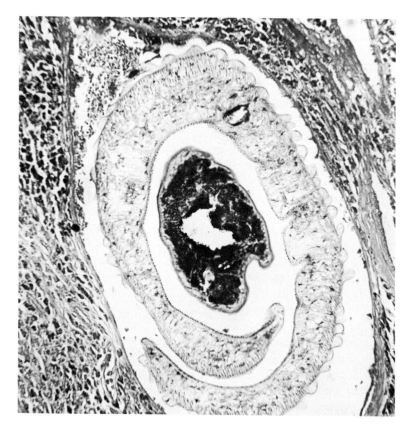

Fig. 7. Female and male in copulation in a mesenteric vein. There is a moderate periphlebitis. H&E. × 200.

CLINICOPATHOLOGIC CORRELATIONS. The clinical manifestations of *acute schistosomiasis* [32-34] begin in sudden fashion. Intermittent or remittent fever (101–104°F), lasting from 1 to 10 weeks, chills, profuse perspiration, headaches, and generalized aches and pains are observed associated with epigastric pain and bloody, mucous diarrhea, sometimes accompanied by tenesmus. The diarrhea lasts from one week to three or more months and may merge with the more chronic intestinal complaints of the later phase. Practically all patients suffer from a dry hacking cough. Physical examination reveals generalized lymphadenopathy, a moderately enlarged spleen, and a large, soft, tender liver. In some instances edema of the face and eyelids and urticarial rashes of the skin and mucous membranes are seen. The blood shows moderate anemia and normal or increased leukocytic counts, with eosinophilia ranging from 20 to 80 per cent. Liver function tests are usually normal, although some retention of bromsulphalein and elevated cephalin flocculation tests may be observed. There is marked hypergammaglobulinemia. Jaundice is not present. Radiologic examination of the chest reveals patchy infiltrates suggesting bronchopneumonia; this usually clears within a few days and has the morphologic appearance and evanscent character of eosinophilic pneumonitis.

In the initial stages of illness, schistosome eggs may or may not be seen in stools and biopsy material; however, they are usually found after the thirty-fifth day postinfection.

The clinical manifestations of the acute stage are attributed by most authors to the onset of oviposition and are regarded as allergic phenomena instigated in the host by the live miracidium and its metabolic products. In favor of this hypothesis are the marked hyperplasia of lymph nodes and spleen, the hypergammaglobulinemia, pronounced eosinophilia, the enanthematous reaction of the intestinal mucosa, and the urticarial rashes and edema of face and eyelids which may reach the proportions of angioneurotic edema. However, there is evidence in favor of the toxic effect produced by the immature worms which may be operative in the pathogenesis of the early illness. Koppisch [72] observed in experimental animals an intense eosinophilia of the portal spaces and polypoid endophlebitis even before oviposition had started. The endophlebitic process becomes more severe as the worm matures and is thought to be caused by metabolic products of the worm. But the most damaging effect results from the presence of eggs in the venules of the mucosa and submucosa of the intestine and bladder and in the liver and lungs. The inflammatory response is caused by toxic products excreted by the miracidium (probably enzymatic substances akin to those observed in cercariae), and its severity is proportional to the number of eggs deposited at one site.

In the *intestine* the phase of oviposition is characterized clinically by persistent diarrhea, with crampy abdominal pain and mucus and blood in the stools. Sigmoidoscopic examination reveals a reddened, granular mucosa with pinpoint yellowish elevations giving it a sandlike appearance. Shallow irregular ulcers averaging 3 mm in diameter are seen, sometimes becoming confluent and forming large areas of ulceration. The adjacent mucosa is hyperemic, studded with petechiae, and bleeds easily on contact. In *S. japonicum* infections the female deposits large numbers of eggs at once, whereas with *S. mansoni* and *S. haematobium* oviposition occurs individually or in small clumps. Single eggs or clumps of them are trapped in the smaller venules, occluding their lumens and causing congestion and hemorrhages which in conjunction with the lytic secretions of the embryo facilitate their extrusion into the adjacent stroma. Although it has been suggested that the lateral or terminal spines may act by perforating the vascular wall, extrusion of the egg is more likely related to destruction of the venule by the mechanism just mentioned. Kohlschütter and Koppisch [71] also observed proliferation of endothelial cells which surround the egg and eventually place it in an extraluminal position.

The inflammatory response is characterized by an outpouring of neutrophils and eosinophils which surround the egg forming a microabscess.[73,99] Histiocytes and multinucleated giant cells migrate into the area and encircle the egg, which is often seen within the cytoplasm of a giant cell. In *S. japonicum* infections the greater number of eggs deposited at one site results in the formation of larger abscesses with central necrosis, ischemia of the overlying mucosa, and development of a craterlike ulceration. The edema and inflammation impair the plasticity of the mucous membrane which is more easily traumatized by the peristaltic action of the gut and the passage of fecal matter, a mechanism probably contributing significantly to the discharge of eggs into the intestinal lumen (Fig. 8).

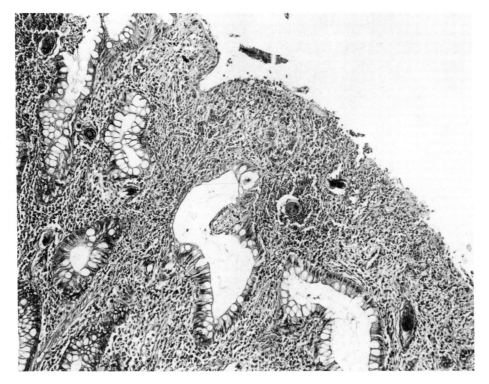

Fig. 8. Section of a sessile rectal polyp showing erosion of the surface epithelium, inflammatory infiltrate in lamina propria, and scattered eggs without pseudotubercle formation. H&E. × 125.

Ova located more deeply in the mucosa and submucosa are surrounded by a cuff of eosinophils and neutrophils, plasma cells, fibroblasts, and multinucleated giant cells. The latter are frequently seen engulfing the egg and are of the foreign body type. The miracidium lives three weeks or longer thereafter,[93,151] the acute inflammatory response subsides, and the lesion is eventually replaced by fibroblasts with layering of reticulin fibers and finally hyalinization. Continuous oviposition in immediately adjacent areas accounts for the presence side by side of acute lesions with others in various stages of healing. Conglomeration of pseudotubercles (Fig. 9), focal scarring, together with adjacent areas of edema and inflammation, make the mucosa bulge into the intestinal lumen in the form of sessile or pedunculated masses, wrongly referred to as "papillomas" or "adenomas." These polyps are actually inflammatory lesions, with a smooth or cauliflower-like appearance, of variable size. They are made up of granulation tissue, eggs in different stages of degeneration, pseudotubercles, and foci of acute inflammation interspersed with zones of fibrosis; the epithelium plays little or no part in their structure and is, more often than not, atrophic or ulcerated at the summit of the lesion. The granulomatous

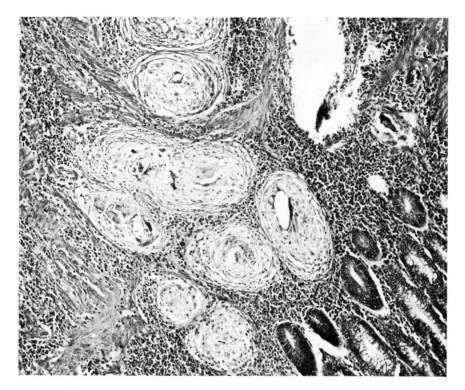

Fig. 9. Conglomerate of pseudotubercles in submucosa of intestine. Note shrunken eggs and eggshells within the lesions. H&E. × 130.

process affects also the muscularis and the serosa. Serosal or subserosal granulomas are associated with a focal exudative peritonitis leading to the fibrous adhesions which bind adjacent loops of the intestine.[17] Cicatrization of the inflammatory process causes the intestinal wall to become narrowed or even stenotic,[105] rigid, and inelastic. In *S. japonicum* infections such fibrosis may involve the entire length of the colon and segments of the small bowel; the mesentery is thickened and retracted with the expected hindrance to intestinal dynamics. In *S. mansoni* and *S. haematobium* infections the lesions are usually limited to the rectum and descending colon. Occasionally adult worms may induce a proliferative and exudative vasculitis with further impairment of regional circulation (Fig. 10).

Ischiorectal and anorectal abscesses and fistulas, anal fissures, and tags (inflammatory fibroepithelial polyps) contribute to complicate the picture (Fig. 11). Intestinal pseudopolyps may be numerous and sometimes of considerable size, causing obstruction or rectal prolapse. Tumorlike masses may be felt in the cecum or elsewhere in the colon, suggesting malignancy. Appendicitis is not an uncommon complication. There is no evidence to suggest that intestinal schistosomiasis predisposes to cancer;[54] the occasional reports in which cancer of the colon coexisted with schistosomiasis can be explained best as a chance occurrence (Fig. 12).

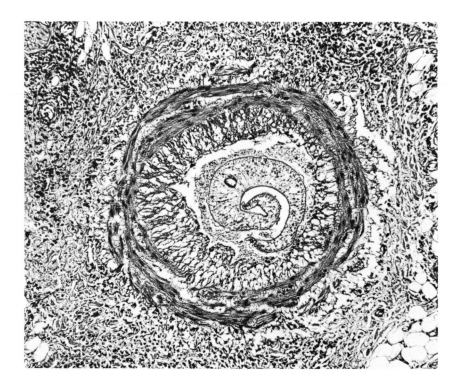

Fig. 10.   Adult worm in lumen of mesenteric vessel with marked edema of endothelial and subendothelial layers and, to a lesser extent, of muscularis. There is marked inflammatory reaction about vessel and in fat. H&E. × 130.

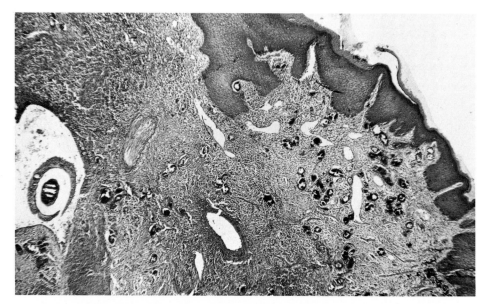

Fig. 11. Fibroepithelial inflammatory polyp of anus. Worms in copulation are seen in a vessel to the left. Numerous calcified eggs are scattered throughout the lesion. H&E. × 40.

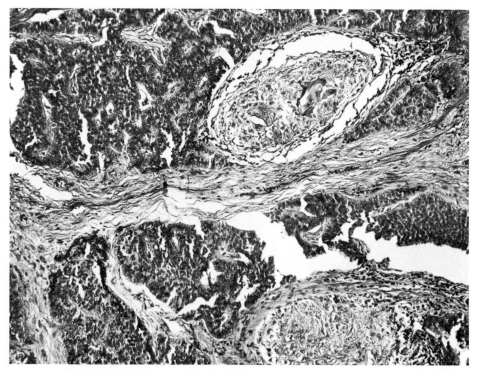

Fig. 12. Rectal carcinoid with several pseudotubercles containing remnants of eggs. H&E. × 130.

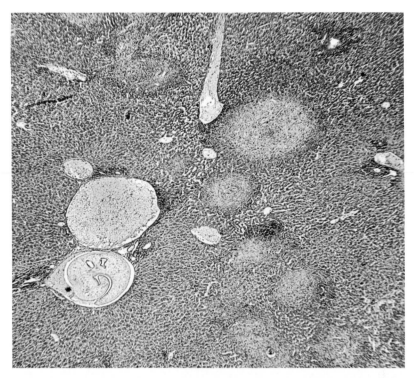

Fig. 13. Liver of mouse 45 days after infection. An adult worm is seen in an intrahepatic portal vein radicle. Numerous pseudotubercles are noted in other portal spaces. H&E. × 60.

As the worms move continuously within the mesenteric veins seeking adequate places to oviposit, eggs are swept by the blood stream and carried to the liver or lungs (Fig. 13). In the liver the eggs [26,124] become trapped in the intrahepatic portal venules, sometimes reaching the hepatic sinusoidal system.[1,72] In *S. mansoni* infections, eggs are trapped singly, inciting a proliferation of the endothelium which surrounds them. Neutrophils, eosinophils, epithelioid and multinucleated giant cells appear with formation of the characteristic pseudotubercle (Fig. 14). The endothelial lining becomes swollen, detached, and the inflammatory process destroys the vascular wall partly or completely (Fig. 15). In *S. japonicum* infections the eggs may appear conglutinated by a transparent substance probably of parasitic origin.[99] The greater number of eggs and, possibly, the more toxic effects produced by this species induce the development of large abscesses with prolonged delay in the formation of pseudotubercles. Around the eggs (more often in *S. japonicum* than in *S. mansoni* or *S. haematobium* infections) a fringe of fibrinoid material is noted spreading from the shell.[57,72,99] This material is thought to represent antigen–antibody complexes. Experimental studies carried out by a number of authors employing immunocytochemical techniques have demonstrated antibodies and antigen–antibody complexes in the granulomas and portal tracts.[5,83,90]

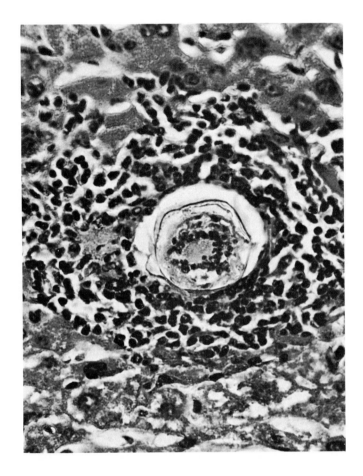

Fig. 14A. Mouse liver with a focus of early inflammation about a schistosome egg. The cells are predominantly neutrophils and eosinophils. H&E. × 400.

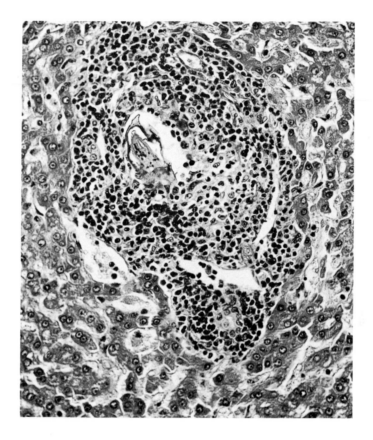

Fig. 14B. Granulomatous inflammation about a partly degenerated egg; the cells are predominantly histiocytes with neutrophils and eosinophils. H&E. × 325.

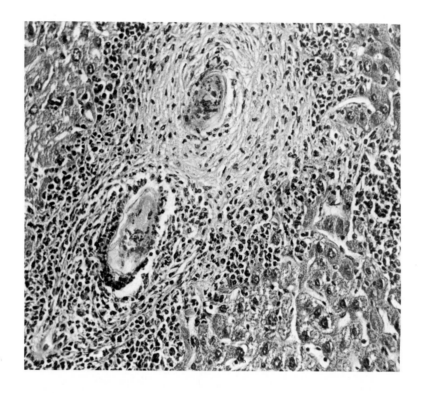

Fig. 14C. Mouse liver with two pseudotubercles. One (above) shows marked fibroblastic reaction with only scanty inflammatory cells. The other shows an earlier stage of the inflammatory response with a fringe of neutrophils and eosinophils about the live embryo. H&E. × 300.

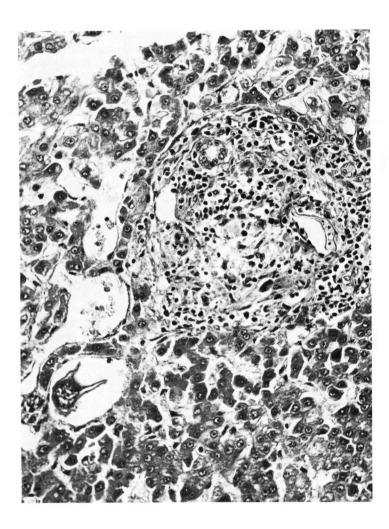

Fig. 15A. Granulomatous focus with complete replacement of portal venule; a shrunken eggshell is seen to the right. An egg is noted in a sinusoid at the left lower corner. Note compression of adjacent cell plates. H&E. × 325.

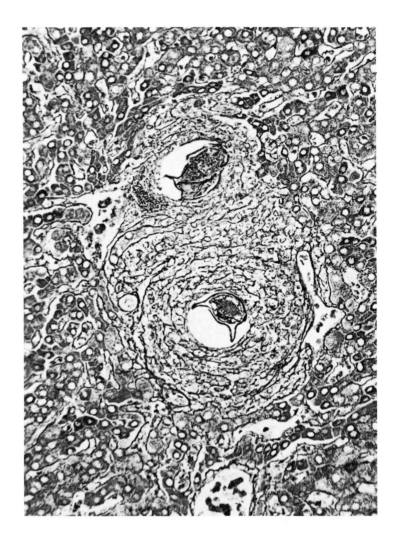

Fig. 15B. Two pseudotubercles, one filling and distending a portal venule which is widened; observe the abundant reticulin fibers. Another is in an extravascular position. Wilder's reticulin stain. × 300.

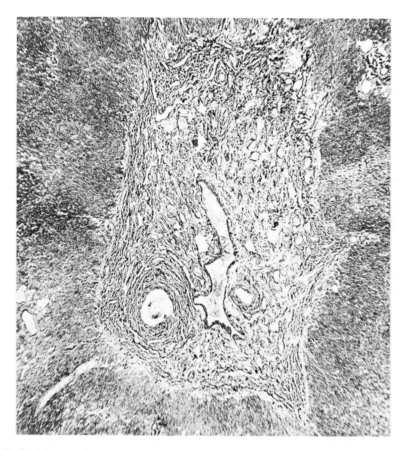

Fig. 16. Portal space in advanced schistosomal fibrosis. The portal vein is irregular in contour; numerous vascular channels permeate the broadened portal space. There is narrowing of a hepatic artery and foci of parenchymatous hemorrhage. Wilder's reticulin stain.
× 60.

With the death of the miracidium the inflammation subsides, the egg shells
become phagocytosed, and finally the pseudotubercle is replaced by fibroblasts with
deposition of reticulin fibers and ultimately hyalinization. Repetition of the inflammatory insults leads to progressive enlargment of the portal spaces which appear
as broad, stellate bands consisting of dense collagenized connective tissue [72,82,99,131]
(Fig. 16). Hypertrophic nerve trunks, bile ducts, and intrahepatic arterioles with
narrowed lumens, medial hypertrophy, and subendothelial thickening are noted
(Fig. 17). The portal veins may be difficult to discern; they are replaced by a
granulomatous process containing eggs in different stages of resorption, pseudo-

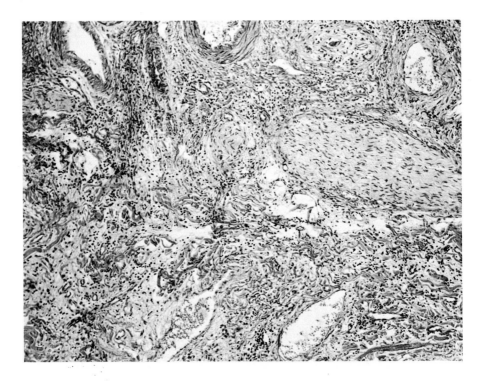

Fig. 17. High power view of a portal area showing hypertrophy of nerves, sclerosis of hepatic arteries, and replacement of portal vein by vascularized connective tissue. H&E. × 130.

tubercles, eosinophils, and other inflammatory cells which extend and partly or completely destroy the vein wall. The elastic fibers are fragmented and the smooth muscle cells isolated in small clumps or degenerated. Other veins show narrowing or obliteration of the lumen by fibrous connective tissue containing numerous thin wall vascular channels interconnecting among themselves and with those of the adjacent tissue (Fig. 18). Still other portal spaces have numerous widely dilated and congested vascular channels reminiscent of a cavernous hemangioma (Fig. 19). Not infrequently this engorgement and vascular dilatation extend to the sinusoidal system [26,31] (Fig. 20).

The liver parenchyma is well preserved, although it is not rare to encounter areas of liver cell necrosis. Foci of intraparenchymatous hemorrhages are not un-usual. There is proliferation and hyperplasia of Kupffer's cells which often contain hematoidin excreted by the adult worms.[72,73,99] Intralobular fibrosis is not seen unless the process is complicated by nutritional deficiencies or viral hepatitis or perhaps as the result of repeated bouts of ischemia (Fig. 21).

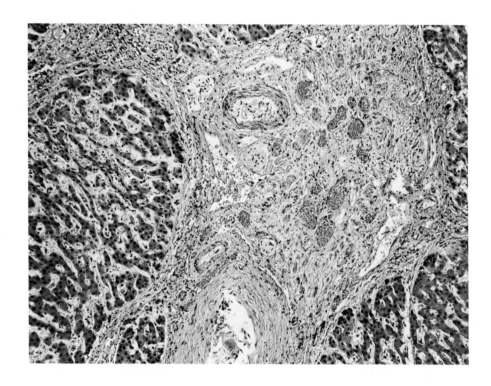

Fig. 18. Angiomatoid transformation of portal space. Note narrowing of hepatic artery and phlebosclerosis of portal vein (lower midfield). Pseudotubercles are no longer seen. There is perilobular fibrosis. H&E. $\times$ 130.

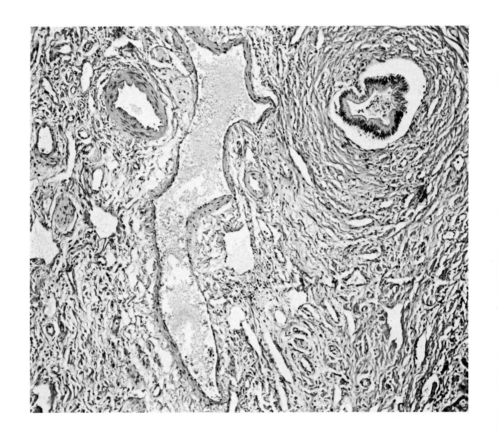

Fig. 19. Angiomatoid appearance of portal space with extensive collagenization. H&E.
× 150.

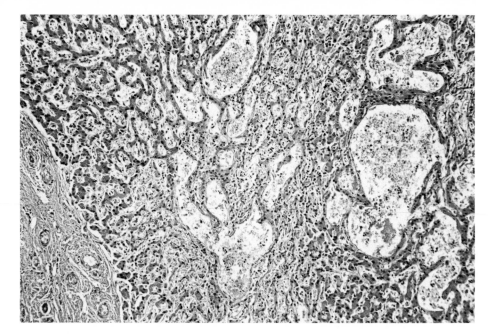

Fig. 20. Fibrosis and angiomatoid changes in a portal space (left lower corner) and marked dilatation of sinusoidal spaces with compression and focal disorganization of liver cell plates. H&E. × 130.

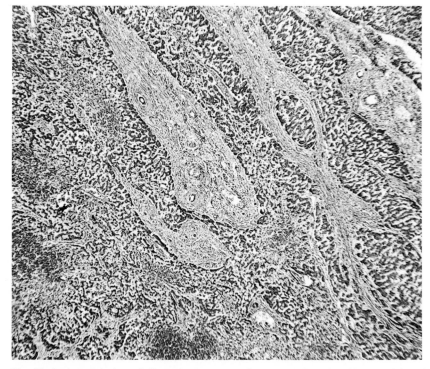

Fig. 21. Marked nodulation of liver due to extensive portal fibrosis. Observe fairly large areas of parenchymatous hemorrhages. H&E. × 60.

185

Grossly the liver may be small (Fig. 22), enlarged, or of normal size; its weight ranges from 700 to 2,500 g, and its consistency from firm to hard, cutting like rubbery material.[118] The capsule usually shows a fine or coarse nodularity, not as striking as that of Laennec's or postnecrotic cirrhosis. It is often bosselated. Occasionally, it may be quite smooth. The cut surface is characteristic. Symmers [149] first described the gross appearance of schistosomal liver fibrosis and likened it to "a number of white clay-pipe stems having been thrust at various angles into the organ." The larger branches of the portal vein are surrounded by mantles of white or pink fibrous tissue which diminish in width toward the periphery. The appearance frequently suggests a mosaic pattern, with round, ovoid, or irregularly outlined nodules separated by depressed fibrous areas. The portal spaces may show widely dilated gaping veins or complete obliteration of the normal structure. The nodules of parenchymal tissue vary from pinkish brown to gray, with zones having a darker brown or reddish color. In some cases the portal fibrosis is less conspicuous and affects the organ in a more diffuse manner.

Intrahepatic blockage of the portal circulation results in portal hypertension and development of a massive collateral venous circulation [52,74,103] (Fig. 23). In some patients thrombosis of the portal vein with extension to the splenic occurs. The *spleen* is usually greatly enlarged and may weigh 1,800 g or more.[135] The capsule is thickened and may contain whitish irregular plaques. Its consistency is increased, and the cut surface shows a dark red appearance with irregular nodules or fibrous bands. Occasionally, irregular zones of hemorrhagic infarction may be detected macroscopically. Histologically, there is fibrous thickening of the septa, hyperplasia of reticuloendothelial cells, diminution or disappearance of lymphoid follicles, and massive congestion, with scattered areas of fresh and old hemorrhage. Siderocalcific structures (Gandy–Gamna nodules) are readily seen (Fig. 24).

Clinically the patients tend to be predominantly in the second to third decades of life,[37,46] younger than those afflicted with portal hypertension secondary to cirrhosis.[132] The most common complaint is hemorrhage: hematemesis, melena, or both. The liver is usually readily palpable, firm to hard, and nontender. Jaundice is rarely seen. Spider angiomas, gynecomastia, testicular atrophy, and loss of body hair occur rarely. Edema of legs and ascites may be present especially in the terminal stages of the disease. In keeping with the well-preserved liver cells, the liver function tests are usually normal or only slightly impaired. As a rule the abnormal tests are those which indicate disturbed protein metabolism.[125] Thus, cephalin flocculation and thymol turbidity tests are frequently abnormal, and bromsulphalein retention is increased in 50 per cent of cases. On the other hand serum glutamic oxalacetic and pyruvic transaminases are normal, and the prothrombin time, if impaired, can be readily corrected by administration of vitamin K. Hypoalbuminemia is found in one fourth of the patients, and hypergammaglobulinemia is a constant finding. Serum potassium and sodium levels are normal unless the patient has ascites. Rodriguez found normal liver function tests in 40 per cent of his patients,[135] and El-Ghoulmy et al. in 75 per cent of their series.[37]

Hypersplenism (leukopenia, thrombocytopenia) may be observed; anemia when present is related to bleeding episodes and is of the hypochromic microcytic type.[15,19]

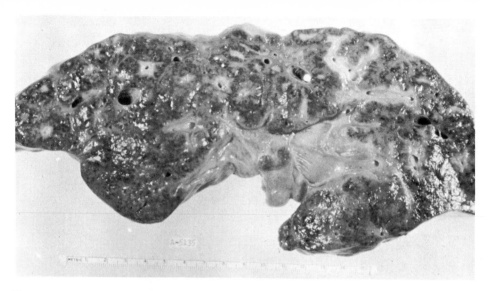

Fig. 22. Bosselation of the liver surface is prominent. Note the whitish cuffs surrounding portal veins. (Courtesy of Dr. R. A. Marcial-Rojas.)

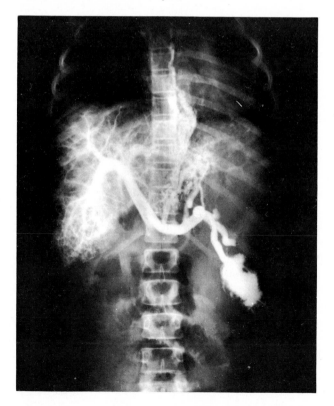

Fig. 23. Splenoportogram in a patient with schistosomal hepatolienal syndrome. The prominence of anastomotic channels along the stomach and lower esophagus is shown by the corkscrew appearance of dilated collateral communications. (Courtesy of D Morales and Hector M. Vallés.)

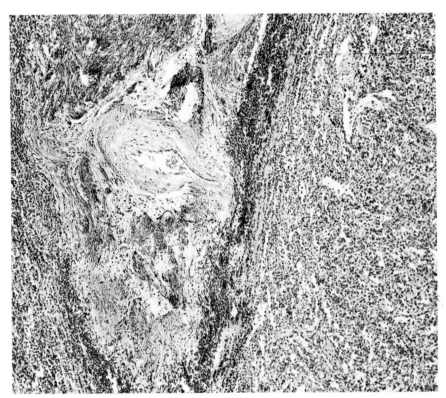

Fig. 24. Spleen in schistosomal portal hypertension showing congestion, hyperplasia of reticuloendothelial cells, and a large siderocalcific body (Gamna–Gandy body). H&E. ×130.

Wedge intrahepatic venous pressures are consistent with a presinusoidal portal vein blockage.[16,126] Andrade et al.[6] have recently reported on a group of patients with schistosomal hepatolienal syndrome and ascites, which they explained by finding histologic evidence of postnecrotic cirrhosis. They considered this lesion to be the result of either repeated bouts of ischemia subsequent to bleeding episodes or to a chronic immunologic response instigated by schistosomal antigens, by liver cell breakdown products, or both. There is increasing evidence that in a considerable number of cases the vaso-occlusive disease caused by schistosomes is further complicated by factors such as nutritional deficiencies or viral hepatitis. Erfan et al.[38,39] in 180 cases of portal hypertension found schistosomiasis to be the sole cause of the syndrome in 36 per cent; in 34 per cent it was associated with Laennec's cirrhosis or viral hepatitis.

It is generally accepted that from 5 to 10 per cent of patients with schistosomiasis develop portal hypertension;[45] in the remainder isolated granulomas or mild to moderate degrees of portal fibrosis are accidentally found by needle biopsy or at necropsy.[7,46,73]

Pulmonary lesions occur when eggs embolize to the pulmonary arterial system.[28,38,40,114,129] Although they may reach the lungs by way of pre-existing

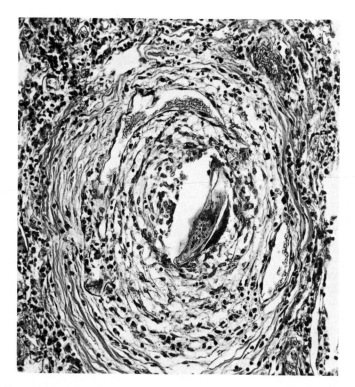

Fig. 25. Well-developed pseudotubercle with degenerated egg filling a pulmonary alveolar space. H&E. × 140.

intrahepatic anastomotic channels,[123] undoubtedly the large majority are carried by the blood along collateral venous communications secondary to portal hypertension. The incidence of pulmonary lesions varies; Koppisch [73] found granulomas in only 2 of his 147 autopsies, whereas Shaw and Ghareeb [143] encountered them in 33 per cent of their 282 cases. Lopes de Faria [84] in 180 cases observed pulmonary lesions in 18 instances.

Eggs become impacted in pulmonary arterioles ranging from 50 to 200 microns in diameter.[84,85] Then they are extruded into the adjacent stroma where pseudotubercles form (Fig. 25), having caused little or no damage to the arterial wall. The pseudotubercles measure from 0.5 to 1 ml and appear grossly as tiny, whitish gray firm nodules, bulging on the cut surface and arranged in rows or isolated along the branches of the pulmonary artery. The granuloma may fill an alveolar space or bulge into the lumen of a bronchiole; healing occurs by fibrous replacement, leaving a minute scar which may contain a calcified egg. This type of lesion is asymptomatic.

In approximately 2 to 6 per cent of patients with pulmonary lesions a process

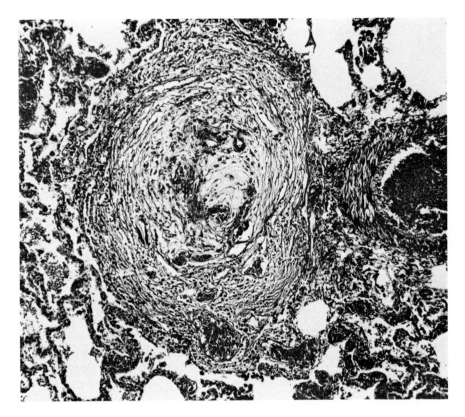

Fig. 26. Thrombosed pulmonary artery with organization and irregular recanalization of vessel. Note a distended vein at the lower margin. Remnants of eggs are seen in the former lumen of the vessel. H&E. × 140.

of much greater severity develops. The eggs trapped in the lumen of an arteriole induce an intense granulomatous inflammation resulting in vascular occlusion (Fig. 26). At first the eggs are surrounded by eosinophils, neutrophils, and hyaline thrombi; soon mononuclear cells move in and a pseudotubercle with multinucleated giant cells engulfing the egg is formed. The endothelium degenerates, fibroblasts invade the area, and the lesion is slowly replaced by collagenized connective tissue containing numerous slitlike, irregular channels lined with endothelial cells (Fig. 27). The diameter of the vessel is increased and there is subintimal fibrosis which may extend to the media, but the elastic membranes are intact. Within the original lumen of the vessel an incomplete attempt at recanalization leads to the formation of an angiomatoid lesion. Were it not for the presence of granulomas and of eggs or fragments thereof, the lesion would be indistinguishable, by ordinary staining techniques, from that encountered in recanalized thrombi of different etiology.

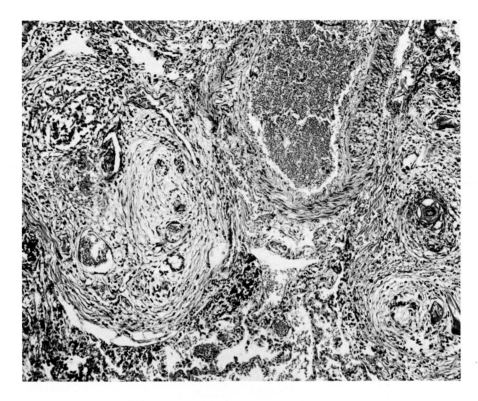

Fig. 27. Intravascular angiomatoid (left) and extravascular pseudotubercles about live eggs or shells (righthand corner). The unobstructed portion of the pulmonary artery at top shows endothelial swelling and focal edema of the wall. H&E. × 130.

In other lesions the granulomatous process extends to the wall of the vessel which is focally destroyed (Fig. 28). Eosinophils, neutrophils, and histiocytes surrounding the egg move across the arteriolar wall, inducing a necrotizing arteritis, until the egg reaches an extravascular location. The elastic membranes are pushed ahead of the granuloma, becoming frayed and finally disrupted, and leading to the formation of a dumbbell-shaped pseudoaneurysm (Fig. 29). The lumen of the vessel is occluded by an organizing thrombus, while the periadventitial tissues show a granulomatous process involving adjacent venous channels which become partly or completely thrombosed. The granulomatous process is ultimately replaced by fibrous tissue (Fig. 30). Newly formed blood vessels permeate the area with the development of tortuous dilated venous channels that communicate through the wall with the angiomatoid lesion of the arterial lumen and result in arteriovenous fistulas (Fig. 31).

The incidence of widespread pulmonary arterial lesions varies from 2 per cent to 5.5 per cent. When patients with schistosomal liver fibrosis alone are considered the incidence reaches 12 per cent.

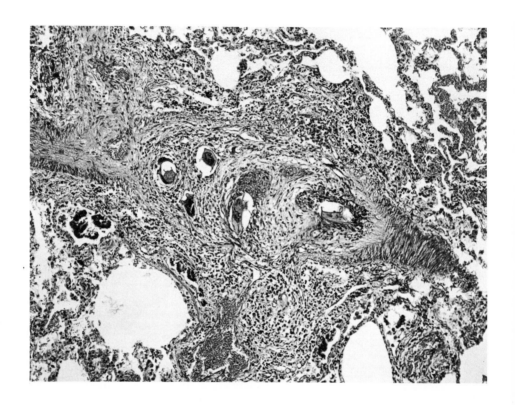

Fig. 28. Section of pulmonary artery showing complete segmental destruction by a granulomatous process around eggs. Note involvement of adjacent vein which is partly occluded
with distal dilatation. H&E. × 120.

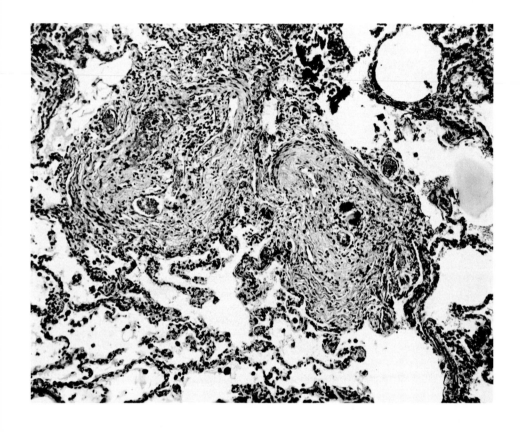

Fig. 29. Obliterative pulmonary endarteritis with incipient recanalization. The vessel on right shows a pseudoaneurysmal pouch and several multinucleated giant cells containing eggshells. H&E. × 130.

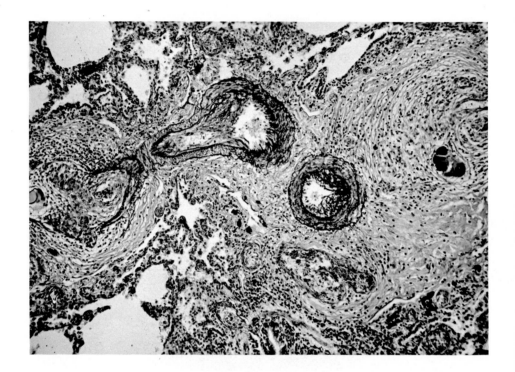

Fig. 30. The pulmonary arteries show severe proliferative endarteritis. Toward the left the vessel is occluded by a granulomatous process with remnants of eggs. The elastic lamellae are destroyed. Toward the right are several extravascular pseudotubercles. Beneath the cross section of the narrowed pulmonary arterial branch there is an extravascular angiomatoid area. Weigert's reticulin stain. × 130.

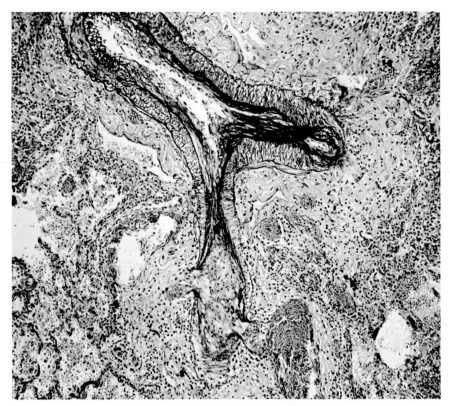

Fig. 31. Arteriovenous anastomosis secondary to schistosomal granulomatous vasculitis. Weigert's reticulin stain. × 120.

Lopes de Faria [84] has described another vascular lesion involving predominantly pulmonary arteries of less than 200 microns in diameter which he considers to be caused not by ova but by focal reactivity in a previously damaged vessel, induced by toxic products of the parasite. The lesion is characterized by edema, swelling, and hyperplasia of endothelial cells, a necrotizing panarteritis with destruction of the media and elastic membranes, and the presence in the lumen of polypoid eosinophilic masses partly covered with endothelial cells that form irregular narrow channels. Fibrosis and hyalinization eventually lead to occlusion or marked narrowing of the affected vessel, with resulting increased resistance in the pulmonary circulation.

Pulmonary atheromatosis of the arteries and subendothelial concentric proliferation of the arterioles with medial hypertrophy are also observed and considered to be the result of increased pulmonary pressure.

Occasionally adult parasites may reach the pulmonary vessels (Fig. 32). Although mild or no inflammation may be seen in the vessel where the live worm

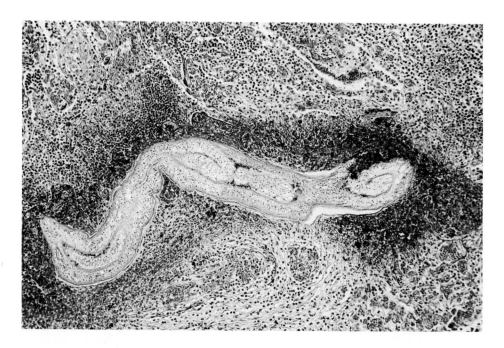

Fig. 32. Dead adult worm trapped in a pulmonary vessel. There is extensive necrosis of the wall and adjacent pulmonary parenchyma. H&E. × 130.

lodges, death of the parasite induces a necrotizing pneumonitis which appears grossly as round or elliptical, whitish gray patches of consolidation measuring from 0.1 to 0.5 cm with the worm in the center. There is infiltration by eosinophils and neutrophils, which are eventually replaced by epithelioid cells forming layered rows about the fragments of the partly preserved worm. Calcium incrustation of the parasite may occur.

As a result of the granulomatous or allergic arteritis, the formation of pseudo-aneurysm and the arteriovenous anastomosis, there is pulmonary hypertension leading to cor pulmonale.[65] The patients are usually young individuals, predominantly males, who complain of shortness of breath of relatively short duration, with engorgement of neck vessels, precordial and chest pain on exertion, right upper quadrant pain, and edema of the legs or anasarca. Heart murmurs may be absent, but when present they are loud and heard predominantly over the pulmonic and mitral areas.

Occasionally diastolic murmurs may be heard in both areas and when transmitted to the apex may suggest rheumatic heart disease. Clubbing of the fingers is rare and cyanosis uncommon because of the absence of lesions of pulmonary capillaries.

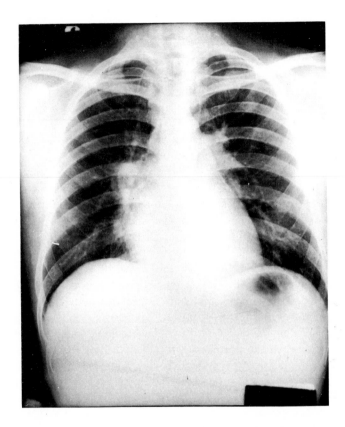

Fig. 33. Radiograph showing pulmonary peripheral arterial occlusive disease due to schistosoma eggs. There is dilatation of right ventricle and pulmonary artery (early cor pulmonale). (Courtesy of Drs. F. Hernandez-Morales and Hector M. Vallés.)

Radiologic studies show marked enlargment and dilatation of the right ventricle (Fig. 33) and dilatation of the pulmonary artery which may reach aneurysmal proportions.[62] A fine nodular mottling of the pulmonary parenchyma may also be detected. The radiologic picture suggests mitral stenosis or congenital heart defects. Angiocardiographic studies fail to demonstrate septal defects, although a displacement of the interventricular septum toward the left (reverse Bernheim syndrome) may be noted.[46] Electrocardiographic studies show right axis deviation and right ventricular hypertrophy; occasionally incomplete right bundle branch block may be noted. Catheterization studies show normal oxygen saturation, and pulmonary function studies are normal. On the other hand, pressure studies show marked elevation of the pulmonary arterial pressure with normal wedge pressures. There is increased systemic and pulmonary vascular resistance and decreased cardiac output.[134]

Hemoptyses are rare.[133] Over 90 per cent of patients with Manson's schistosomiasis suffering from cardiopulmonary manifestations also have advanced portal hypertension. Because of the frequent association of portal and vascular lesions, it has been suggested that this clinicopathologic complex be labeled "portopulmonary obstructive syndrome." This is a hardly tenable suggestion, considering that extensive pulmonary lesions are also found in *S. haematobium* infections, while concomitant portal hypertension is seen in less than 3 per cent of such patients.

At autopsy the right ventricle is dilated and hypertrophied, measuring 1.0 cm or more in thickness. The pulmonic valve diameter may measure twice as much or more that of the mitral. The left ventricle appears dwarfed by comparison with the right.

Recently attention has been called to another syndrome associated with pulmonary schistosomiasis characterized by rather sudden onset of progressive cyanosis, slight elevation in pulmonary arterial pressure and mild or absent cor pulmonale.[87,88,96,106] Partial pressures of pCO_2 and pO_2 in alveolar air were found to be low, and the blood was unsaturated after breathing a mixture of 98 per cent oxygen for 10 minutes. Angiocardiographic studies showed rapid filling of the pulmonary veins and left atrium, suggesting arteriovenous fistulas.[157] Clubbing of the fingers was a prominent feature of the syndrome. Whereas Lopes de Faria [86,87] feels that the arteriovenous fistulas are the result of abnormal communications created by the action of the ova reaching and involving small pulmonary veins, Marchand et al.[96] believe that the shunts are not related directly to the schistosomal infection but are rather the result of portal hypertension and are similar to those found in cirrhosis. Calabresi and Abelman [23] have demonstrated normally occurring communications between the portal and intrathoracic veins as well as between the portal and the pulmonary venous system. Rydell and Hoffbauer [139] have suggested that pulmonary arteriovenous shunts may develop in patients with cirrhosis under the influence of factors similar to those operative in spider angiomas. According to this hypothesis, the increase in portal venous pressure forces blood to flow into the pulmonary venous circuit thus creating high levels of oxygen unsaturation.

As mentioned above, *S. haematobium* lodges in the vesical and pelvic venous plexuses where oviposition occurs.[56,58] The female schistosome, containing about 30 eggs in its uterus at one time, deposits them in rows or small clumps within the venules of the submucosa and the vesical wall (Fig. 34). After they pass into the perivascular tissue, necrosis and abscesses are formed, causing sloughing of the mucous membrane and discharge of ova, pus, and blood into the lumen. The earliest clinical manifestation is a painless, post-micturition hematuria which may be microscopic or overt.[2,55,56,58] However, several months may elapse between deposition of eggs in the bladder wall and their identification in urine.[42] The mucosa is hyperplastic, edematous, reddened, and contains small irregular shallow ulcers more abundant in the lower portion and around the urethral orifice. Small polypoid masses composed of granulation tissue and either live or calcified ova are noted. Later granulations and sandy patches are noticeable throughout the mucosal surface.[156] The bladder wall becomes fibrosed and contracted. Dysuria, frequency, pollakiuria, and a burning sensation down the urethra are common complaints; occasionally suprapubic pressure or pain are noted.

Calcium oxalate and calcium phosphate concretions develop around masses of eggs or sloughed off fragments of the mucosa. Cystoscopic examination becomes difficult or impossible to carry out. The number of calcified ova embedded in the

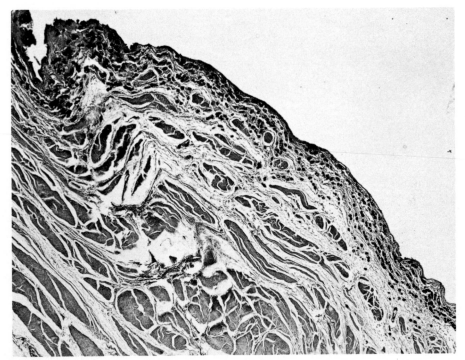

Fig. 34. Section of bladder showing multiple calcified eggs beneath the mucosa. H&E. × 25. (Section courtesy of Dr. G. W. Hunter, III.)

submucosa and vesical wall may be so great that the bladder casts a definite shadow on plain x-ray films of the abdomen. Makar [92] has stated that linear, lamellated, wavy calcifications can be seen in 60 per cent of individuals suffering from chronic bilharzial cystitis; in patients with added carcinoma the calcific shadows are more irregular, dense, tend to be localized to one area of the organ, and are detected in 84 per cent of the cases. Foci of leukoplakia and cystitis glandularis are common findings on biopsy or necropsy.

There is a great deal of controversy regarding whether schistosomal cystitis predisposes to bladder cancer.[92,104,122] Chronic inflammation and irritation in conjunction with endogenous and exogenous factors as yet unspecified have been invoked to explain the relatively high incidence of bladder cancer in certain geographic areas. Inadequate or controversial statistical reports and the prevalence of this infection in the populations studied have cast doubts as to the causal relationship. However, cancer of the bladder occurs in a much younger age group in endemic than in nonendemic areas. In Makar's series [92] of 380 cancers of the bladder, 150 developed in individuals under 40 years of age. Another peculiarity is the predominant histologic type. Thus, squamous cell carcinoma represents about 10 per cent of all bladder cancers in Europe and the United States, whereas in Africa Prates and Gillman [122] observed squamous cell carcinoma in 59 per cent of

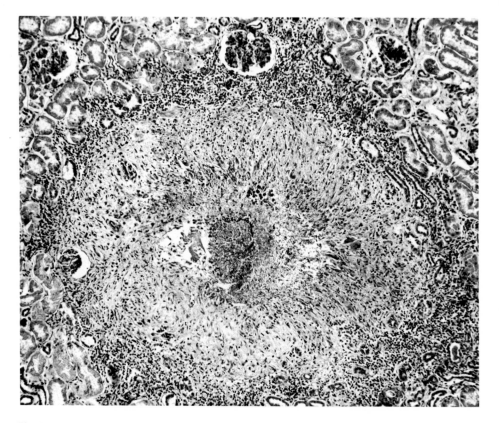

Fig. 35. Large granulomatous focus in renal parenchyma with central eosinophilic necrosis, most likely secondary to a trapped adult worm. H&E. × 125.

their 139 cases; 21 per cent were papillary transitional cell tumors, and the remainder were anaplastic or solid transitional cell cancers.

The ureters are also involved in a large number of patients. Hervé and Piganiol [56] found ureteropelvic involvement in 34 of 100 patients with schistosomal cystitis. This involvement is bilateral in 75 per cent of patients. Grossly the ureter is rigid, tortuous, elongated, and either dilated or stenosed. The mucosa is granular and reddened. Although most of the eggs are observed in the submucosa, they can also be found in the muscularis and adventitia. Fibrosis leads to destruction of the muscle coat, impairment or cessation of peristaltic activity, and hydronephrosis. Pyelonephritis is common. Ureteral involvement may cause severe colicky pain indistinguishable from that caused by a passing stone.

Occasionally, the parasites may enter the interlobular veins of the kidney where after their death they stimulate an acute necrotizing lesion (Fig. 35), in the center of which remnants of the parasite and abundant eosinophilic material are seen; surrounding the central area there are abundant epithelioid cells. Healing occurs by fibrous replacement. Occasionally eggs are seen in afferent arterioles or in the

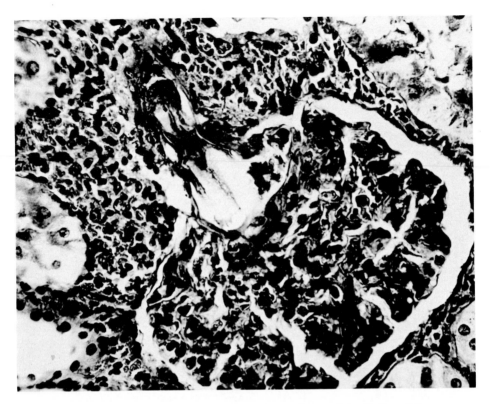

Fig. 36. Eggshell lodged in an afferent glomerular arteriole. H&E. × 400.

center of the pseudotubercles after having reached the kidney through the systemic circulation (Fig. 36).[8,141]

Prostatic involvement is not common and occurs more often in *S. haematobium* infections than with either of the other two species.[8,13] Makar has classified the prostatic lesions into two groups: 1, an early or congestive type characterized clinically by dysuria, pollakiuria, and a firm, enlarged gland and 2, a late or atrophic type showing stony hard consistency, nodularity, and decreased size. Histologically there are scattered pseudotubercles (Fig. 37) containing live eggs, egg shells, or calcified ova. Involvement of seminal vesicles (Fig. 38) is often observed when the prostate is affected. Their glands are large, nodular, and cystic and cause aspermia, hemospermia, and painful ejaculation. The inflammatory reaction may be mild, although the gland is studded with myriads of calcified eggs. It is unusual to observe

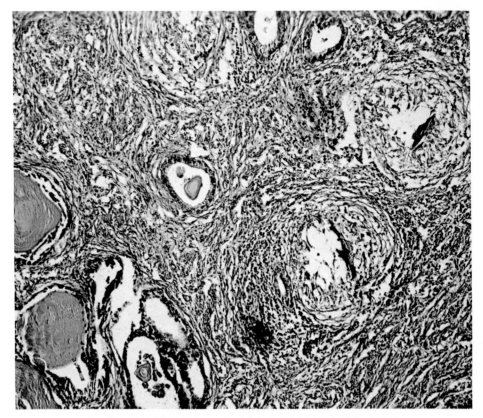

Fig. 37. Schistosomal pseudotubercles in prostate. H&E. × 125.

orchio-epididymitis. In one instance bilateral testicular infarction followed extensive involvement of the spermatic cord.[66]

Penile lesions with a verrucous appearance, ulcerations involving the skin of the penis or scrotum, and elephantiasis are rare complications.[109]

The parasites reach the genital organs by way of anastomoses between the hemorrhoidal and hypogastric veins. The valvular system of these vessels, being imperfectly developed, offers no hindrance to their migration. Makar[91] has also shown that communications exist between the spermatic and mesenteric veins. As the ovarian veins are the female counterpart of the spermatic vessels, migration along these channels allows the parasites to lodge in organs not habitually inhabited by them. Mature and immature parasites have been demonstrated a number of times.[8,109]

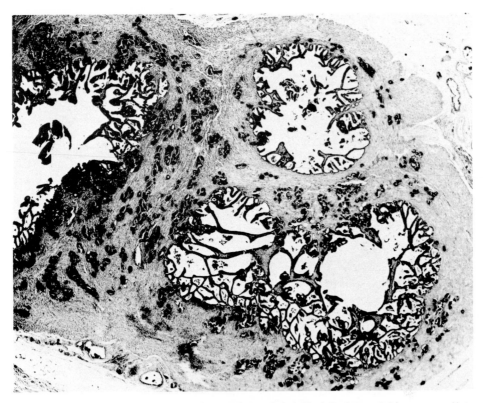

Fig. 38. Seminal vesicles riddled with myriads of calcified S. haematobium eggs. Note absence of inflammatory reaction. H&E. × 25. (Section courtesy of Dr. G. W. Hunter, III.)

The most common complications affecting the female genital organs are those involving the fallopian tube and ovaries.[9,25,55,109,142] Salpingitis and salpingo-oophoritis although more common with *S. haematobium* are also encountered occasionally in *S. mansoni* and *S. japonicum* infections. Clinically the symptoms and signs are consistent with pelvic inflammatory disease; sometimes they suggest the presence of a cystic tumor. The lesions are chiefly encountered in the submucosa of the tube, causing narrowing of the lumen (Fig. 39), segmental dilatation, and extensive adhesions to the ovary and pelvic wall. Sometimes the distal portion of the tube is distended and filled with hemorrhagic, granular material. Charlewood et al.[25] state that in *S. haematobium* infection the lesions involve preferentially the wall, leaving the mucosa undamaged. As the lumen remains patent insemination of the ovum may occur, although rigidity of the wall due to the granulomatous process

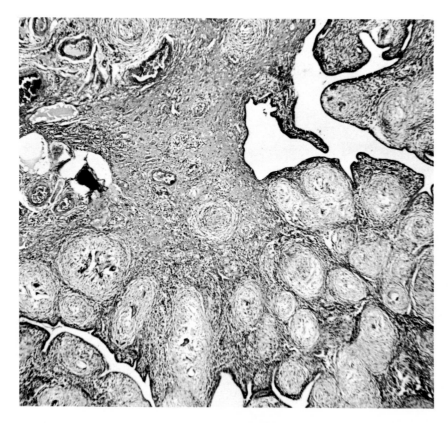

Fig. 39. S. mansoni granulomatous salpingitis. Most pseudotubercles contain live or fragmented eggs. Note distortion of lumen. H&E. × 60.

may interfere with its migration into the endometrial cavity. Apparently ectopic tubal pregnancy secondary to schistosomal salpingitis is not uncommon in Africa.[36,108] Irregularities in the menstrual cycle seem to be related to the systemic effects of the disease rather than to lesions of the endometrium or ovaries. Large regions of granulomatous inflammation and abscess formation may be found in ovaries (Fig. 40), but the process seldom is extensive enough to result in functional incompetence. Granulomas have been observed also in the vulva, endometrium, myometrium, and cervix (Fig. 41).[9,102] In massive infections schistosomal lesions of variable severity may be seen in practically all organs, e.g., thyroid,[81] adrenals,[51] myocardium,[12,48,81] bone marrow, and skin of the anterior abdominal wall.[11,12,14,22,107]

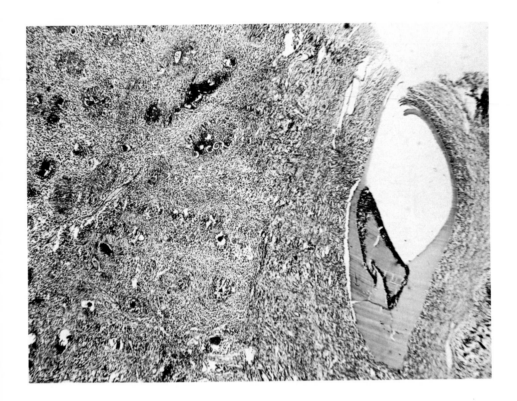

Fig. 40. A section of ovary showing many granulomas due to S. mansoni. H&E. × 60.

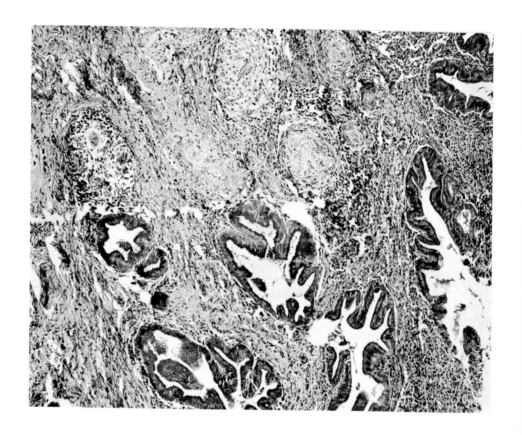

Fig. 41. Section of uterine cervix with pseudotubercles, some containing remnants of egg-shells. H&E. × 125.

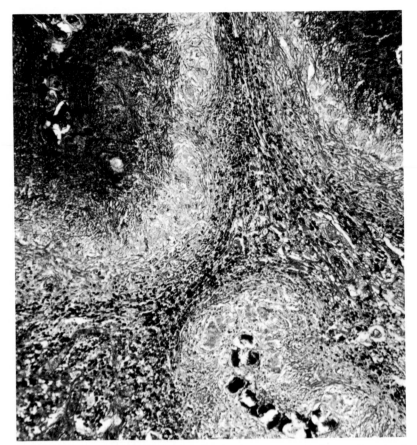

Fig. 42. Section of brain illustrating large foci of granulomatous inflammation about numerous partly calcified S. japonicum eggs. H&E. × 130.

Among the rarest but most severe of complications are those resulting from involvement of the central nervous system.[10,18,98,144] *S. japonicum* is by far the species most frequently responsible, although isolated cases caused by *S. mansoni* and *S. haematobium* have been reported.[98,100] Clinically,[53,70] the symptoms are of sudden onset. Violent headaches sometimes localized to the affected zone, mental confusion, convulsive seizures followed by transitory motor or sensory defects, hyperreflexia, coma, and disturbances in visual acuity are noted in variable degrees. In general, the symptomatology does not differ from that caused by rapidly expanding intracranial tumor. Grossly the meninges are roughened or thickened with adhesions between dura and arachnoid. A grayish exudate is noted along the cortical vessels and tiny pinpoint gray or yellow nodules are scattered over the cortex in the involved area. The size of the lesions varies considerably; some have been described as large as an orange. Not infrequently they have a racemose appearance. They are friable or rubbery, partly calcified, and centrally necrotic. Histologically (Fig. 42) there are large numbers of eggs in the center of the

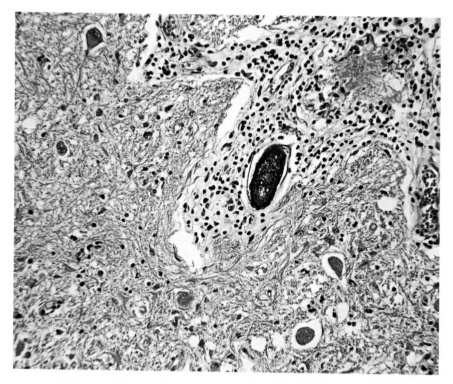

Fig. 43. S. mansoni egg trapped in a venule of spinal cord. Observe foci of inflammation and fibrinoid necrosis (upper part of field). Adjacent neurons are unaffected. H&E. ×325. (Section courtesy of Dr. R. A. Marcial-Rojas.)

lesion where necrotic cells, eosinophils, neutrophils, and multinucleated giant cells are seen. A peripheral multilayered zone of epithelioid cells with scattered lymphocytes and eosinophils surrounds the area. In the periphery there is proliferation of fibroblasts with deposition of connective tissue fibers and hyperplasia of glial cells. The adjacent neurons are degenerated; occasionally thrombosis or obliterative angiitis is noted. Adult worms have never been observed within the intracerebral lesions, although Monteiro de Barros et al.[100] have observed one patient with several adult male and female worms in the leptomeninges.

Ova may also embolize to the vessels of the spinal cord, causing transverse myelitis (Fig. 43). They lodge in venules where an expanding granulomatous process develops with compression of the adjacent ganglion cells and tracts.[59,98,117]

Not all eggs reaching the central nervous system cause lesions. Gelfand[47] by means of a digestion technique of brain tissue was able to find eggs in over 50 per cent of his cases, although there was no clinical or macroscopic evidence of neurologic impairment.

It is still questionable how schistosoma eggs reach the central nervous system. Greenfield[50] supported the hypothesis that they were deposited in situ by stray female worms. Fujinami[44] afforded some experimental evidence in support of this theory by finding adult worms in the cerebral veins of a monkey exposed to a heavy

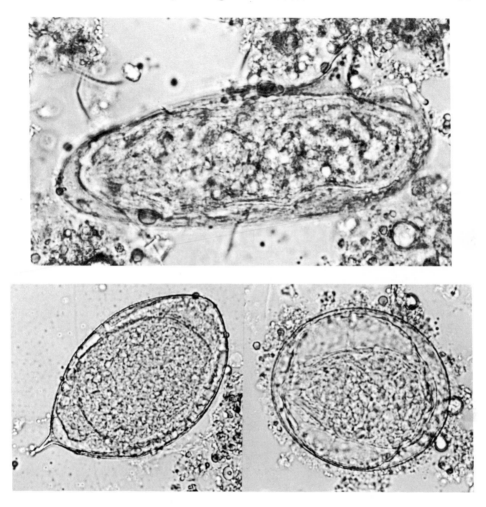

Fig. 44. Top, S. mansoni with lateral spine (feces); fresh preparation. × 450. Bottom left, S. haematobium egg in fecal matter; note characteristic terminal spine. Fresh preparation. × 450. Bottom right, S. japonicum with a rounder shape; knob is not detected in this specimen (fecal matter). Fresh preparation. × 450.

concentration of cercariae. More recently Monteiro de Barros et al.[100] found adults in the leptomeninges of one of their patients, and Raper [127] identified what he considered to be a degenerated and partly calcified worm in the cord. Others believe that eggs are embolized from distant areas either through the paravertebral venous plexuses or, in some instances, via the systemic circulation.[70]

DIAGNOSIS.   The diagnosis is based on the demonstration of ova in stools, urine, or biopsy samples (Table 1) (Fig. 44).[43,61] Shedding of eggs begins shortly after the fifth week postinfection, although in urinary bilharziasis several months may elapse before eggs are encountered in the urine.[43] The ova are readily seen in the mucous material intermingled or covering the fecal matter, especially in patients

Table 1

Species	Length microns	Width microns	Special Features
S. haematobium	112–170	40–70	Terminal spine
S. mansoni	114–175	45–70	Lateral spine
S. japonicum	70–100	50–65	Lateral knob usually not detected

with dysenteric symptoms. At least three consecutive samples should be studied before ruling out the presence of eggs. Urine should be collected at or near the end of micturition and the specimen let stand or centrifuged. The sediment is then smeared onto a slide and examined. When eggs are scanty, especially in chronic infections, it may be necessary to employ concentration methods (e.g., formalin-ether, acid-sodium sulphate-Triton-ether) [43,61] prior to rendering a negative diagnosis. Materials must be studied fresh, under the low power of the microscope and with attention paid to whether embryos are alive or dead; only the presence of live eggs should be interpreted as indicative of active infection. Concentration methods often kill the embryo.[61]

Ottolina [113] has shown that direct examination of biopsy specimens obtained proctoscopically is an excellent means for establishing the diagnosis. The tissue should be secured after proper preparation of the bowel.[128] Samples are taken from suspicious areas or zones of edematous hyperemic mucosa, placed on a slide, teased apart, and flattened.[155] A drop of water is then added to the sample which is gently compressed between two slides; examination is carried out immediately under low power. The technique is positive in 65 per cent of cases. Turner [150] has suggested the use of scrapings employing a spoon-shaped curette; mucus and superficial epithelium are removed and examined directly. Apparently the results obtained by this method are as good as those after biopsy. In addition scrapings are done with less difficulty or complication; after biopsy hemorrhages may require fulguration of the site.

Needle biopsy of the liver is a valuable adjunct in the diagnosis. Because of the focal character of the lesions, the core of tissue may not show the pathognomonic pseudotubercle and egg. Ishak et al.[63] have obtained positive results in 41.7 per cent of 61 patients with hepatic schistosomiasis who at the time of biopsy were excreting no eggs in the stools. In 12 others they found lesions suggestive but not diagnostic for this infection. Dimmette [35] in 189 patients obtained better results with wedge than with needle biopsy specimens. He found diagnostic lesions in 45 per cent and adult worms in 7.3 per cent of the cases. Rosenberg and Black [137] advise using part of the biopsy specimen for direct examination by compression between two glass slides; they quote Yoshizumi having found, by this method, positive results in 60 per cent of 113 individuals with negative stools. Latty et al.[76] in a comparative study of various laboratory procedures found that in some patients stools may be positive while rectal biopsies are negative and vice versa. For these reasons they advise a thorough examination of three stool samples as the first step, followed if necessary by rectal or liver biopsies.

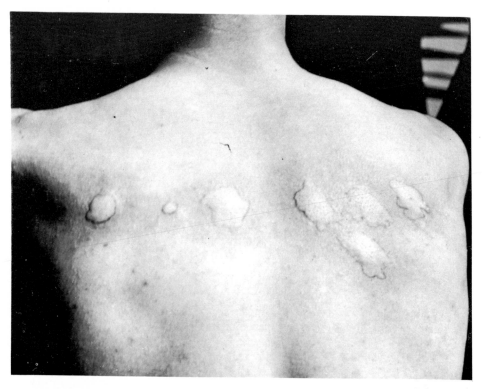

Fig. 45. Skin tests using schistosomal antigens of various nitrogen concentrations; observe large wheals with pseudopod formation and erythema. Control second from left. (Courtesy of Dr. Irving G. Kagan.)

Immunologic methods are of great value in the diagnosis of schistosomiasis. Intradermal skin test,[68,69] when carried out employing suitable antigens, gives positive results in approximately 90 per cent of adult patients. Results are not as good in children. Positivity is greater in males than in females. Positive results are also greater when the skin of the back rather than the forearm is injected. The antigen of choice is made of adult schistosomes, and the dose employed varied from 0.01 to 0.05 ml of an antigen containing 20 to 60 micrograms N per ml. The response is of the immediate type and must be read within 15 minutes. Positive reactions are characterized by the formation of a wheal with irregular edges and pseudopods measuring more than 1.1 cm (Fig. 45).

The complement-fixation test [116] employing either adult or other schistosomal antigens gives positive results in 75 to 95 per cent of patients with both acute and chronic infections. The sensitivity of the test decreases in chronic infections. Positive results can also be obtained using pleural or peritoneal exudates instead of serum. The test becomes positive early in the course of the disease; results obtained compare favorably with those following intradermal tests.

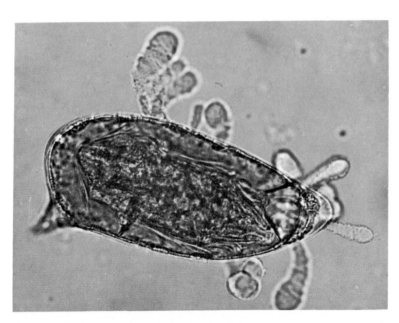

Fig. 46. S. mansoni egg incubated in immune serum showing the features of the circumoval precipitin test. × 400. (Courtesy of Dr. Irving G. Kagan.)

In the circumoval precipitin test (Oliver-Gonzalez),[110,136] schistosome eggs incubated at 37° C for two hours in serial dilutions of inactivated serum will cause the formation of globular or chainlike precipitates of various sizes around the egg shell (Fig. 46). Previous absorption of serum with live or lyophilized eggs will prevent the formation of precipitates, although absorption with cercarial or adult antigens will not interfere with the reaction. The test is species specific.[111] There is no cross reaction when eggs of *S. haematobium* or *S. japonicum* are used, and only a slight precipitate forms around *S. mansoni* eggs when used against serum of individuals infected with *S. japonicum* or *S. haematobium*. This test is also valuable in the evaluation of therapeutic cure;[112] it decreases within two months after initiation of therapy and becomes negative six months after therapy. The test gives a higher percentage of reactors in chronic than in acute infections.

The cercaria–Hüllen reaction (CHR) of Vogel and Minning[152] is characterized by the formation of a thick membrane or envelope around cercariae incubated in serum of patients with schistosomiasis. Stirewalt and Evans[146] studied the phenomenon under the phase microscope and demonstrated that the normal cuticle covering the cercariae is composed of two membranes separated from one another by a clear space about 2 to 3 microns wide. Shortly after the cercariae are exposed to the action of immune serum this space expands so that within 60 minutes it completely surrounds the entire cercarial body. Positive results are obtained in about 80 per cent of patients and the reaction becomes negative six months after therapy.

The cercarial agglutination test is based on the agglutinating properties of serum of infected patients against cercariae. Its positivity coincides with the appearance of eggs in feces. Maximum titers are achieved about 80 days postinfection.[69] Apparently the titer decreases with chronicity of the disease.

Precipitin,[69] hemagglutination,[69] flocculation,[4] and miracidial immobilization tests [69] have been used to a much lesser extent in the diagnosis of human schistosomiasis.

Recently Kagan et al.[67] have evaluated the fluorescent antibody test in the diagnosis of schistosomiasis and concluded that although it is a sensitive technique for measuring antibody to cercariae and adult schistosomes, its specificity is low due to many false positive results.

References

1. Aidaros, S.M., and Soliman, L.A.M. Portal vascular changes in human bilharzial cirrhosis. J. Path. Bact., 82:19, 1961.
2. Allen, J.F. Parasitic hematuria or bloody urine. Practitioner, 40:310, 1888.
3. Alves, W. Bilharziasis in Africa. Cent. Afr. J. Med., 3:123, 1957.
4. Anderson, R.I. Serologic diagnosis of Schistosoma mansoni infections. I. Development of a cercarial antigen slide flocculation test. Amer. J. Trop. Med., 9:299, 1960.
5. Andrade, Z.A., Paronetto, F., and Popper, H. Immunocytochemical studies in schistosomiasis. Amer. J. Path., 39:589, 1961.
6. ———— Santana, S., and Rubin, E. Hepatic changes in advanced schistosomiasis. Gastroenterology, 42:393, 1962.
7. ———— and Prata, A. Asymptomatic schistosomiasis studied by needle biopsy of the liver. Amer. J. Trop. Med., 12:854, 1963.
8. Areán, V.M. Lesions caused by Schistosoma mansoni in the genitourinary tract of men. Amer. J. Clin. Path., 26:1010, 1956.
9. ———— Manson's schistosomiasis of the female genital tract. Amer. J. Obstet. Gynec., 72:1038, 1956.
10. Ariizumi, M. Cerebral schistosomiasis japonica: Report of one operated case and fifty clinical cases. Amer. J. Trop. Med., 12:40, 1963.
11. Armbrust, A. de F. Esquistossomose da vesicula biliar. O Hospital, Rio de Janeiro, 35:467, 1949.
12. ———— Miocardite esquistossomótica (forma granulomatosa). O Hospital, 36:213, 1949.
13. ———— Lesoes geniturinárias na esquistossomosis mansoni. O Hospital, Rio de Janeiro, 38:177, 1950.
14. ———— Rare histopathologic aspects of Manson's schistosomiasis. Amer. J. Trop. Med., 6:731, 1957.
15. Ata, A. el-Hi. Hematological study of bilharzial hepatolienal fibrosis. J. Egypt. Med. Ass., 42:285, 1959.
16. Aufses, A.H., Schaffner, F., Rosenthal, W.S., and Herman, B.E. Portal venous pressure in "pipe-stem" fibrosis of the liver due to schistosomes. Amer. J. Med., 27:807, 1959.
17. Azar, J.E., Schraibman, I.G., and Pitchford, R.J. Some observations on Schistosoma haematobium in the human rectum and sigmoid. Trans. Roy. Soc. Trop. Med. Hyg., 52:562, 1958.
18. Basset, R.C., and Lowenberg, K. Cerebral schistosomiasis. J. Neuropath. Exp. Neurol., 8:220, 1949.
19. Bibawi, E. Intrasplenic pressure in course of diffuse bilharzial hepatic fibrosis. Amer. J. Trop. Med., 10:716, 1961.
20. Bilharz, T. Fernere Mitteilungen ueber Distomum Haematobium. Z. Wiss. Zool., 4:454, 1853.

21. Billings, F.L., and Hunninen, A.V. Studies on acute schistosomiasis japonica in the Philippine Islands. Bull. Hopkins Hosp., 78:21, 1946.
22. Cahill, K.M., and El Mofty, A.M.: Extra-genital cutaneous lesions in schistosomiasis. Amer. J. Trop. Med., 13:800, 1964.
23. Calabresi, P., and Abelman, W.H. Porto-caval and porto-pulmonary anastomosis in Laennec's cirrhosis and in heart failure. J. Clin. Invest., 36:1257, 1957.
24. Cerquira Falcão, E. Professor Pirajá da Silva, incontestable discoverer of "Schistosoma mansoni." Z. Tropenmed. Parasit., 10:146, 1959.
25. Charleswood, G.P., Shippel, S., and Renton, H. Schistosomiasis in gynecology, J. Obstet. Gynaec. Brit. Emp., 56:367, 1949.
26. Cheever, A.W. A comparative study of *Schistosoma mansoni* infections in mice, gerbils, multimammate rats and hamsters. Amer. J. Trop. Med., 14:211, 227, 1965.
27. Cheng, C., Chiang, S., Chang, K., Yeh, L., Li, S., Lin, C., Kuo, C., Liu, Y., and Hsiao, C. Schistosomal hypophyseal dwarfism—Study of 72 cases. Chin. Med. J., 79:26, 1959.
28. Clark, E., and Graef, I. Chronic pulmonary arteritis in schistosomiasis mansoni associated with right ventriculary hypertrophy. Amer. J. Path., 11:693, 1935.
29. Cobbold, T. Entozoa: An Introduction to the Study of Helminthology with Reference more Particularly to Internal Parasites of Man. London, Gombridge and Sons, 1864.
30. Cort, W.W. The development of the Japanese blood-fluke, *Schistosoma japonicum*, Katsurada, in its final host. Amer. J. Hyg., 1:1, 1921.
31. DeWitt, H.B., and Warren, K.S. Hepato-splenic schistosomiasis in mice. Amer. J. Trop. Med., 8:440, 1959.
32. Diaz-Rivera, R.S., Ramos-Morales, F., Koppisch, E., Garcia-Palmieri, M.R., Cintrón-Rivera, A.A., Marchand, E.J., Gonzalez, O., and Torregrosa, M.V. Acute Manson's schistosomiasis. Amer. J. Med., 21:918, 1956.
33. ———— Ramos-Morales, F., Garcia-Palmieri, M.R., and Gonzalez, O. La Esquistosomiasis aguda de Manson. El cuadro clinico. Bol. Asoc. Med. P. Rico, 49:155, 1957.
34. ———— Koppisch, E., Ramos-Morales, F., Garcia-Palmieri, M.R., and Torregrosa, M.V. La esquistosomiasis mansónica aguda. Patogénesis. Bol. Asoc. Med. P. Rico, 49:201, 1957.
35. Dimmette, R.M. Liver biopsy in clinical schistosomiasis. Gastroenterology, 29:219, 1959.
36. El-Bedri, L. Ectopic pregnancy caused by *Schistosoma haematobium* infection of the fallopian tube. Amer. J. Obstet. Gynec., 76:515, 1958.
37. El-Ghoulmy, A., Nabawy, M., Mondough, G., Aidaros, S., and Omar, A. Hepatic schistosomiasis in children. J. Trop. Med. Hyg., 58:25, 1955.
38. Erfan, M. Pulmonary schistosomiasis. Trans. Roy. Soc. Trop. Med. Hyg., 42:109, 1948.
39. ———— Erfan, H., Mousa, A.M., and Deeb, A.A. Pulmonary schistosomiasis. Trans. Roy. Soc. Trop. Med. Hyg., 42:477, 1949.
40. Farid, Z., Greer, J.W., Ishak, K.G., El Nagah, A.M., LeGolvan, P.C., and Mousa, A.H. Chronic pulmonary schistosomiasis. Amer. Rev. Tuberc. Pulm. Dis., 79:119, 1959.
41. Faust, E.C., and Meleney, H.E. Studies on schistosomiasis japonica. Monograph. Ser. Amer. J. Hyg., No. 3, 1924.
42. ———— Jones, C.A., and Hoffman, W.A. Studies on schistosomiasis mansoni in Puerto Rico. III. Biological studies. 2. The mammalian phase of the life cycle. Puerto Rico J. Pub. Health Trop. Med., 10:133, 1934.
43. ———— and Russell, P.F. Clinical Parasitology, 7th ed. Philadelphia, Lea & Febiger, 1964, Ch. 27.
44. Fujinami. Quoted by Shimidzu, K. Arch. Klin. Chir., 182:401, 1935.
45. Garcia-Palmieri, M.R., Rafucci, F.L., Diaz-Bonnet, L.A., and Bernal-Rosa, J.F.

Shunt surgery for portal hypertension due to *Schistosoma mansoni:* evaluation and management in 41 cases. J.A.M.A., 171:268, 1959.

46. Garcia-Palmieri, M.R., and Marcial-Rojas, R.A. The protein manifestations of schistosomiasis mansoni: A clinicopathologic evaluation. Ann. Intern. Med., 57:763, 1962.

47. Gelfand, M. Schistosomiasis in South Central Africa. The Postgraduate. Cape Town and Johannesburg, Pross-Juta and Co., Ltd., 1950.

48. ———— Alves, W., and Woods, R.W. The frequency of schistosomal ovideposition in the heart. Trans. Roy. Soc. Trop. Med. Hyg., 53:282, 1959.

49. Gonzalez Martinez, I. Refiriendo a un estudio de la bilharzia hematobium y bilharziosis en Puerto Rico. Rev. Med. Trop., Havana, 5:193, 1904.

50. Greenfield, J.G., and Pritchard, B. Cerebral infection with *Schistosoma japonica.* Brain, 60:361, 1937.

51. Guirguis, S., and El-Kateb, H. Bilharziasis of the adrenal glands. J. Trop. Med. Hyg., 62:103, 1959.

52. Hamilton, P.K., Hutchison, H.S., Jamison, P.W., and Jones, H.L. The pathology and pathogenesis of hepatosplenic disease associated with schistosomiasis. Amer. J. Clin. Path., 32:18, 1959.

53. Hammarsten, J.F. Diagnosis of cerebral schistosomiasis. Arch. Neurol. Psych., 79:132, 1957.

54. Haubrick, W.S., and Wells, R.M. Carcinoma coexisting with Manson's schistosomiasis. Amer. J. Dig. Dis., 2:335, 1957.

55. Hervé, P.A., Piganiol, G., and Tyssandier. Les complications genitales de la bilharziose urinaire chez l'homme. Bull. Soc. Path. Exot., 50:567, 1957.

56. ———— and Piganiol, G. Données récents dans la bilharziose urinaire. Ann. Inst. Med. Trop. (Lisboa), 15:647, 1958.

57. Hoeppli, R. Histological observations in experimental schistosoma japonicum. Chin. Med. J., 46:1179, 1932.

58. Honey, M., and Gelfant, M. Urological aspects of bilharziasis in Rhodesia. Cent. Afr. J. Med., 6:1, 58, 109, 153, 199, 248, 1960.

59. Horrax, G., Rodriguez, J.M.R., and Castillo, R. Lesiones medulares de origen bilharziano. Gaz. Med. Caracas, 64:253, 1956.

60. Huang, M., Chiang, S., and Lu, C. Schistosomiasis dwarfism. Chin. Med. J., 80:437, 1960.

61. Hunter, G.W., Frye, W.W., and Swartzwelder, J.C. A Manual of Tropical Medicine, 3rd ed. Philadelphia, W.B. Saunders Co., 1960.

62. Ibrahim, M., and Girgis, B. Bilharzial cor pulmonale: A clinico-pathological report of 50 cases. J. Trop. Med. Hyg., 63:55, 1960.

63. Ishak, K.G., LeGolvan, P.C., Salib, M., Sabour, M., and Nooman, Z. Needle biopsy of the liver and spleen in schistosomiasis. Amer. J. Clin. Path., 31:46, 1959.

64. Jackson, J.H. Bilharzia. A background to its endemicity and control in Africa, with particular reference to irrigation schemes. S. Afr. J. Lab. Clin. Med., 4:1, 1958.

65. Jawahiry, K.I., and Karpas, C.M. Pulmonary schistosomiasis: Detailed clinico-pathologic study. Amer. Rev. Resp. Dis., 88:517, 1963.

66. Joshi, R.A. Bilateral total infarction of the testis due to schistosomiasis of the spermatic cord. Amer. J. Trop. Med., 11:357, 1962.

67. Kagan, I.G., Sulzer, A.J., and Carver, K. An evaluation of the fluorescent antibody test for the diagnosis of schistosomiasis. Amer. J. Epidemiol., 81:63, 1965.

68. ———— Pellegrino, J., and Memoria, J.M.P. Studies on the standardization of the intradermal test for the diagnosis of bilharziasis. Amer. J. Trop. Med., 10:200, 1961.

69. ———— and Pellegrino, J. A critical review of immunological methods for the diagnosis of bilharziasis. Bull. W.H.O., 25:611, 1961.

70. Kane, C.A., and Most, H. Schistosomiasis of the central nervous system. Experiences in World War II and a review of the literature. Arch. Neurol. Psych., 59:141, 1948.

71. Kohlschütter, E., and Koppisch, E. On the mode of extrusion of schistosome ova from the blood vessel into the tissues. Schweiz. Z. Path. Bakt., 4:357, 1941.

72. Koppisch, E. Estudios sobre la esquistosomiasis de Manson en Puerto Rico. IV. Alteraciones anatomopathologicas en el conejo y rata albina inoculados experimentalmente con el S. mansoni. Puerto Rican J. Pub. Health. Trop. Med., 13:55, 1937.

73. ——— Studies on schistosomiasis mansoni in Puerto Rico. VI. Morbid anatomy of the disease as found in Puerto Ricans. Puerto Rican J. Pub. Health Trop. Med., 16:395, 1940–1941.

74. Krakower, C., Hoffman, W.A., and Axmayer, J.H. Portal-systemic collateral veins in the guinea pig with schistosomal cirrhosis of the liver. Arch. Path., 36:39, 1943.

75. Lanoix, J.M. Relation between irrigation engineering and bilharziasis. Bull. W.H.O., 18:1011, 1958.

76. Latty, S.G., Hunter, G.W., Moon, A.P., Sullivan, B.H., Burke, J.C., and Sproat, H.F. Studies on schistosomiasis. X. Comparison of stool examination, skin test, rectal biopsy and liver biopsy for detection of *Schistosoma mansoni*. Gastroenterology, 27:324, 1954.

77. Leiper, R.T. Report on the results of the Bilharzia Mission in Egypt. J. Roy. Army Med. Corps, 25:1, 1915.

78. Letulle, M. Un cas de bilharziase intestinale contracté a la Martinique. Rev. Med. d'Hyg. Trop., 1:46, 1904.

79. Lewert, R.M., and Lee, C.L. Studies on the passage of helminth larvae through host tissues. I. Histochemical studies on extracellular changes caused by penetrating larvae. II. Enzymatic activity of larvae in vitro and in vivo. J. Infect. Dis., 95:13, 1954.

80. ——— Invasiveness of helminth larvae. Rice Institute Pamphlet, 45:97, 1958.

81. ——— and Mandlowitz, S. Innate immunity to *Schistosoma mansoni* relative to the state of connective tissue. Ann. N.Y. Acad. Sci., 113:54, 1963.

82. Lichtenberg, F. Lesions of intrahepatic portal radicles in Manson's schistosomiasis. Amer. J. Path., 31:757, 1955.

83. ——— Studies on granuloma formation. III. Antigen sequestration and destruction in the schistosome pseudotubercle. Amer. J. Path., 45:75, 1964.

84. Lopes de Faria, J. Cor pulmonale in Manson's schistosomiasis. I. Frequency in necropsy material; pulmonary vascular changes caused by schistosome ova. Amer. J. Path., 30:167, 1954.

85. ——— Pulmonary vascular changes in schistosomal cor pulmonale. J. Path. Bact., 68:589, 1954.

86. ——— Pulmonary arterio-venous fistula and arterial distribution of eggs of *Schistosoma mansoni*. Amer. J. Trop. Med., 5:860, 1956.

87. ——— Czapski, J.M., Leite, M.O.R., Penna, D. de O., Fujioka, T., and Cintra, A.B. de U. Cyanosis in Manson's schistosomiasis: role of pulmonary schistosomatic arteriovenous fistulas. Amer. Heart J., 54:196, 1957.

88. ——— Barbas, J.V., Fujioka, T., Lion, M.F., Silva, U. de A., and Decourt, L.V. Pulmonary schistosomatic arteriovenous fistulas producing a new cyanotic syndrome in Manson's schistosomiasis. Amer. J. Hyg., 58:556, 1959.

89. Lutz, A. Schistosomum mansoni e a schistomatose segundo observações feitas no Brazil, Mem. Inst. Oswald Cruz, 11:121, 1919.

90. Magalhaes, H.M., Filho, A., Krupp, I.M., and Malek, E.A. Localization of antigen and presence of antibody in tissues of mice infected with *S. mansoni* as indicated by fluorescent antibody techniques. Amer. J. Trop. Med., 14:84, 1965.

91. Makar, N. Some surgical aspects of bilharziasis. Xéme. Cong. Soc. Intern. Chirurg., Cairo, 3:561, 1935.

92. ——— A note on the pathogenesis of cancer in the bilharzial bladder. Brit. J. Surg., 45:240, 1957.

93. Maldonado, J.F. The longevity of the unhatched miracidium of *S. mansoni* in the liver of mice. Amer. J. Trop. Med., 8:16, 1959.

94. ——— The host parasite relationships in schistosomiasis mansoni. Bol. Asoc. Med. P. Rico, 51:228, 1959.

95. Manson, P. Report of a case of bilharzia from the West Indies. J. Trop. Med., 5:384, 1902.

96. Marchand, E.J., Marcial-Rojas, R.A., Rodriguez, R., Polanco, G., and Diaz-Rivera, R.S. The pulmonary obstruction syndrome in *Schistosoma mansoni* pulmonary endarteritis. Arch. Intern. Med., 100:965, 1957.

97. ——— de Jesus, M., and Biaschoechea, Z.A.R. Cyanotic syndrome in portal hypertension in hepato-splenic schistosomiasis and portal cirrhosis. Amer. J. Cardiol., 10:496, 1962.

98. Marcial-Rojas, R.A., and Fiol, R.E. Neurologic complications of schistosomiasis. Review of the literature and report of two cases of transverse myelitis due to *S. mansoni*. Ann. Intern. Med., 59:215, 1963.

99. Meleney, H.E., Sandground, J.H., Moore, D.V., Most, H., and Carney, B.H. The histopathology of experimental schistosomiasis. II. Bisexual infections with *S. mansoni, S. japonicum,* and *S. hematobium.* Amer. J. Trop. Med., 2:883, 1953.

100. Monteiro de Barros, O., Giannoni, F.G., Marigo, C., and Frizzo, F.J. Cor pulmonale é miocardite esquistosomóticos. Arq. Hosp. Santa Casa de São Paulo, 2:33, 1956.

101. Most, H., and Levine, D.I. Schistosomiasis in American tourists. J.A.M.A., 186:453, 1963.

102. Motta, L. da C., and Elejalde, G. Presença de ovos de esquistosomo de Manson em fibroma uterino. Ann. Fac. Med. Univ. São Paulo, 19:253, 1943.

103. Mousa, A.H., and El-Garem, A. The haemodynamic study of Egyptian hepato-splenic bilharziosis. J. Egypt. Med. Ass., 42:444, 1959.

104. Mustachi, P., and Shimkin, M.B. Cancer of the bladder and infestation with *Schistosoma hematobium.* J. Nat. Cancer Inst., 20:825, 1958.

105. Mynors, J.M. Infestational schistosomiasis resembling regional ileitis. Trans. Roy. Soc. Trop. Med. Hyg., 51:45, 1957.

106. Naeye, R.L. Advanced pulmonary vascular changes in schistosomal cor pulmonale. Amer. J. Trop. Med., 10:191, 1961.

107. Nagaty, H.F., Moawa, D., and Salem, S. Papular skin lesions in which schistosome eggs were found. Amer. J. Trop. Med., 6:266, 1957.

108. Nayat, M.G.H. Ectopic pregnancy in a tube infested with bilharzia. S. Afr. Med. J., 33:219, 1959.

109. Nosny, Y. La bilharziose génito-urinaire (etude anatomopathologique). Bull. Soc. Path. Exot., 56:999, 1963.

110. Oliver-Gonzalez, J. Anti-egg precipitin in the serum of humans infested with *S. mansoni.* J. Infect. Dis., 95:86, 1954.

111. ——— Bauman, P.M., and Benenson, A.S. Species specificity of the anti-egg precipitin in schistosome serums. J. Infect. Dis., 96:95, 1955.

112. ——— Ramos, F.L., and Coker, C.M. Serological reactions against egg antigens as an aid in the evaluation of therapy in schistosomiasis. Amer. J. Trop. Med., 4:908, 1955.

113. Ottolina, C. The rectoscopic biopsy by transparency. A new diagnostic method for schistosomiasis mansoni. Amer. J. Trop. Med., 27:603, 1947.

114. Paul, R. Pulmonary schistosomiasis. Cent. Afr. J. Med., 2:355, 1956.

115. Pautrizel, R., Tribouley, J., and Duret, J. L'activité transaminasique du serum chez des sujets bilharziennes avant et après traitement par le dimercapto-suceinate d'antimoine sodique. Bull. Soc. Path. Exot., 56:992, 1963.

116. Pellegrino, J., and Pedreira de Freitas, J.L. Quantitative complement fixation test in schistosomiasis mansoni. Amer. J. Trop. Med., 10:537, 1961.

117. Pepler, W.J., and Lombard, C.M. Spinal cord granuloma due to *Schistoma haematobium.* J. Neuropath. Exp. Neurol., 17:656, 1958.

118. Perez, V., and Schaffner, F. Pathologic features of pipe-stem fibrosis of the liver due to schistosomiasis. J. Mount Sinai Hosp., N.Y., 26:544, 1959.

119. Pinto, C., and Almeida, A.F. Schistosomiasis mansoni no Brazil. Rio de Janeiro, Imprensa Nacional, 1948.
120. Pirajá da Silva, M. Contribucão para o estudo da eschistosomiase na Bahia. Brazil. Med., 22:281, 1908.
121. ——— La eschistosomose a Bahia. Arch. Parasit. Paris, 13:283, 1909.
122. Prates, M.D., and Gillman, J. Carcinoma of the urinary bladder in the Portuguese East African, with special reference to bilharzial cystitis and pre-neoplastic reactions. S. Afr. J. Med., 24:13, 1959.
123. Prinzmetal, M., Ornitz, E.M., Simkin, B., and Bergman, H.C. Arterio-venous anastomoses in liver, spleen and lung. Amer. J. Physiol., 152:48, 1948.
124. Ragheb, M. Schistosomiasis of the liver. Clinical, pathologic, and laboratory studies in Egyptian cases. Gastroenterology, 30:631, 1956.
125. Ramirez, E.A., Rivera, A., Serrano, D., and Cancio, M. Electrophoretic serum protein studies in chronic human Manson's schistosomiasis. Amer. J. Trop. Med., 10:530, 1961.
126. Ramos, O.L., Saad, F., and Leser, W.P. Portal hemodynamics and liver cell function in hepatic schistosomiasis. Gastroenterology, 47:241, 1964.
127. Raper, A.B. Cerebral schistosomiasis. E. Afr. Med. J., 25:262, 1948.
128. Recio, P.M. The diagnosis and treatment of colorectal schistosomiasis. Dis. Colon Rectum, 30:110, 1958.
129. Richert, J.H., and Krakauer, R.B. Diffuse pulmonary schistosomiasis. Report of two cases proved by lung biopsy. J.A.M.A., 169:1302, 1959.
130. Ritchie, L.S., and Jachowski, L.A. "Bilharzia": A military hazard in Puerto Rico. Milit. Med., 125:253, 1960.
131. Rivera, R.S.D., Morales, F.R., Sotomayor, Z.R., Lichtenberg, F., Garcia-Palmieri, M.R., Rivera, A.A.C., and Marchand, E.J. The pathogenesis of Manson's schistosomiasis. Ann. Intern. Med., 47:1082, 1957.
132. Rodgriguez, H.F., Garcia-Palmieri, M.R., Rivera, J.V., and Rodriguez-Molina, R. A comparative study of portal and bilharzial cirrhosis. Gastroenterology, 29:235, 1955.
133. ——— and Rivera, E. Pulmonary schistosomiasis. New Eng. J. Med., 258:1196, 1958.
134. ——— Fernandez-Durán, A., Garcia-Moliner, L., and Rivera, E. Cardiopulmonary schistosomiasis. Amer. Heart J., 65:253, 1963.
135. ——— Schistosomal hepato-splenomegaly. Bol. Asoc. Med. P. Rico, 48:393, 1956.
136. Rodriguez-Molina, R., Oliver-Gonzalez, J., and Serrano, D.G. Studies on the immunity of schistosomiasis mansoni: evaluation of the circumoval precipitin tests as a diagnostic procedure in clinical schistosomiasis mansoni. Report of 46 cases. Bol. Asoc. Med. P. Rico, 48:389, 1956.
137. Rosenberg, E., and Black, H. The value of biopsy cores of fresh hepatic tissue in the diagnosis of schistosomiasis. Amer. J. Clin. Path., 32:472, 1959.
138. Ruffer, M.A. Remarks on the histology and pathological anatomy of Egyptian mummies. Cairo Scient. J., 4:3, 1910.
139. Rydell, R., and Hoffbauer, W.W. Multiple pulmonary arteriovenous fistulas in juvenile cirrhosis. Amer. J. Med., 21:450, 1956.
140. Sambon, L.W. What is *Schistosoma mansoni?* Sambon J. Trop. Med. Hyg., 12:1, 1909.
141. Sanjurjo, L.A., and Koppisch, E. Manson's schistosomiasis with unilateral involvement of the kidney. J. Urol., 66:298, 1951.
142. Seif-Eldin, D. Bilharziasis of the fallopian tubes and ovaries. J. Obstet. Gynaec. Brit. Emp., 65:457, 1958.
143. Shaw, A.F., and Ghareeb, A.A. The pathogenesis of pulmonary schistosomiasis in Egypt with special reference to Ayerza's disease. J. Path. Bact., 46:401, 1938.
144. Shimidzu, K. An operated case of schistosomiasis cerebri. Arch. Klin. Chir., 182:401, 1935.

145. Soto, V.R. Naturaleza de la disenteria en Caracas. Tésis Doctoral en Ciencias Médicas, Univ. de Caracas, 1906.
146. Stirewalt, M.A., and Evans, A.S. Serological reactions in *Schistosoma mansoni* infections. I. Cercarial, precipitation, agglutination and CHR phenomena. Exp. Parasit., 4:123, 1955.
147. ——— and Kruidenier, F.J. Activity of the acetabular secretory apparatus of cercariae of *Schistosoma mansoni* under experimental conditions. Exp. Parasit., 11:191, 1961.
148. ——— Chemical biology of secretions of larval helminths. Ann. N.Y. Acad. Sci., 113:36, 1963.
149. Symmers, W.S.C. Note on a new form of liver cirrhosis due to the presence of the ova of *Bilharzia haematobiae*. J. Path. Bact., 9:237, 1904.
150. Turner, J.A. Diagnosis of *Schistosoma mansoni* infection by rectal scrapings: a comparison with rectal biopsy and fecal examination. Amer. J. Trop. Med., 11:620, 1962.
151. Vogel, H. Uber Entwicklung, Lebensdauer und Tod der Eier von *Bilharzia japonicum* im Wirtsgewebe. Deutsch. Tropenmed. Z., 46:57, 1942.
152. ——— and Minning, W. Hüllenbildung bei Bilharziacercarien im Serum bilharziainfizierter Tiere und Menschen. Zbl. Bakt., Parasitenk., Abt. I. Orig., 153:91, 1949.
153. Wallerstein, R.S. Longevity of *Schistosoma mansoni:* observations found on one case. Amer. J. Trop. Med., 29:717, 1949.
154. Walters, J.H., and Mody, V.R. The incubation period of *Schistosoma mansoni* in man. Trans. Roy. Soc. Trop. Med. Hyg., 56:250, 1962.
155. Warner, B.W. The role of the proctologist in the diagnosis of schistosomiasis mansoni by sigmoidoscopy and rectal biopsy. New York J. Med., 56:3137, 1956.
156. Weir, J.M. The unconquered plague. Confidential Report. Rockefeller Institute, 1961.
157. Zaher, M.F., Badr, M.M., and Fawzy, R.M. Bilharzial urinary fistula. J. Egypt. Med. Ass., 42:412, 1959.
158. Zaky, H.A., El-Heneidy, A.R., Tawfick, I.M., Gemei, Y., and Khadr, A.A. Bronchopulmonary shunts in schistosomal cor pulmonale. Dis. Chest., 39:164, 1959.

Addendum

There has been a voluminous literature published on schistosomiasis during the past decade. Limitations in space will permit only a brief summary of the most salient achievements; the interested reader should consult the pertinent references for detailed information.

It is now firmly established that the severity of the granulomatous reaction in schistosomiasis is dependent foremost on the number of eggs deposited by the parasite;[1-4] although other factors (species of schistosome involved, variability in degree of virulence of different strains, reactivity of the host, etc)[5,6] play an important role, the close relationship between egg burden and extent of histologic changes has been corroborated in experimental animals whereby antischistosomal therapy given early in the course of the infection prevents the development of permanent lesions. The bilharzial granuloma has been studied by

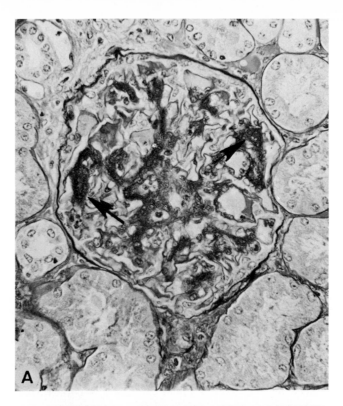

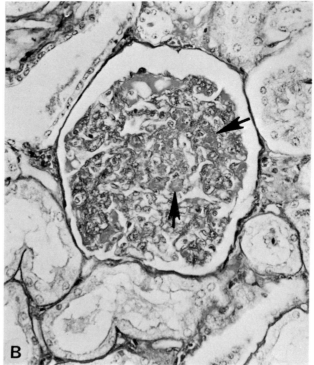

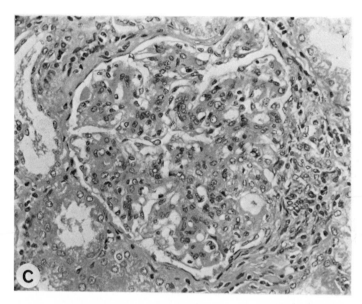

Fig. 1. A. Glomerulus of a chimpanzee exhibiting increase in mesangial matrix and mesangial cell hypercellularity (arrows). The mesangial matrix is comprised of large numbers of PAS-positive fibrils. There is narrowing of some capillary loops and wrinkling of glomerular basement membranes. PAS. Approximately × 250. B. Glomerulus with marked proliferation of cells. Numerous PAS-positive droplets (arrows) are evident. The capillary lumen is reduced in most peripheral loops. PAS. Approximately × 250. C. Glomerulus showing mesangial hypercellularity, sclerosis, and thickening of capillary loops. Periglomerular inflammation and capsular fibrosis are evident. H&E. Approximately × 220. (Courtesy, Dr. Tito Cavallo, Am J Pathol 76:433, 1974).

multidisciplinary methods at various stages of its evolution.[7-10] The chronic phase of this granuloma is believed to be a manifestation of cell-mediated immunity.[5, 11-15]

The development of experimental animal models with schistosomal lesions resembling or identical with those found in human infections [2, 3, 16-19] has greatly enhanced our understanding of the pathophysiology of schistosomiasis and proven singularly helpful in the evaluation of chemotherapeutic antischistosomal drugs.[20, 21]

Vinyl casts of the hepatic vasculature made from human autopsy material have demonstrated pronounced distortion and obstructive lesions of the portal branches especially marked at the periphery of the liver.[18, 22-25] Angiographic studies in human and experimental material have supplemented these observations.[26] Also found was a rich venous network in the portal tracts arising from the peribiliary venous system, as well as an increase in the size and number of intrahepatic-arterial vessels. The last finding explains why patients with hepatosplenic schistosomiasis and portal hypertension have normal hepatic blood flow and normal function tests.[27] On the other hand, the liver in these patients is highly dependent upon arterial blood supply, and any serious drop in systemic blood pressure may result in focal extensive hepatocellular coagulative necrosis.

Glomerular lesions similar to those described in patients with liver cirrhosis [28-30] have been observed also in hepatosplenic schistosomiasis. In a review of 80 autopsies of patients with this syndrome, 36 percent were noted to have glomerular changes characterized by fibrillary, PAS-positive thickening of the mesangial stalks involving diffusely the vascular pole and decreasing in severity toward the periphery of the tufts. The basement membrane was normal or focally thickened. These observations have been confirmed by other investigators in both clinical and experimental material.[9, 31-36] The severity of the glomerular lesions is proportional to the degree of hepatic fibrosis and the intensity of the infection. In the early stages only occasional glomeruli show an increase in mesangial matrix expansion and mesangial cell proliferation with hyaline droplets (Fig. 1). As the disease progresses, the glomeruli become enlarged and there is proliferation of capsular epithelium, thickening of basement membrane, and eventually capsular adhesions, glomerular scars, and epithelial crescents. Antischistosomal therapy stops the progression of these lesions (Fig. 2). In patients with hepatosplenic schistosomiasis without clinical evidence of renal disease, light microscopy may show no obvious changes although ultrastructurally there is deposition of electron dense material and laminated bodies near mesangial cells (Fig. 3). Immunofluorescent studies have demonstrated IgG along glomerular capillary walls and occasionally IgM and B1C. Neither in humans nor in experimental animals have schistosomal antigens been demonstrated in glomerular lesions. Schistosomal antigens have been demonstrated in urine of animals with heavy infections.[37] The findings of circulating DNA and DNA antibodies in patients and experimental animals with heavy schistosomal infections and the recent demonstration of increased amounts in the kidneys of animals with schistosomiasis suggest a possible role of DNA–anti DNA antibody complexes in the pathogenesis of these lesions.

In areas of great endemicity, the incidence of urinary complications (hydronephrosis, hydroureter, pyelonephritis) is extremely high, with 37 percent of schoolchildren showing irreversible lesions.[38, 39] There is sound clinical and experimental evidence that antischistosomal therapy induces regression of lesions in a good many patients.

Schistosomiasis due to *S. intercalatum* has been described in Zaire, Gabon, Central Africa Republic, the Cameroons, and probably exists in Upper Volta, Nigeria, and Chad.[40] The infection may be asymptomatic or cause abdominal pain, blood and mucus in stool, and weight loss. Liver involvement is rare. The eggs are longer and more slender than those of *S. haematobium* and possess a long terminal spine. They are more often found in feces than in urine and may be seen in snip biopsies of the intestinal mucosa. They are acid fast positive, whereas ova of *S. haematobium*, with which they may be confused, are nonacid fast. The parasite seems to induce a lesser degree of antibody response than other species. The indirect fluorescent antibody technic has proven to be most sensitive and reliable when adequate cryostat sections of adult worm are employed.

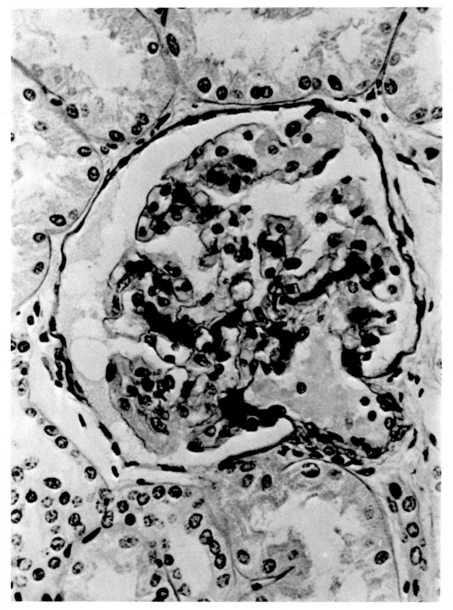

Fig. 2. Glomerulus of a chimpanzee treated within three months postinoculation and killed 16 months after. Note focal distribution of mesangial expansion and normal basement membrane. PAS. × 185. (Courtesy, Dr. Franz von Lichtenberg, in Am J Trop Med Hyg 23:639, 1974.)

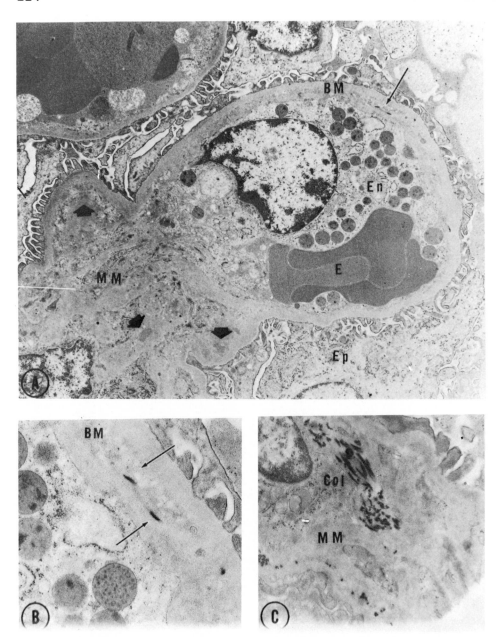

Fig. 3. All photomicrographs are from the same glomerulus. A. A portion of glomerulus with marked mesangial expansion and irregular masses of granular electron-dense material (short arrows) in the mesangial matrix (MM). Collagen fibers (long arrow) are present in a thickened basement membrane (BM). Approximately × 13,500. B. Detail of A showing collagen fibers (arrows) between layers of basement membrane (BM). Approximately × 19,550. C. Mature collagen (Col) present in the mesangial matrix (MM). Approximately × 20,400.

References

1. Block EH, Wahab MFA, Warren KS: In vivo microscopic observations of the pathology and pathophysiology of hepatosplenic schistosomiasis in the mouse liver. Am J Trop Med Hyg 21:546, 1972
2. Cheever AW: A comparative study of Schistosoma mansoni infections in mice, gerbils, multimammate rats and hamsters. I. The relationship of portal hypertension to size of hepatic granulomas. Am J Trop Med Hyg 14:211, 1965; II. Qualitative pathological differences. Am J Trop Med Hyg 14:227, 1965
3. Cheever AW, Erickson DG, Sadun EH, von Lichtenberg F: Schistosoma japonicum infection in monkeys and baboons: parasitological and pathological findings. Am J Trop Med Hyg 23:51, 1974
4. Erickson DG, Jones CE, Tan DB: Schistosomiasis in hamsters: the relationship of egg concentration in the liver to disease. Am J Trop Med Hyg 23:449, 1974
5. Warren KS: The immunopathogenesis of schistosomiasis: a multidisciplinary approach. Trans R Soc Trop Med Hyg 66:416, 1972
6. Warren KS: A comparison of Puerto Rican, Brazilian, Egyptian and Tansanian strains of Schistosoma mansoni in mice. Trans R Soc Trop Med Hyg 61:795, 1967
7. Bogitsh BJ, Wikel SK: Schistosoma mansoni: ultrastructural observations on the small intestine of the murine host. Exp Parasitol 35:68, 1974
8. Li Hsu, Hsu HF, Lost GK, Davis JR: Organized epithelioid cell granulomata elicited by Schistosoma eggs in experimental animals. J Reticuloendothel Soc 12:418, 1972
9. Race GJ, Martin JH, Moore DV, Larsch JE: Scanning and transmission electron-microscopy of the Schistosoma mansoni eggs, cercariae and adults. Am J Trop Med Hyg 22:914, 1972
10. von Lichtenberg F, Smith JH, Cheever AW: The Hoeppli phenomenon in schistosomiasis: comparative pathology and morphology. Am J Trop Med Hyg 15:886, 1966
11. Boros DL, Warren KS: Delayed hypersensitivity type granuloma formation and dermal reaction induced and elicited by a soluble factor isolated from Schistosoma mansoni eggs. J Exp Med 132:488, 1970
12. Domingo EO, Warren KS: The inhibition of granuloma formation around Schistosoma mansoni eggs. Am J Pathol 51:757, 1967
13. Dunsford HA, Lucia HL, Doughty BL, von Lichtenberg F: Artificial granulomas using bentonite and latex carrier particles. Am J Trop Med Hyg 23:203, 1974
14. Stenger RJ, Warren KS, Johnson EA: An ultrastructural study of hepatic granulomas and schistosoma egg shells in murine hepatosplenic Schistosomiasis mansoni. Exp Parasitol 7:116, 1967
15. Warren KS, Domingo EO, Cowan BT: Granuloma formation around Schistosoma eggs and a manifestation of delayed hypersensitivity. Am J Pathol 51:735, 1967
16. Sadun EH, von Lichtenberg F, Hickman RL, et al: Schistosoma mansoni in the chimpanzee: parasitological, clinical, serological, pathological and radiological observations. Am J Trop Med Hyg 15:496, 1966
17. Sadun EH, Cheever AW, Erickson DG, Hickman RL: Experimental infection with Schistosoma haematobium in chimpanzees: parasitological, clinical, serological, and pathological observations. Am J Trop Med Hyg 19:427, 1970
18. von Lichtenberg F, Sadun EH: Experimental production of bilharzial pipe-stem fibrosis in the chimpanzee. Exp Parasitol 22:264, 1968
19. Warren KS: The pathology of "clay stem-pipe cirrhosis" in mice with chronic schistosomiasis mansoni with a note on the longevity of the schistosome. Am J Pathol 49:477, 1966
20. Cheever AW, deWitt WB, Warren KS: Repeated infections and treatment of mice with schistosomiasis mansoni: functional anatomic and immunologic observations. Am J Trop Med Hyg 14:239, 1965

21. Sadun EH, von Lichtenberg F, Erickson DG, et al: Effects of chemotherapy on the evolution of Schistosoma japonicum in chimpanzees. Am J Trop Med Hyg 23:639, 1974

22. Andrade ZA, Cheever AW: Alterations in the intrahepatic vasculature in hepatosplenic schistosomiasis mansoni. Am J Trop Med Hyg 2:425, 1971

23. Cheever AW, Warren KS: Hepatic blood flow in mice with acute hepatosplenic schistosomiasis. Trans R Soc Trop Med Hyg 58:496, 1964

24. Cheever AW, Kunz RE, Myers BJ, et al: Schistosoma haematobium in African hamadryas and gelada baboons. Am J Trop Med Hyg 23:429, 1974

25. von Lichtenberg F, Sadun EH, Cheever AW, et al: Experimental infection with Schistosoma japonicum in chimpanzees. Am J Trop Med Hyg 20:850, 1971

26. Hillyer GV, Lewert RM: Studies on renal pathology in hamsters infected with Schistosoma mansoni and japonicum. Am J Trop Med Hyg 23:404, 1974

27. Ramos-Morales F, Sotomayor ZR, Diaz-Rivera RS, Correa Ramos R: Manson's schistosomiasis in Puerto Rico: clinical analysis of 1845 untreated patients. Bull NY Acad Med 44:316, 1968

28. Bloodworth JMB Jr., Sommers SC: "Cirrhotic glomerulosclerosis," a renal lesion associated with hepatic cirrhosis. Lab Invest 8:962, 1959

29. Fisher ER, Perez-Stable E: Cirrhotic lobular glomerulosclerosis: a correlation of ultrastructure and clinical features. Am J Pathol 52:869, 1968

30. Sakaguchi H, Dachs S, Grishman E, et al: Hepatic glomerulosclerosis: an electron microscopic study of renal biopsies in liver disease. Lab Invest 15:533, 1965

31. Andrade ZA, Andrade SG, Sagigursky M: Renal changes in patients with hepatosplenic schistosomiasis. Am J Trop Med Hyg 20:77, 1971

32. Andrade ZA, Susin M: Renal changes in mice infected with Schistosoma mansoni. Am J Trop Med Hyg 23:400, 1974

33. Brito T, Gunji J, Camargo ME, et al: Advanced kidney disease in patients with hepatosplenic schistosomiasis. Rev Inst Med Trop Sao Paulo 12:225, 1970

34. Cavallo T, Galvanek ES, Ward PA, von Lichtenberg F: The nephropathy of experimental schistosomiasis. Am J Pathol 76:433, 1974

35. Queivos FP, Brito E, Martinelli R, Rocha H: Nephrotic syndrome in patients with Schistosoma mansoni infections. Am J Trop Med Hyg 22:622, 1972

36. Silva LC, Brito T, Camargo M, et al: Kidney biopsy in the hepatosplenic form of infection with Schistosoma mansoni in man. Bull WHO 42:907, 1970

37. Berggren WL, Weller T: Immunoelectrophoresis demonstration of specific antigen in animals infected with Schistosoma mansoni. Am J Trop Med Hyg 16:606, 1967

38. Forsyth DM, McDonald G: Urological complications of endemic schistosomiasis in school children. Trans R Soc Trop Med Hyg 59:171, 1965

39. Lehman JS, Farrid Z, Bassily S, Kent DC: Hydronephrosis and bacteriuria and maximal urine concentration in urinary schistosomiasis. Ann Intern Med 75:49, 1971

40. Wolfe MS: Schistosoma intercalatum infection in an American family. Am J Trop Med Hyg 23:45, 1974

THE DIFFERENTIAL DIAGNOSIS OF COLITIS

VINCENT J. McGOVERN

The colon may be involved in a large number of inflammatory and ulcerative processes, many of which are erroneously labelled ulcerative colitis. Among those most frequently confused with ulcerative colitis are Crohn's (granulomatous) colitis, ischemic colitis, and pseudomembranous colitis. Each of these has distinct pathologic features, and it is important that they be recognized since each condition requires its own specific management and therapy.

Ulcerative Colitis

Acute Ulcerative Colitis

In acute ulcerative colitis prior to ulceration, the mucosa is congested and edematous, often with pinpoints of hemorrhage (Figs. 1, 2). The submucosa is thickened by congestion and edema, and even the muscular coat may be thicker than normal. In very acute or fulminant cases, the bowel may be dilated so that the edema is not obvious. Surprisingly, the serosa in ulcerative colitis seldom gives much indication of the florid disease that becomes apparent when the bowel is opened. Ulcers tend to be orientated in a longitudinal fashion, overlying the taeniae and may extend down to the muscle coat. Transverse ulcers are also formed and penetrate to a variable depth. Mucosal tags and bridges are formed by undermining ulceration, and this process can result in large areas of denudation. Perforations occur mainly in the dilated bowel of the acute or fulminant disease.

Naked eye diagnosis depends upon recognizing that the unulcerated mucosa throughout the affected bowel is not normal. Even when it is not reddened it is thickened and velvety, having lost the bright sheen of normal mucosa. It is from

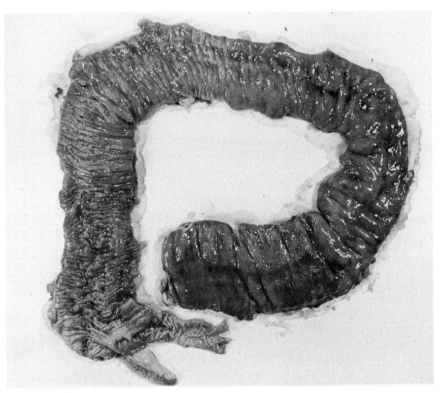

Fig. 1. Resected colon from a 32-year-old female patient with clinically fulminant colitis of 18 days duration. It is edematous, and there are pinpoint hemorrhages but no ulcers.

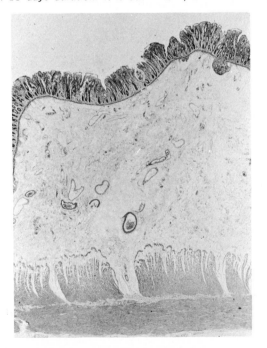

Fig. 2. Photomicrograph of whole thickness of bowel in Figure 1. Submucosal edema is the most prominent feature. H&E. X8.

the unulcerated mucosa that sigmoidoscopic biopsies should be obtained, for this is where the definitive pathologic changes are first manifested.

DIAGNOSIS BY SIGMOIDOSCOPIC BIOPSY.   The features of acute ulcerative colitis to be sought in rectal biopsies are: edematous thickening of the lamina propria; increased cellularity of the lamina propria, consisting mainly of plasma cells; diminished mucus content of the crypt epithelium; and focal degeneration of the crypt epithelium.

The first three of these criteria may occur in other acute diseases in which diarrhea is a symptom, but when there is degeneration of the crypt epithelium in addition, a confident diagnosis of ulcerative colitis can be made (Figs. 3, 4, 5). Degeneration of crypt epithelium follows a certain pattern. In the beginning there is a focal dilatation of the crypt with thinning of the epithelial cells and an accumulation of polymorphonuclear neutrophils both around the affected segment and within it to form the so-called "crypt abscess." This focal degeneration of the crypt epithelium can occur in any part of the tubule in contrast to the crypt degeneration in Crohn's disease in which it is confined to the basal cells. An important point of difference between the two disorders is that there is no significant diminution of mucus content in Crohn's disease, the remainder of an affected crypt is often normal in appearance, and adjacent tubules also appear normal.

The early recognition of ulcerative colitis by rectal biopsy means that the patient can be treated immediately. The rapidity with which adequate therapy may reverse the process in the early stages is well illustrated in the following case. A male aged 75 years developed severe diarrhea clinically diagnosed as fulminant colitis. No ulceration was seen on sigmoidoscopy, but the mucosa was red and

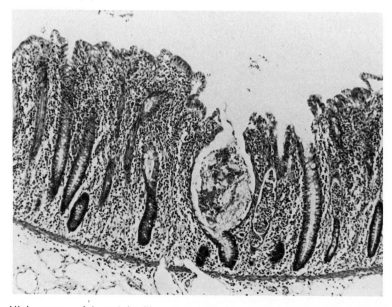

Fig. 3.   High power of bowel in Figures 1 and 2, showing increased cellularity of the lamina propria, diminished mucus content of the crypts, and degenerating crypts with leukocytes within their lumina. H&E. X75.

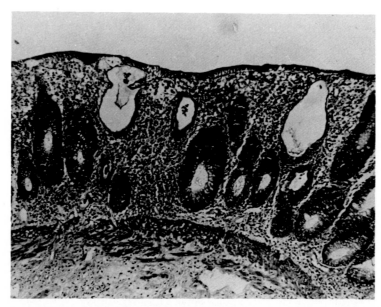

Fig. 4. Rectal biopsy from a 57-year-old male with diarrhea of three weeks duration. No ulceration was seen at sigmoidoscopy, but the diagnosis of acute ulcerative colitis was made on this biopsy because of increased cellularity of the lamina propria, diminished mucus content, and segmental dilatation of crypts with degeneration of epithelial cells. H&E. X75.

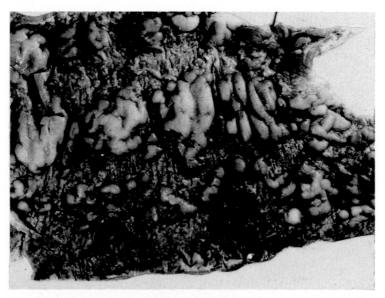

Fig. 5. Patient whose biopsy is illustrated in Figure 4 was found to have gas under the diaphragm on x-ray and was immediately submitted to colonic resection. Deep ulceration was present in the ascending, transverse, and descending colon but not in the recto-sigmoid region. Perforation had occurred in the transverse colon.

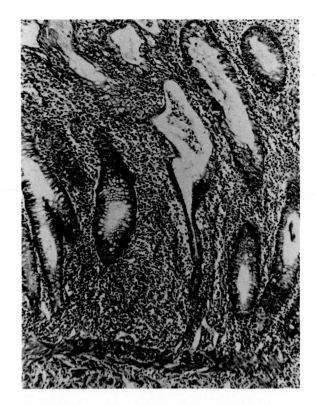

Fig. 6. Rectal biopsy showing the criteria for diagnosis of acute ulcerative colitis: increased cellularity of the lamina propria, diminished mucus content of the crypt epithelium, and segmental degeneration of crypts. H&E. X75.

edematous and bled on contact. A biopsy showed the typical changes of ulcerative colitis (Fig. 6), and this was confirmed radiologically (Fig. 7). With treatment, the symptoms abated, and on sigmoidoscopy 4 weeks later, the mucosa appeared normal. A further biopsy showed almost complete return to normal (Fig. 8), and there was radiologic regression also (Fig. 9). This case illustrates the validity of the diagnosis of ulcerative colitis by rectal biopsy and also serves as a reminder that ulcerative colitis can make its first clinical appearance in old age.

ULCER FORMATION.   Ulcers are formed in several ways. Damage to the epithelial cells can affect normal cell regeneration so that obsolete cells are not replaced, and eventually the lamina propria, denuded of its epithelial protection, becomes vulnerable to bacterial infection. Nodules of granulation tissue may be formed which may eventually be covered with epithelium. Ulceration of this type also occurs in Crohn's disease through destruction of the basal cells from which all the epithelial cells of the crypt are derived.

Degeneration of the basal portions of tubules with the formation of "crypt abscesses" is often followed by undermining of adjacent mucosa, which is then shed. This seems to be the way in which large ulcers are formed (Fig. 10).

Deep ulcers in acute and fulminant cases extend to the muscle coat. The mechanism by which they are formed is not clear. Their coincidence with the longitudinal muscle of the colonic wall is possibly related to the fact that the submucosa over the taeniae may be compared to the creases in the skin of the hand where the skin is bound down to the deeper tissues. Similarly, transverse ulcers tend to occur

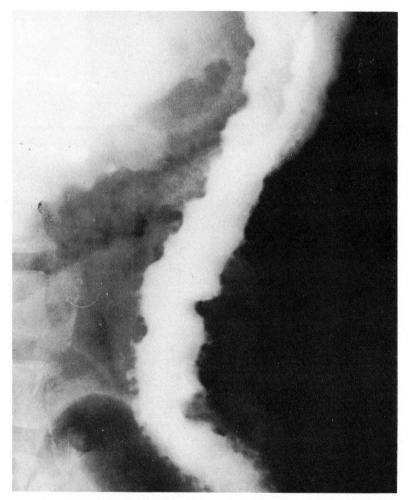

Fig. 7. Barium enema performed at same time as the biopsy in Figure 6 was taken. Deep ulcers of acute ulcerative colitis are present.

in the troughs between the rugae. The presence of ulcers, whether superficial or deep, is not necessary for diagonsis. The diagnostic features are all within the unulcerated mucosa.

Chronic Ulcerative Colitis

There is little difficulty in the diagnosis of chronic ulcerative colitis. The bowel is shortened, its wall is thickened, and the lumen is reduced in caliber. The mucosal surface has lost its normal rugosity, and its surface is irregular, often with no visible ulcers to the naked eye. Excrescences from the mucosal surface may be mucosal tags or polypoidal nodules of mucosal hyperplasia. Microscopically the mucosa exhibits changes similar to those seen in the acute disease but at a lower intensity. Mucus content of the mucosa may be diminished, but in some areas it may even be en-

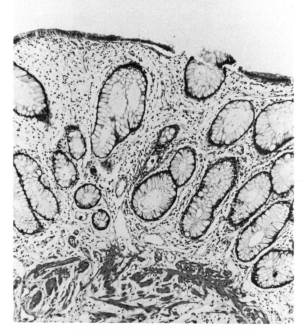

Fig. 8. Rectal biopsy of the same patient represented in Figures 6 and 7 after one month of treatment. The edema has subsided, and the cellularity has diminished. Crypts, though irregular, are close to normal and contain normal amounts of mucus. One degenerate crypt suggests that the disease is still present though suppressed. H&E. X75.

hanced. In areas of previous ulceration the mucosa may be reconstituted almost to the normal state, but if the muscularis mucosae has been disrupted or destroyed regeneration is always very irregular. Ulcers vary in number and in type, and deep ulcers penetrating to the muscle coat may be present.

Except when ulceration has destroyed the muscularis mucosae, fibrosis is not a prominent feature of ulcerative colitis, and stenosis seems to be due more often to muscle spasm than anything else (Figs. 11, 12). This accounts for the radiologic disappearance of what a few weeks or months earlier had been thought to be a stricture.

The rectal biopsy in low-grade, or chronic, ulcerative colitis often reveals edema of the mucosa with increased numbers of plasma cells and an irregular pattern of the crypts, often with diminished mucus content. As in the acute form of ulcerative colitis, actual degeneration of crypt epithelium must be present before the diagnosis can be made.

Malignancy in Ulcerative Colitis

A certain percentage of patients with ulcerative colitis develop carcinoma of the colon, which is often multicentric. The incidence is not high enough to warrant proctocolectomy for every patient with the disease; consequently, patients with chronic ulcerative colitis must be kept under constant surveillance for signs of impending malignancy. The tendency to multicentric carcinomas means that foci of premalignant change can often be recognized in sigmoidoscopic biopsies. Morson and Pang[29] found two types of premalignant change. One consisted of adenomatous and villous polyps in which the usual criteria for carcinoma in situ should be sought.

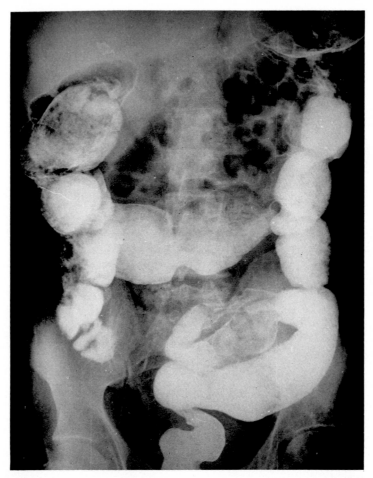

Fig. 9.   Barium enema performed at same time as the biopsy in Figure 8 shows return towards normal.

The other type of change occurred in flat mucosa and consisted of irregular hyperplasia with increased mitotic rate. The presence of Paneth cells did not exclude the diagnosis, and in some instances mucus secretion was increased in amount (Fig. 13).

Crohn's (Granulomatous) Colitis

For many years there was scepticism concerning the existence of Crohn's disease of the colon, although regional colitis had been recorded by a number of writers including Dr. Crohn himself.[3] Eventually, due to the studies of Lockhart-Mummery and Morson,[20, 21, 28] the concept of Crohn's disease of the colon became generally accepted.

Crohn's colitis may simulate ulcerative colitis in both its clinical and radiologic appearances. Deep longitudinal ulcers overlying the taeniae may resemble those of ulcerative colitis, but the normal appearance of the mucosa between the ulcers auto-

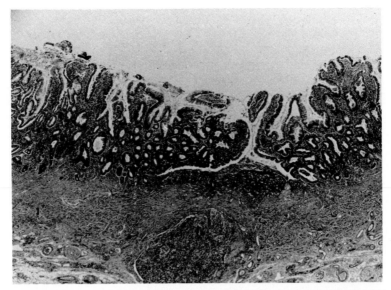

Fig. 10.   Formation of ulcer by undermining in ulcerative colitis. H&E. X60.

matically excludes that diagnosis and in conjunction with the thickened bowel wall is highly suggestive of Crohn's disease (Fig. 14). The classical cobblestone pattern of the mucosa is due to transverse ulcers between the rugae in addition to longitudinal ulceration, but if there is much muscular spasm the appearance may be more polypoid than cobblestone (Fig. 15).

In the majority of cases, the pathologist has little difficulty in arriving at the correct diagnosis. The presence of tuberculoid granulomas is usually considered to be diagnostic. They are found in all coats of the bowel wall but are most frequently present in the submucosa (Table 1).[24] They may also be found in regional lymph nodes and in anal skin tags (Fig. 16).

Table 1.   Crohn's Colitis: Granulomas*

	NUMBER	PERCENTAGE
Resected specimens	30	100
Mucosa	3	10
Submucosa	15	50
Muscle	10	33
Subserosa	9	30
Anal	6	20
Lymph nodes	6	20
Total	23	77

* From McGovern, V.J., and Goulston, S.J.M. *Gut,* 9:164, 1968.

In approximately 25 percent of cases, however, granulomas are either absent or so scarce that they are not found in ordinary routine sections. In such cases, one must rely on other criteria for diagnosis. The most helpful diagnostic features are the characteristic lymphoid aggregates, the fibrosis, and the mode of ulcer formation.

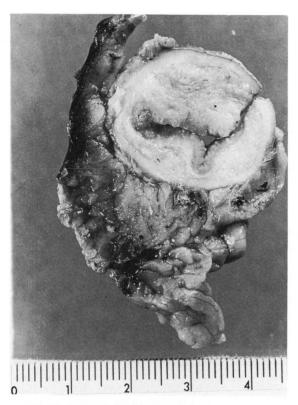

Fig. 11. "Stricture" of colon in chronic ulcerative colitis.

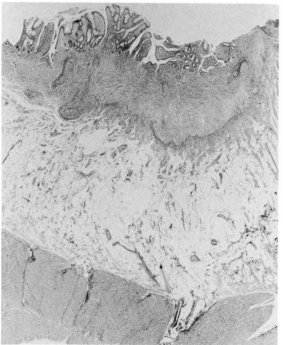

Fig. 12. Microscopic appearances of the stricture in Figure 11. The mucosa is irregular; the muscularis mucosae is greatly hypertrophied with delineation of the two layers; the submucosa is composed of adipose tissue and the muscle coat is hypertrophied. H&E. X8.

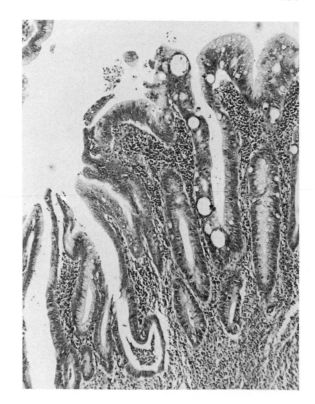

Fig. 13. Precarcinomatous focus in a patient with chronic ulcerative colitis who had an established carcinoma in the cecum and another in the transverse colon. There is epithelial atypia, and mitoses are present high in the crypts instead of being confined to the basal regions. H&E. X75.

LYMPHOID AGGREGATES. Lymphoid tissue is normally present in the bowel wall and usually consists of follicular aggregates with or without germinal centres. They may be confined to the lamina propria or they may be partly in the submucosa. In any chronic inflammatory condition, lymphoid tissue in the vicinity of the muscularis mucosae may be increased in quantity and exhibit prominent germinal centres, but in Crohn's disease the typical lymphoid aggregates are situated in the deeper portions of the submucosa and do not have germinal centres (Fig. 17). Lymphoid aggregates in Crohn's disease may be found in all layers of the bowel wall, but they are found most consistently in the submucosa (Table 2).

Table 2. Crohn's Colitis: Lymphoid Aggregates*

	NUMBER	PERCENTAGE
Resected specimens	30	100
Submucosa	30	100
Muscle	19	63
Subserosa	24	80

* From McGovern, V.J., and Goulston, S.J.M. *Gut,* 9:164, 1968.

FIBROSIS. Fibrosis is invariably present in the submucosa of affected segments but may also be found in the other coats (Fig. 17, Table 3). It does not have the dense cicatricial quality found in benign strictures of ischemic origin, but it can be fairly firm and in the resected specimen is often visible to the naked eye. Fibrotic strictures

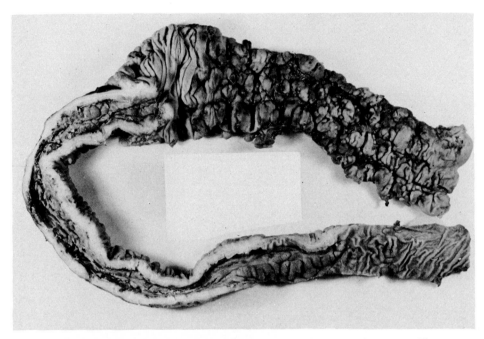

Fig. 14. Crohn's disease of the terminal ileum and of the ascending colon. The cecum appears to be unaffected. Between the ulcers, the colonic mucosa appears normal.

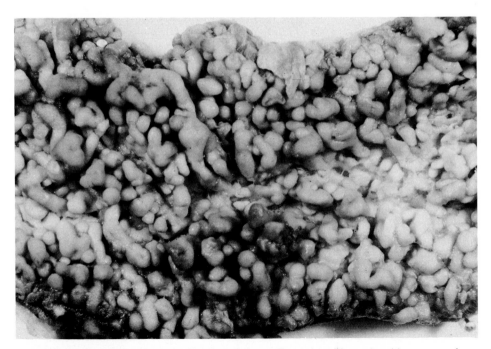

Fig. 15. Long standing Crohn's disease of the entire colon. The polypoid mucosa simulates ulcerative colitis.

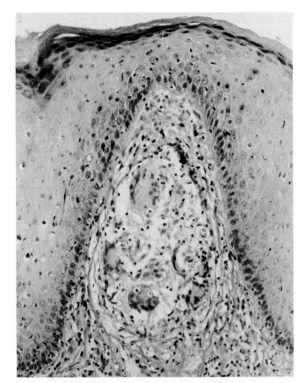

Fig. 16. Anal granuloma from the patient whose colon is illustrated in Figure 15. H&E. X150.

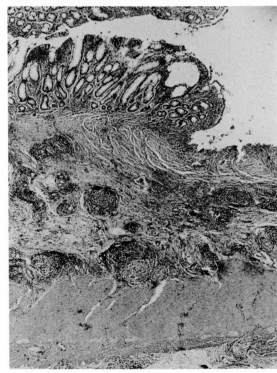

Fig. 17. Whole thickness of bowel wall in Crohn's disease showing the margin of an ulcer, fibrosis of the submucosa, and lymphoid aggregates. There are tuberculoid granulomas just above the muscle coat. H&E. X22.

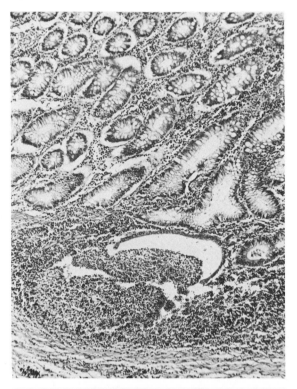

Fig. 18. Destruction of the base of a crypt with the formation of an abscess. The overlying crypt epithelium appears normal. H&E. X60.

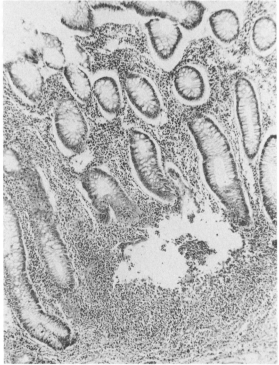

Fig. 19. Destruction of the bases of crypts with abscess formation. A granulomatous reaction is developing in the deeper portion. H&E. X60.

Table 3. Crohn's Colitis: Fibrosis*

	NUMBER	PERCENTAGE
Resected specimens	30	100
Submucosa	30	100
Muscle	18	60
Subserosa	13	43

* From McGovern, V.J., and Goulston, S.J.M. *Gut,* 9:164, 1968.

of the colon occasionally complicate pulmonary tuberculosis. These two conditions can be differentiated from Crohn's disease because they lack the characteristic lymphoid aggregations and the typical patterns of ulcer formation.

ULCER FORMATION. Aggregates of lymphocytes are present in the bases of ulcers in the earliest stages of formation. Whereas degeneration of crypt epithelium starts at any level in ulcerative colitis, it always starts in the basal cells of the crypts in Crohn's disease and never in the absence of lymphocytic aggregates (Fig. 18). Lymphocytes, however, are sometimes replaced by a granulomatous reaction in the base of an ulcer (Fig. 19). Neutrophils and other leucocytes accumulate around the affected crypt cells, often in the form of a "crypt abscess," while the more superficial portions of these tubules are unaffected. When a complete crypt is involved, however, an oblique cut may show only a superficial crypt abscess. The mucosal epithelium surrounding an ulcer may be quite normal in contrast to what is found in ulcerative colitis.

Once the process of cell degeneration starts, ulcers form in the same way as in ulcerative colitis, by undermining or by loss of tubules from the lamina propria. Another kind of ulceration takes the form of clefts, which extend into the submucosa in an oblique undermining fashion or penetrate directly through the bowel wall in the form of fistulas (Fig. 20). In very acute lesions, the affected portion of mucosa may be replaced by a mass of fissured leucocytic exudate from which fistulous abscesses track through the bowel wall.

When healing occurs, mucosa may grow down a fistulous track into the submucosa and produce the appearance which has been described as "colitis cystica profunda."[9]

DIAGNOSIS. The diagnosis of Crohn's disease of the colon is readily made when the characteristic macroscopic appearances are accompanied by the presence of tuberculoid granulomas. When granulomas are absent, one can still make the diagnosis on the presence of submucosal fibrosis with lymphoid aggregates and normal mucosal epithelium in the unulcerated areas. The main diagnostic features are presented in Table 4. Irregularity of the mucosal pattern, which results from healing

Table 4. Crohn's Colitis: Diagnosis*

	PERCENTAGE
Submucosal lymphoid aggregates	100
Submucosal fibrosis	100
Granulomas	76
Fissured ulcers	59

* From McGovern, V.J., and Goulston, S.J.M. *Gut,* 9:164, 1968.

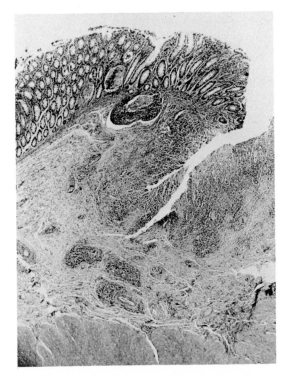

Fig. 20. Splitlike fissure extending into the submucosa. Typical fibrosis and lymphoid aggregates are present in the submucosa. H&E. X17.

of an ulcer in which there had been disruption or destruction of the muscularis mucosae, may suggest the diagnosis of ulcerative colitis, but the normality of the epithelial cells is an important distinguishing feature.

Cleftlike ulcers extending obliquely into the submucosa are highly suggestive of Crohn's disease when they are present, but the most characteristic features of ulcer formation are the collections of lymphocytes in the deepest part of the lamina propria with subsequent degeneration of the basal cells of the overlying crypts.

Rectal biopsy is regarded by Lockhart-Mummery and Morson[21] as a valuable aid to diagnosis, and in 16 of the 19 cases in which rectal biopsy was performed, tuberculoid granulomas were found. These authors emphasize that care must be exercised in selecting the site for the biopsy. Mindful of the fact that Crohn's disease is patchy and that normal bowel is present between the affected areas, Lockhart-Mummery and Morson recommend that the edge of an ulcer is a suitable site for biopsy provided that a good deal of submucosal tissue be obtained.

Anal lesions are common in Crohn's disease, and a high percentage of these have tuberculoid granulomas.[21] Furthermore, granulomas in anal lesions such as fistulas, fissures, and tags have been found to antecede the clinical and radiologic manifestations of Crohn's disease in some cases.[13]

Ischemic Enterocolitis

Ischemic enterocolitis is the name given to a disorder which has been variously described in the past as hemorrhagic enterocolitis,[42] uremic enterocolitis,[16] acute postoperative enterocolitis,[31] and even staphylococcal enterocolitis. It is now known to be a specific entity caused by transient ischemia of the alimentary tract, which is insufficient to cause full-thickness infarction of the bowel.[23] There is an acute form which affects the whole or only a portion of the intestinal tract, and a chronic form which affects only a segment of the gut, usually in the region of the splenic flexure and upper part of the descending colon.

PRECIPITATING FACTORS. The chief precipitating factors in the causation of ischemic enterocolitis are: hypotension; splanchnic vasoconstriction; mesenteric vascular occlusion; and cardiac and aortic surgical operations.

Hypotension is a component of the shock syndrome and is encountered in a large variety of disorders both medical and surgical, the commonest being myocardial infarction. Septicemia, acute hemorrhagic pancreatitis, acute hemorrhage, and syncope are other fairly common conditions which precipitate ischemic enterocolitis through hypotension.

Splanchnic vasoconstriction occurs when there is a fall in the effective circulating blood volume, as in congestive cardiac failure. Digitalis also causes splanchnic vasoconstriction,[10] and this probably accounts for the occasional case of ischemic enterocolitis in patients under treatment for congestive cardiac failure. Other agents causing splanchnic vasoconstriction are catecholamines and gram-negative bacterial endotoxins.[41] The splanchnic blood flow is also reduced by halothane and cyclopropane anesthesia,[6] and while this is not of clinical importance in most subjects, it is possibly significant in patients who have sustained blood loss or who are hypotensive.

Mesenteric vascular occlusion occurs in a variety of ways. The commonest is atheromatous occlusion of the mesenteric vessels at their origin. Embolus is the next most frequent cause of occlusion, and thrombosis leading to ischemic enterocolitis has occasionally been observed in patients with polyarteritis nodosa and with aortic arteritis (Takayasu's disease). Ischemic enterocolitis is also seen in dissecting aneurysm and atheromatous aneurysm of the abdominal aorta.

During *cardiac operations or operations involving the aorta,* the blood supply to the gut is often temporarily suspended or reduced in volume. At autopsy, these patients frequently exhibit ischemic enterocolitis and other visceral manifestations of the shock syndrome.

Most cases fit into the categories just mentioned, but there is a small group in which there is no clear-cut history or objective evidence of a precipitating cause. Sometimes the precipitating cause is revealed at a later date by the discovery of unsuspected cardiovascular disease. A case of this type was that of a 46-year-old psychiatric patient with ischemic colitis who was eventually found to be subject to attacks of atrial fibrillation accompanied by severe hypotension. There are others, however, in which the precipitating cause remains a mystery.

PREDISPOSING FACTORS. The majority of patients who become severely hypotensive or who suffer from congestive cardiac failure do not develop ischemic disease of the intestinal tract. Conditions which predispose to ischemic enterocolitis are: atheromatous disease of the mesenteric arteries; respiratory insufficiency; anemia; and inadequate mesenteric arterial anastomoses.

In the presence of one of these factors, the gut may have insufficient reserves to withstand any further reduction of blood supply by an episode of hypotension, arteriolar vasoconstriction, or sudden vascular occlusion. Ischemic enterocolitis or even infarction of the gut may ensue.

An important predisposing factor in the development of ischemic enterocolitis is the relatively poor vascular anastomosis in some persons, in the vicinity of the splenic flexure and descending colon (Fig. 21). This area is supplied by an accessory from the middle colic branch of the superior mesenteric artery anastomosing with the left colic branch of the inferior mesenteric artery. Whereas the rest of the alimentary tract has a continuous system of vascular arcades, this is not always the case in this region which is thereby rendered particularly vulnerable to any reduction in blood supply or in oxygen tension. Reiner[35] showed that the mesenteric system can be readily filled through the superior mesenteric artery but less easily through the inferior mesenteric. Occlusion of the superior mesenteric artery is thus likely to have more far-reaching and serious consequences than occlusion of the inferior mesenteric, but, in either case, the portion of the gut most likely to be affected is the splenic flexure and the upper part of the descending colon.

In a few cases hypotension alone, without any discoverable predisposing cause, has been responsible for fatal ischemic enterocolitis.[23]

PRIMARY DISEASE.   Ischemic enterocolitis complicates a variety of disorders but the most common are those of the cardiovascular system, particularly myocardial

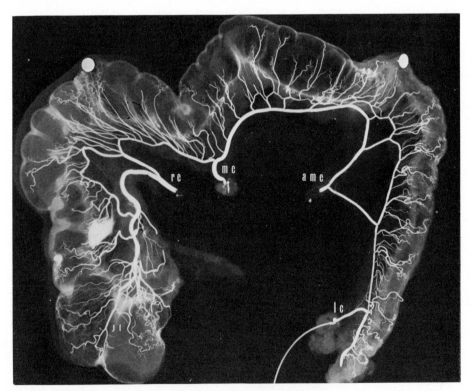

Fig. 21.   X-ray of injected autopsy specimen of large bowel showing the anastomotic pattern. The descending colon is supplied by an accessory branch (amc) of the middle colic artery (mc) which anastomoses with the left colic (lc) artery.

infarction and congestive cardiac failure. These patients often have atheromatous narrowing of the mouths of their mesenteric vessels and are thereby predisposed to development of ischemic enterocolitis by the shocked state in myocardial infarction, or by splanchnic vasoconstriction in congestive cardiac failure.

Because of its association with degenerative cardiovascular disease, ischemic enterocolitis is most frequently seen in older persons. Nevertheless, it can occur at any age, even infancy. We have seen it in a New Guinea child whose bowel was predisposed by healing polyarteritis. The precipitating factor in this case was not determined.

Other primary disorders commonly associated with ischemic enterocolitis have been rheumatoid disease and pulmonary emphysema.

PATHOLOGY. The affected portion of gut in acute ischemic enterocolitis is intensely congested, frequently hemorrhagic, with free blood in the lumen. The serosa may be congested and discolored, but often it appears quite normal. Ulcers are very irregularly distributed and may encircle the lumen, or in the colon they may have a longitudinal orientation overlying the *taeniae coli* (Fig. 22). Perforation of ulcers is more common in the small intestine than in the large.

Microscopically, hemorrhages are found in the mucosa and, in severe cases, in the submucosa also. Fibrin thrombi in mucosal capillaries are characteristic of

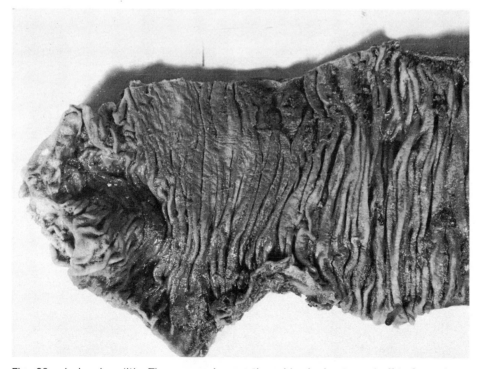

Fig. 22.   Ischemic colitis. The mucosa is necrotic and beginning to peel off to form ulcers. The patient was a 79-year-old female who had involvement of the terminal ileum, ascending colon, and part of the transverse colon ascribed to kinking of the ileo-colic artery by adhesions.

ischemic enterocolitis; in severe cases, they extend into the submucosal venules and veins. Sometimes there is actual necrosis of venules even when they do not contain thrombi. Apart from capillaries, the vessels affected are always veins and venules, never arteries or arterioles (Figs. 23, 24). The mucosa rapidly becomes necrotic

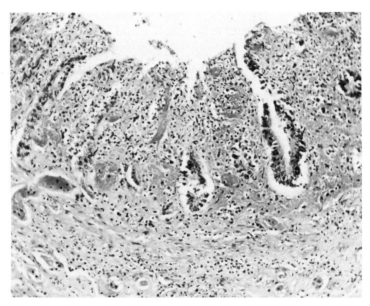

Fig. 23. Ischemic colitis resulting from hypotension due to fatal hemorrhagic pancreatitis. There are fibrin thrombi in the mucosa which also shows inflammation and early mucosal necrosis. Hemorrhage was minimal. H&E. X150.

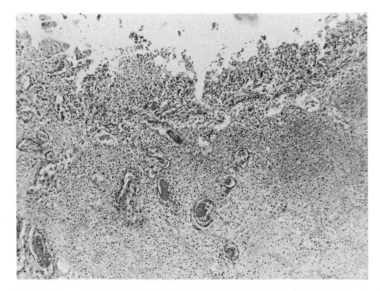

Fig. 24. Ulcer with necrotic surface. There is hemorrhage and inflammation in the submucosa. Fibrin thrombi are present in the remnants of the mucosa and in the submucosal venules. The patient had severe hypotension from myocardial infarction which occurred four days before death. H&E. X60.

and after three or four days undergoes dissolution, leaving an ulcer. Healing may be rapid if the disorder is of mild degree, but perforation may occur. When the ulceration extends through the muscularis mucosae, healing is by cicatrizing granulation tissue, and at this stage one may refer to the disorder as chronic.

Acute ischemic enterocolitis due to hypotension or splanchnic vasoconstriction usually complicates some disorder that is already likely to be fatal. Consequently, it tends to be diagnosed more frequently at autopsy than in the living patient. Should the patient survive, healing of deep ulcerations can lead to benign strictures simulating neoplastic disease when confined to single short segments.

When a vessel is occluded, there may be temporary ischemia pending the development of anastomotic compensation. In the large bowel, the segment of bowel affected is usually where the anastomoses are least effective, in particular the splenic flexure and descending colon. If infarction does not occur, a localized area of ischemic enteritis or colitis results, which may then progress to cicatricial stenosis (Figs. 25, 26, 27).

Ischemic colitis may be said to be chronic when ulcers persist beyond six weeks from the onset of the condition. By that time, if the lesion is severe enough to be causing symptoms, there should be cicatricial narrowing of the affected portion of colon (Fig. 28). The luminal surface is covered with a fibrinous exudate, and fibrous thickening of the wall can be seen with the naked eye.

Microscopically, the fibrosis is more dense than that seen in any other disease of the colon. It may be confined to the submucosa, but in some cases it will be found replacing the muscle coat. At an earlier stage, one may find organizing thrombi within veins and venules of the submucosa, but by the time stenosis of the gut has occurred, one has to rely on the criterion of Marston, et al.,[26] namely the presence of hemosiderin-containing phagocytes in the submucosa, for confirmation of diagnosis.

DIFFERENTIAL DIAGNOSIS. Sigmoidoscopic biopsy can be most helpful in distinguishing between acute ischemic colitis and acute ulcerative colitis. Ulcerative colitis almost invariably involves the rectosigmoid region, and it would be very unusual for a normal biopsy in the acute disease. Ischemic colitis sometimes affects the sigmoid colon, and the presence of hemorrhage in the lamina propria or even fibrin thrombi may then be found.

Chronic ischemic colitis is an obstructive lesion and is therefore most likely to be confused clinically with carcinoma or Crohn's disease. It is usually beyond the range of the sigmoidoscope, and the diagnosis can only be made with certainty after the specimen has been removed. The absence of granulomas and lymphoid accumulations and the presence of dense cicatrization and hemosiderin-containing phagocytes in the submucosa indicate that the stenosing lesion is of ischemic origin. The possibility of ischemic stricture of the colon should already have been suspected because of the site of the lesion and perhaps the history.

Pseudomembranous Colitis

Pseudomembranous colitis is a pathologic entity of uncertain etiology, characterized by sudden onset of profound shock due to severe watery diarrhea.

The bowel is usually dilated and has lost its normal mucosal pattern. Yellow

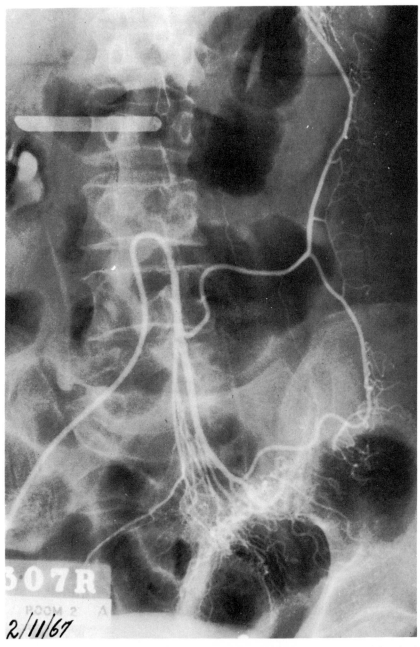

Fig. 25.   Angiogram of 67-year-old woman who was awakened by severe abdominal pain accompanied by distension and passage of blood per rectum. A catheter is in the inferior mesenteric artery. Filling of the hemorrhoidal vessels is good, but there is defective filling in the distribution of the left colic artery.

or greenish bile-stained plaques a few millimeters in diameter may be sparsely scattered over the mucosa of a small segment of the large bowel, or there may be numerous plaques involving the entire large bowel and sometimes a portion of the

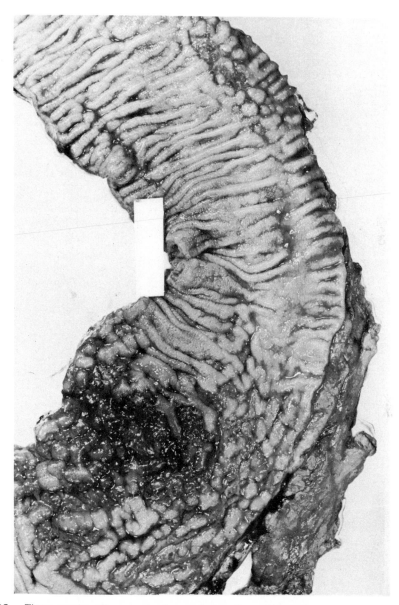

Fig. 26.   Three weeks after onset of symptoms, the patient whose angiogram is reproduced in Figure 25 had a left hemicolectomy. There are linear ulcers in the upper part of the descending colon and a large irregular ulcerated area in the lower part.

small bowel. The appearance in the more florid cases has been likened to the cracked moss-covered bark of a tree (Fig. 29). The consistency of the plaques varies from gelatinous and semitranslucent to opaque and firm, according to the relative proportions of mucus and fibrin in their composition. The ileum may be involved to a certain extent, but the disease affects the colon much more frequently. The serosa usually appears normal.

Microscopically, there is a characteristic appearance. The earliest lesion con-

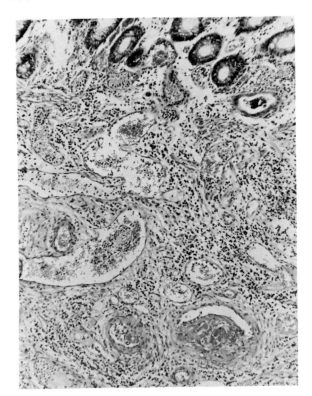

Fig. 27. The ischemic nature of the ulcers in the colon illustrated in Figure 26 is confirmed by the presence of organizing venular thrombi in the submucosa. H&E. X75.

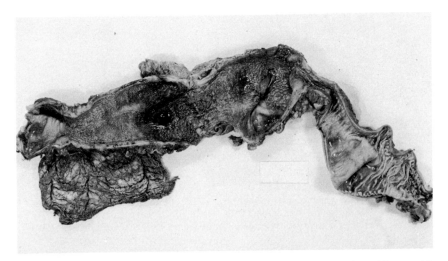

Fig. 28.   Resected portion of transverse colon and descending colon in a 46-year-old male showing stenosis, which is particularly marked in the descending colon. The colon was resected 12 weeks after the sudden onset of diarrhea. Histologically this specimen showed dense cicatrization with hemosiderin-containing phagocytes in the granulation tissue. The patient died from a cardiomyopathy of unknown cause, and an elongated thrombus attached at one end to the arch of the aorta was found at autopsy. The ischemia of the colon was presumably due to embolus.

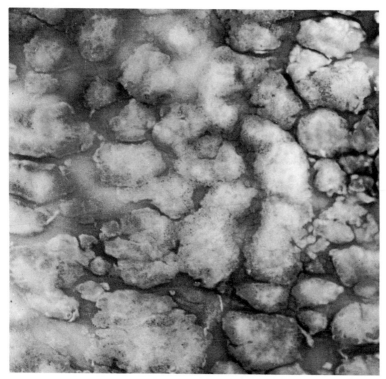

Fig. 29.   Portion of the colon showing the typical plaques of pseudomembranous colitis. X 2.5.

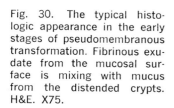

Fig. 30. The typical histologic appearance in the early
stages of pseudomembranous
transformation. Fibrinous exudate from the mucosal surface is mixing with mucus
from the distended crypts.
H&E. X75.

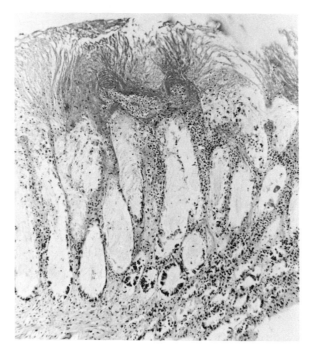

sists of foci of fibrinoid necrosis of the mucosal surface, while the subjacent crypt epithelium produces excessive amounts of mucus. Fibrin erupts from the surface and mixes with the mucus to form a jelly-like mucofibrinous exudate which fuses with the necrotic surface of the mucosa (Fig. 30). Between the plaques of pseudomembranous transformation, the mucosa is quite normal.

There is marked edema of the submucosa, but cellular infiltration is absent. Polymorphonuclear leucocytes in moderate numbers may be found in the surface exudate only.

In the early stages the exudate can be scraped off the bowel surface with a knife, but later it is firmly incorporated into the mucosa and cannot be easily removed. Eventually, if the patient survives long enough, the affected mucosa is discarded, and ulcers may result if the whole thickness of mucosa has become necrotic.

ETIOLOGY. Pseudomembranous enterocolitis occurs most commonly in association with obstructive lesions of the colon, but it is also found in cardiorenal conditions in which it may be precipitated by uremia, cardiac failure, or pneumonia. Of 94 patients who developed the condition postoperatively, 41 were being treated for carcinoma of the colon (Pettet, et al.[32]); of 14 patients in whom the condition was not preceded by surgical operation, 5 had colonic obstruction due to carcinoma of the colon, and cardiac disease was the next most common accompanying disorder (Kleckner, et al.[19]); 5 of the 14 patients described by Goulston and McGovern[12] had colonic obstruction, while cardiac and renal disease were the commonest disorders in the remainder.

Foci of pseudomembranous change too small to cause clinical manifestations are common in obstructive conditions and have been observed by the writer even on the surface of an adenomatous polyp of the colon.

The cause of pseudomembranous colitis is obscure. Possible causes suggested by previous authors have been antibiotic therapy,[34] surgical operations,[32] staphylococcal enterotoxin,[1, 39, 40] and ischemia.[14, 25] None of these factors can be a sole cause, since the disorder occurred prior to the antibiotic era[32] and occurs in patients who have never undergone a surgical operation.[2, 12, 19] Furthermore, a staphylococcus is recovered from the stools of only a minority of patients with pseudomembranous enterocolitis,[4] and ischemia produces specific lesions which we have already discussed.

From the histologic appearances, it seems that pseudomembranous colitis is due to a soluble toxin which diminishes in intensity as it penetrates the bowel wall. Where it is most concentrated at the mucosal surface, it causes necrosis; in lesser concentration it stimulates the crypt epithelium to excess mucus secretion; in the submucosa it causes increased permeability and edema. In all probability, the changes of pseudomembranous colitis can be elicited by a variety of toxins present in the lumen when the bowel is rendered susceptible by obstruction, chronic cardiorenal disease, or other debilitating disorders.

Necrotizing Enterocolitis

In 1947, Jeckeln[17] in Germany reported a necrotizing enteritis which he called *Darmbrand,* literally "gut burn" and analogous to "heart burn." This was later shown by Zeissler and Rassfield-Sternberg[43] and by Fick and Wolken[11] to be due to the beta toxin of *Clostridium welchii* Type F (now recommended to be included in Type C[38]). A similar disorder, described by Murrell and Roth,[30] affects the jejunum of New Guinea natives and is due to pork infected with *C. welchii* Type C.[8]

Involvement of the colon by the same type of necrotizing process has also been reported by Killingback and Williams,[18] Duncan,[7] Renwick, McGovern, and Spence.[36] Case 6 of Renwick, et al. points to the likelihood of *C. welchii* being responsible in these cases also. This was the case of a 55-year-old man with acute myeloblastic leukemia who was admitted to hospital with obvious clinical septicemia, abdominal pain, and absent bowel sounds. *C. welchii* of undetermined type was grown from his blood. The patient died 12 hours after admission, and at autopsy there was typical necrotizing colitis.

Clinically, necrotizing colitis presents with acute onset of abdominal pain which suggests an intra-abdominal emergency requiring immediate surgery.

PATHOLOGY. The entire colon may be affected or the process may be restricted to a small segment; in either case, the small intestine may be involved in some part. The affected bowel is dilated and has patchy greenish-brown foci of necrosis along its length. These may be plainly visible on opening the peritoneal cavity, but the extent of the disease is usually greater on the mucosal than the serosal surface. Microscopically, there is coagulative necrosis of the mucosa and, to a certain extent, of the submucosa also. There may be an infiltrate of polymorphonuclear neutrophil leucocytes at the junction of the necrotic and nonnecrotic zones, but at a later stage leucocytes infiltrate the necrotic tissue also. Killingback and Williams[18] stress the finding of gram-positive bacilli in the necrotic tissue. The significance of this is doubtful, as bacteria tend to invade any necrotic intestinal mucosa. Ulcers are formed when necrotic mucosal tissue is discarded; there is then the danger of perforation.

The histologic diagnosis of necrotizing enterocolitis depends upon finding necrosis of the mucosa with none of the characteristics of ischemic disease or other specific forms of colitis. The gross specimen, together with its characteristic clostridial odor, usually presents an obvious diagnosis.

Staphylococcal Enterocolitis

It is well known that certain strains of *Staphylococcus pyogenes* produce an enterotoxin which causes diarrhea and that many of the patients who have diarrhea under tetracycline therapy are in fact suffering from staphylococcal enteritis. This diarrhea, however, subsides with the administration of antibiotics to which the staphylococcus is sensitive.[5, 15]

Apart from simple staphylococcal diarrhea, there is always the possibility that the staphylococcus may invade established lesions of ulcerative colitis, Crohn's disease, or ischemic enterocolitis. This, however, seems to happen very rarely.

Ulcerative lesions of the intestinal tract due to staphylococcus are rare; Powell,[33] in an analysis of 40 autopsy cases in which there had been staphylococcal septicemia, found none. In 22 autopsies in which death had been due to staphylococcal septicemia, the writer found none with enterocolitis. Nevertheless, the staphylococcus should not be dismissed as a possible pathogen for the colon. In a certain proportion of patients with pseudomembranous colitis, *S. pyogenes* has been recovered from the stool as the dominant organism, and staphylococcal enterotoxin may well be one of the toxic agents which produce this reaction.[4] This is difficult to prove, and attempts to reproduce the changes of pseudomembranous enterocolitis in experimental animals by using *S. pyogenes* have not been successful. Inflammations of the alimentary tract have been induced and have been called pseudomembranous enterocolitis, but the illustrations and histologic descriptions have been those of non-specific inflammation with leucocytic infiltration through all coats of the intestinal wall, [1, 37, 39, 40] whereas in pseudomembranous enterocolitis, there is usually no leucocytic infiltration of the bowel wall.

One must conclude that apart from simple staphylococcal enteritis, ulcerative lesions of the intestine due to the staphylococcus are extremely rare.

Colitis Cystica Profunda

Colitis cystica profunda is not a separate entity. It can occur in any ulcerative lesion of the colon and is due to epithelialization of deep ulcers. It is found most frequently in the rectosigmoid region,[9] and there is a danger that it may be mistaken in sigmoidoscopic biopsies for carcinoma. Epstein, et al.[9] were not able to establish the etiology in their four cases, but we have encountered the condition in Crohn's disease, in ulcerative colitis, and in ischemic colitis (Fig. 31).

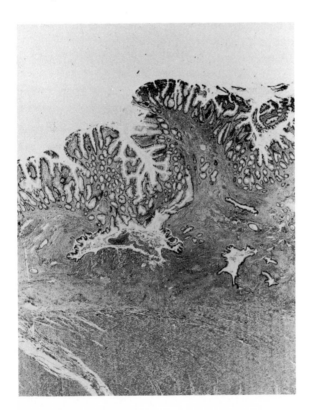

Fig. 31. Downgrowth of epithelium during healing of deep ulcers in ulcerative colitis has produced an appearance that could be mistaken for carcinomatous invasion in a small sigmoidoscopic biopsy. H&E. X60.

Obstructive Colitis

"Colitis and antecedent carcinoma" is the title given by Millar[27] to a condition in which there is a carcinoma of the sigmoid or descending colon associated with a segmental colitis proximal to it. The length of the affected segment varies from a few centimeters to about 25 centimeters. Between the segment of bowel exhibiting the colitis and the carcinoma, there is a zone of normal bowel mucosa varying in length from a few centimeters to about 20 centimeters or longer. This condition may simulate acute ulcerative colitis both clinically and radiologically, and the carcinoma may not be recognized. One of Millar's cases and one of the three cases seen in Royal Prince Alfred Hospital presented in this way (Fig. 32).

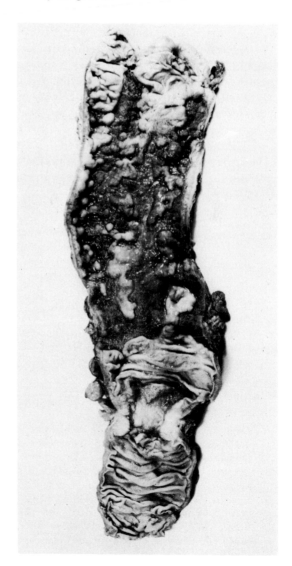

Fig. 32.   Carcinoma of the sigmoid colon with deep ulceration of the bowel proximally. There is a short segment of normal mucosa between the carcinoma and the ulceration.

Macroscopically, there is linear ulceration overlying the *taeniae coli,* while between the ulcers the mucosa appears normal. Microscopically, the bases of the ulcers are lined by granulation tissue, and, although occasional vessels appear to have been occluded by organized thrombus, the pathogenesis of the condition is obscure. Between the ulcers the mucosa appears normal.

Summary

In *ulcerative colitis,* the diagnostic feature is inflammation of the mucosa with degeneration of crypt epithelium beginning at any level of the crypt. The mucosa adjacent to an ulcer is never normal.

The main lesion in *Crohn's disease* is lymphocytic aggregates together with fibrosis of the submucosa. Destruction of crypt epithelium always begins at the crypt base, and the mucosa adjacent to an ulcer is usually normal.

Ischemic colitis is characterized by hemorrhage in the mucosa and fibrin thrombi in mucosal vessels often extending into submucosal vessels. Hemosiderin granules are found in the cicatricial tissue of the chronic lesion.

Pseudomembranous colitis starts with necrosis of the surface epithelium and increased mucus production in the crypts. The fibrinous exudate and mucus coalesce with the necrotic surface epithelium in the form of plaques.

The diagnostic criteria outlined in this essay should enable most cases of colitis to be categorized without much difficulty. Even so, cases will arise from time to time in which the features are not sufficiently explicit for classification.

References

1. Bennett, I.L. Jr., Wood, J.S. Jr., and Yardley, J.H. Staphylococcal pseudo-membranous enterocolitis in chinchillas; a clinico-pathologic study. Trans. Ass. Amer. Physicians, 69:116, 1956.
2. Bloomfield, D.A., and Walters, M.N.I. Pseudo-membranous enterocolitis. Med. J. Aust., 2:854, 1960.
3. Crohn, B.B., and Berg, A.A. Right-sided (regional) colitis. J.A.M.A., 110:32, 1938.
4. Dearing, W.H., Baggenstoss, A.H., and Weed, L.A. Studies on the relationship of *Staphylococcus aureus* to pseudomembranous enteritis and to post-antibiotic enteritis. Gastroenterology, 38:441, 1960.
5. ——— and Heilman, F.R. Micrococcic (staphylococcic) enteritis as a complication of antibiotic therapy: Its response to erythromycin. Proc. Mayo Clin., 28:121, 1953.
6. Deutsch, S. Physiology of the splanchnic circulation and its alteration by general anesthesia and hemorrhage in man. Amer. J. Surg., 114:353, 1967.
7. Duncan, T. Necrotising colitis: Case report. Amer. J. Surg., 108:885, 1964.
8. Egerton, J., and Walker, P. Isolation of *Clostridium perfringens* type C from necrotic enteritis of man in New Guinea. J. Path. Bact., 88:275, 1964.
9. Epstein, S.E., Ascari, W.Q., Ablow, R.C., Seaman, W.B., and Lattes, R. Colitis cystic profunda. Amer. J. Clin. Path., 45:186, 1966.
10. Ferrer, M.I., Bradley, S.E., Wheeler, H.O., Enson, Y., Preisig, R., and Harvey, R.M. The effect of digoxin in the splanchnic circulation in ventricular failure. Circulation, 32:524, 1965.

11. Fick, K., and Wolken, A. Necrotic jejunitis. Lancet, 1:519, 1949.
12. Goulston, S.J.M., and McGovern, V.J. Pseudomembranous colitis. Gut, 6:207, 1965.
13. Gray, G.K., Lockhart-Mummery, H.E., and Morson, B.C. Crohn's disease of the anal region. Gut, 6:515, 1965.
14. Hardaway, R.M., and McKay, D.G. Pseudomembranous enterocolitis. Arch. Surg., 78:446, 1959.
15. Jackson, G.G., Haight, T.H., Kass, E.H., Womack, C.R., Gocke, T.M., and Finland, M. Terramycin therapy of pneumonia: Clinical and bacteriologic studies in 91 cases. Ann. Intern. Med., 35:1175, 1951.
16. Jaffe, R.H., and Laing, D. Changes of digestive tract in uremia; pathologic anatomic study. Arch. Intern. Med., 53:851, 1934.
17. Jeckeln, E. Enteritis necroticans. Deutsch. Med. Wschr., 73:172, 1948.
18. Killingback, M., and Williams, K.L. Necrotising colitis. Brit. J. Surg., 9:175, 1961.
19. Kleckner, M.S., Bargen, J.A., and Baggenstoss, A.H. Pseudomembranous enterocolitis: Clinicopathologic study of 14 cases in which the disease was not preceded by an operation. Gastroenterology, 21:211, 1952.
20. Lockhart-Mummery, H.E., and Morson, B.C. Crohn's disease (regional enteritis) of the large intestine and its distinction from ulcerative colitis. Gut, 1:87, 1960.
21. ———— and Morson, B.C. Crohn's disease of the large intestine. Gut, 5:493, 1964.
22. McGovern, V.J., and Archer, G.T. The pathogenesis of ulcerative colitis. Aust. Ann. Med., 6:68, 1957.
23. ———— and Goulston, S.J.M. Ischaemic enterocolitis. Gut, 6:213, 1965.
24. ———— and Goulston, S.J.M. Crohn's disease of the colon. Gut, 9:164, 1968.
25. Marston, A. The bowel in shock. Lancet, 2:365, 1962.
26 ———— Pheils, M.T., Thomas, M.L., and Morson, B.C. Ischemic colitis. Gut, 7:1, 1966.
27. Millar, D.M. Colitis and antecedent carcinoma. Dis. Colon Rectum, 8:243, 1965.
28. Morson, B.C., and Lockhart-Mummery, H.E. Anal lesions in Crohn's disease. Lancet, 2:1122, 1959.
29. ———— and Pang, L.S.C. Rectal biopsy as an aid to cancer control in ulcerative colitis. Gut, 8:423, 1967.
30. Murrell, T., and Roth, L. Necrotizing jejunitis: A newly discovered disease in the highlands of New Guinea. Med. J. Aust., 1:61, 1963.
31. Penner, A., and Bernheim, A. Acute post-operative enterocolitis. Arch. Path., 27:966, 1939.
32. Pettet, J.D., Baggenstoss, A.H., Dearing, W.H., and Judd, E.S. Postoperative pseudomembranous enterocolitis. Surg. Gynec. Obstet., 98:546, 1954.
33. Powell, D.E.B. Non-suppurative lesions in staphylococcal septicaemia. J. Path. Bact., 82:141, 1961.
34. Reiner, L. Mesenteric vascular occlusion studied by post mortem injection of the mesenteric arterial circulation. In Pathology Annual 1966, Sommers, S.C., ed. New York, Appleton-Century-Crofts, 1966, Vol. 1, p. 193.
35. ———— Schlesinger, J.J., and Miller, G.M. Pseudomembranous colitis following aureomycin and chloramphenicol. Arch. Path., 54:39, 1952.
36. Renwick, S.B., McGovern, V.J., and Spence, J. Necrotizing enterocolitis: A report of six cases. Med. J. Aust., 2:413, 1966.
37. Speare, G.M. Staphylococcus pseudomembranous enterocolitis; a complication of antibiotic therapy. Amer. J. Surg., 88:523, 1954.
38. Sterne, M., and Warrock, G.H. The types of Clostridium perfringens. J. Path. Bact., 88:279, 1964.
39. Tan, T.L., Drake, C.T., Jacobson, M.J., and Van Prohaska, J. The experimental development of pseudomembranous enterocolitis. Surg. Gynec. Obstet., 108:415, 1959.
40. Van Prohaska, J. Pseudo-membranous (staphylococcal) enterocolitis. Arch. Surg., 79:197, 1959.

41. Wilson, G.S., and Miles, A.A. Topley and Wilson's Principles of Bacteriology and Immunity, 5th ed. London, Edward Arnold Ltd., 1964, p. 1240.
42. Wilson, R., and Qualheim, R.E. A form of acute haemorrhagic enterocolitis afflicting chronically ill individuals. Gastroenterology, 27:431, 1954.
43. Zeissler, J., and Rassfeld-Sternberg, L. Enteritis necroticans due to *Clostridium welchii* type F. Brit. Med. J., 1:267, 1949.

Addendum [*]

Ulcerative Colitis

The histologic diagnosis of ulcerative colitis and its distinction from Crohn's disease can be difficult, and no assistance can be obtained from immunofluorescence or electronmicroscopy. Kent [1] found that, in 10 percent of his colitis cases, there was overlapping of criteria, while Glotzer et al [2] found overlapping in a quarter of their cases.

As indicated by Gonzalez-Licea and Yardley, [3] bacillary dysentery may cause lesions in the colonic mucosa identical with those seen in acute ulcerative colitis (Fig. 1). Consequently it is necessary to have negative bacterial cultures before making a definite diagnosis of acute ulcerative colitis.

Carcinoma in Ulcerative Colitis

The experience of Morson and Pang [4] has been amply confirmed at Royal Prince Alfred Hospital, [5] and finding precancerous lesions in rectal biopsies has occasionally resulted in resections of colons containing small invasive carcinomas, which had not been demonstrated radiologically (Fig. 2).

There are certain strict criteria to be followed in the diagnosis of precancerous lesions in sigmoidoscopic specimens. The less active the colitis, the more significant is the presence of cellular atypia, and conversely, one should be more guarded in the interpretation of cellular atypia in the presence of active inflammation. The chief features to be sought are irregularity and lateral branching of the crypts, multilayering of cells both on the mucosal surface and in the crypt walls, irregularity of nuclei, and marked lack of uniformity in mucus content of cells. In our experience, precancerous changes are more frequent in flat mucosa than in polypoidal areas.

Crohn's Disease

It is quite possible that the disorder we call Crohn's disease represents more than one entity. As Lockhart-Mummery [6] has shown, the age incidence is bimodal, there being a peak in the second decade and another in the fifth and sixth decades. Among the most important diagnostic features are its focal nature, transmural inflammation, depth of ulceration, sinus tracts, intramural abscesses, and granu-

* This work was prepared with the assistance of Dr. Bishnu Dutta.

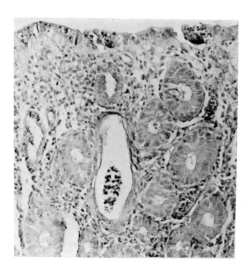

Fig. 1. Rectal biopsy showing acute colitis due to *Shigella flexneri*. There is diminished mucus content of crypts, an early crypt abscess, increased cellularity of the lamina propria, and polymorphonuclear invasion of the surface epithelium. H&E. × 120.

lomas. Glotzer et al [2] found that the presence of microscopic sinuses and/or granulomas correlated significantly with clinical Crohn's disease and their absence with clinical ulcerative colitis, but in one-quarter of cases there was histologic overlapping.

Crohn's disease occurs most frequently in the right side of the colon. Con-

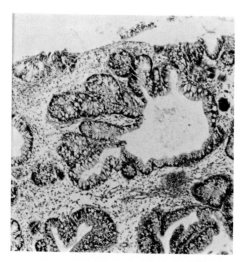

Fig. 2. Rectal biopsy from male aged 40 years with ulcerative colitis that had been quiescent for 20 years. There is lateral branching of the crypts, multilayering of nuclei, and irregularity of mucus secretion. The resected colon had an invasive carcinoma not shown by barium enema. H&E. × 48.

sequently the sigmoidoscopic appearances are often normal. Nevertheless random rectal biopsies may still result in a positive diagnosis.[5] It is our custom to cut serial sections of rectal biopsies and to stain four representative slides each with three or four tissue sections. If, in a case of suspected Crohn's disease, no granulomas are found, all the sections are stained and examined. In this way, granulomas have been found in what appeared to be normal rectal mucosa in about one-third of patients with clinical and radiologic right-sided disease.

Apart from granulomas, the diagnosis can be regarded as certain if there is the characteristic pattern of crypt degeneration. In Crohn's disease there are always small aggregations of lymphocytes at the base of affected crypts. In such cases serial sections may reveal granulomas in addition. When there is only an aggregate of lymphocytes, serial sections will indicate whether there is an associated degenerating crypt or whether it is only part of a normal lymphoid follicle (Fig. 3).

Nonspecific Colitis

In a recent series of 383 sigmoidoscopic biopsies obtained from 290 patients, there were 100 biopsies from 84 patients in which the diagnosis was "nonspecific colitis."[5] In these specimens there was an increase in cellularity of the lamina propria, and in very acute cases there were neutrophil leucocytes present that penetrated into crypt epithelium. Crypt abscesses and destruction of crypts were not uncommon, but the crypts did not have the characteristic flask-shaped dilatations that characterize crypt abscesses in both ulcerative colitis and bacillary dysentery (Fig. 4).

Some patients with these changes in their rectal mucosa gradually evolved

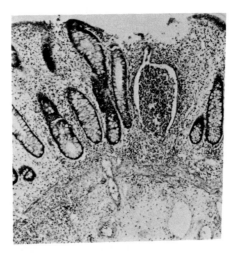

Fig. 3. Rectal biopsy of male aged 23 years with extensive colitis due to Crohn's disease, but almost normal sigmoidoscopic appearances. There is a crypt abscess with a collection of lymphocytes at its base. Adjacent crypts are within normal range. H&E. × 48.

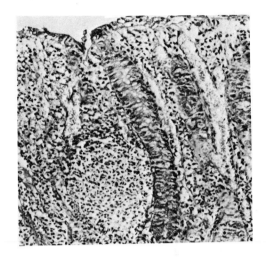

Fig. 4. Rectal biopsy of male aged 27 years with symptoms and radiologic appearances of ulcerative colitis. After one month the radiologic appearances and biopsy had returned to normal and remained so. There is destruction of crypts and replacement of one by an acute abscess. The other crypts have diminished mucus content and the lamina propria is densely infiltrated. H&E. × 48.

into histologically recognizable ulcerative colitis; others recovered completely.

Various salmonellae, in particular *S. typhimurium* and *S. München,* have been recovered from the stools of patients with acute nonspecific colitis, but in the majority of cases no specific etiologic agent was found. Acute proctitis can be caused by *N. gonorrhoea,* but here too no etiologic agent can be found in the majority of cases.

References

1. Kent TH, Ammon RK: Differentiation of ulcerative colitis and regional enteritis of colon. Arch Pathol 89:20, 1970
2. Glotzer DJ, Gardner RC, Goldman H, et al: Comparative features and course of ulcerative and granulomatous colitis. N Engl J Med 282:582, 1970
3. Gonzalez-Licea A, Yardley JH: Nature of the tissue reaction in ulcerative colitis. Gastroenterology 51:825, 1966
4. Morson BC, Pang LSC: Rectal biopsy as an aid to cancer control in ulcerative colitis. Gut 8:423, 1967
5. McGovern VJ: Rectal biopsy in the differential diagnosis of colitis. Rendic.Gastroenterol (Rome) 4:94, 1972
6. Lockhart-Mummery HE: Crohn's disease of the large bowel. Br J Surg 59:823, 1972

THE TECHNIQUE AND INTERPRETATION OF RECTAL BIOPSIES IN INFLAMMATORY BOWEL DISEASE

BASIL C. MORSON

The expression "inflammatory bowel disease" can be used to describe a wide variety of inflammations of the small and large intestine. In Europe and North America ulcerative colitis and Crohn's disease are the most important but these must be distinguished from the dysenteric infections which are very common and widespread in other parts of the world. The differential diagnosis of inflammatory bowel disease also includes the three unrelated disorders: the solitary ulcer syndrome, cathartic colon, and ischaemic enterocolitis.

Rectal biopsy has been used for the diagnosis of tumors of the rectum since shortly after the first World War.[1] Its use in the diagnosis of amebic dysentery was reported in 1957 [2] and the first attempts to define its role in the diagnosis of ulcerative colitis and Crohn's disease of the colon were also described about this time.[3-5] During the past decade there has been an increasing awareness of the value of rectal biopsy in the differential diagnosis of inflammations of the rectum.[6]

The introduction of fiberoscopic colonoscopy has now made it possible to take biopsies from any part of the large bowel, including even the terminal ileum. These samples are currently rather smaller than rectal biopsies but improvement in the technical methods of taking colonoscopic biopsies is producing pieces of tissue which are satisfactory for histologic interpretation, provided they are correctly oriented. From the viewpoint of the histopathologist the technique and interpretation of colonic biopsies are essentially the same as for rectal biopsy. As endoscopy and biopsy of the whole large intestine become routine methods of investigation it is imperative that histopathologists improve their technique of preparation as well as interpretation of biopsy material from inflammatory bowel diseases. However, more accurate histologic criteria will only be developed if there is close co-operation between gastroenterologists, surgeons, and histopathologists.

Technical Methods

Meticulous attention to technique makes interpretation easier and more productive of useful information. Choice of fixative is important but correct micro-anatomic orientation of the biopsy when it is embedded in paraffin wax is essential. The techniques recently developed for the examination of jejunal biopsies are an example.

At the present time the endoscopist will use either a forceps technique or a suction method for rectal biopsy.[6-8] The latter, in my experience, produces pieces of tissue of standard shape and size which are easily oriented correctly at the embedding stage. However, the suction biopsy method has a small but significant complication factor in the form of hemorrhage from the rectum. The biopsy should be treated in the same way regardless of the technique used by the endoscopist.

The piece of tissue obtained should be placed on the operator's finger so that its submucosal surface, which appears as a central white core, is uppermost. A small piece of frosted glass or nylon mesh (not filter paper, which is much less satisfactory) is lightly applied to the submucosal surface of the specimen, which will adhere to it by the specimen's own stickiness. The whole is then dropped into a fixative. Choice of fixative is a controversial issue but in my experience *buffered* formol saline and formol mercury are perfectly satisfactory. After the specimen has been fixed it is removed from the piece of frosted glass or nylon mesh, turned

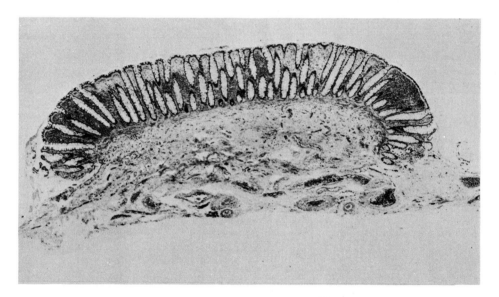

Fig. 1. Suction biopsy specimen of normal rectal mucosa. There is good microanatomic orientation of the mucosa and submucosa. The dark areas in the mucous membrane are artifactual hemorrhage. Hematoxylin and eosin. × 9.5.

on its side, and processed in the usual way. Often it will have floated off spontane-
ously but seldom before it has become fixed in a flat position. The flattening of the
specimen, produced by mounting, allows histologic sections to be cut at right
angles, thus producing correct microanatomic orientation of the biopsy.

The Normal Rectal Mucosa (Figs. 1 and 2)

In the ideal biopsy the epithelial tubules should appear strictly parallel to
one another and in most of them the whole length of the crypt should be under ob-

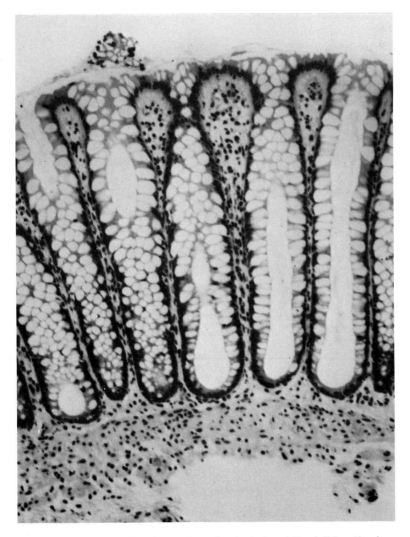

Fig. 2. Normal rectal mucosa. The biopsy is well oriented and the full length of every crypt
is under observation. Note how the base of each crypt rests directly against the muscularis mucosae. Hematoxylin and eosin. × 100.

servation. Loss of parallelism and branching of crypts are abnormal. The crypts are evenly spaced in normal mucosa and the bases rest directly on the muscularis mucosae. Any significant gap between the base of the crypts and the muscularis mucosae is either due to mucosal atrophy or to edema.

The epithelial crypts in normal rectal mucosa are almost wholly lined by goblet cells, but it is normal for some of the surface cells and those at the base of the crypts to be without signs of mucin production. Argentaffin cells are present at the base of many crypts but Paneth cells are not a feature of normal rectal mucosa.

In normal mucosa the epithelial tubules are embedded in a connective tissue stroma or lamina propria which contains a variable quantity of lymphocytes, plasma cells, and macrophages, but very few polymorphonuclear leukocytes. The normal cellular content of the lamina propria is, at present, assessed subjectively from experience.

Hemorrhage into the mucous membrane in the absence of any other abnormality can be an artifact (Fig. 1) and seems to be more common with suction than forceps biopsy. Thickening of the muscularis mucosae is also artifactual in badly oriented biopsies which have been cut tangentially. The distinction between a normal mucosal lymphoid follicle and a focus of lymphocytic infiltration is also made difficult by tangential cutting.

Ulcerative Colitis

Although there are no specific features in the histology of ulcerative colitis, there are patterns of inflammation which are characteristic of the different clinical phases of the disease. Ulcerative colitis is a disease of remissions and exacerbations of varying severity. The histopathologist studying an excised surgical specimen or a single rectal biopsy sees the morphology of the disease only at that particular moment in time, whereas with repeated or sequential biopsies it is possible to monitor the progress of the patient. By comparing sequential biopsies with one another a dynamic "moving" picture of the histology can be established which enables the diagnosis of ulcerative colitis to be made more accurately and also gives valuable information about the histology of the different phases of the disease (Fig. 3).

Fig. 3. A. Ulcerative colitis in an active phase. There is marked mucin depletion of the epithelium and many aggregates of polymorphs are present, some within the crypts and others passing across the epithelial membrane. The content of lymphocytes and plasma cells in the lamina propria is increased. Hematoxylin and eosin. × 65. B. Ulcerative colitis in a resolving phase. Biopsy from the same patient as in Figure 3A one month after treatment with ACTH and steroid enemas. Note the disappearance of polymorphs, restoration of the goblet cell population, and irregularity of the architecture of the crypts. The content of chronic inflammatory cells in the lamina propria remains abnormal. Hematoxylin and eosin. × 65. C. Ulcerative colitis in a resolving phase. Biopsy from the same patient as in Figure 3A and B showing further improvement in the histology two months after treatment. There is still a slight increase in the chronic inflammatory cell content of the lamina propria. Note the branching and irregular architecture of the crypts. Hematoxylin and eosin × 65. D. Ulcerative colitis now in remission. Rectal biopsy in same patient as in Figure 3A–C three months after beginning of treatment. There is no inflammation and no epithelial abnormality except for perhaps a slight irregularity of crypt architecture. Hematoxylin and eosin. × 65.

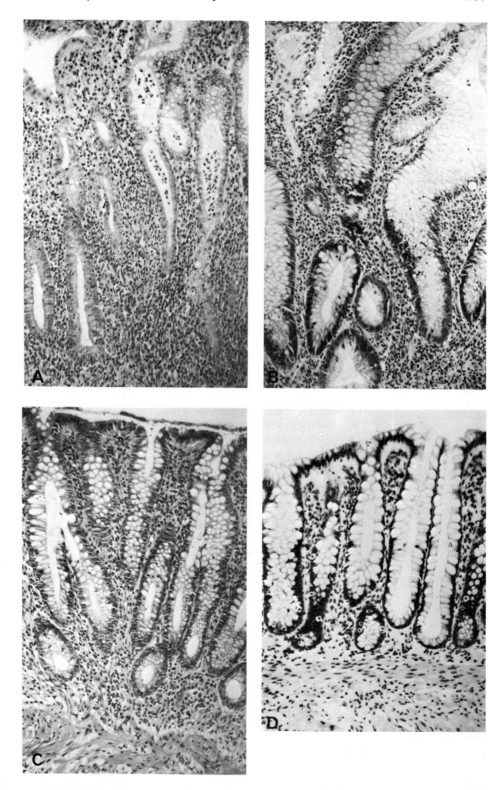

The monitoring of patients with ulcerative colitis by regular rectal biopsy is useful in a number of ways. It can establish the diagnosis, check the accuracy of sigmoidoscopic observations, and identify the phase of the disease and the severity of the mucosal damage. Moreover, it has an important role in the diagnosis of the precancerous phase of ulcerative colitis.

The salient features of the biopsy diagnosis of ulcerative colitis are summarized in Table 1.

TABLE 1.   Rectal Biopsy in Ulcerative Colitis: Salient Features

Active Phase

1. Irregular mucosal surface with luminal pus
2. Loss of epithelium with ulceration
3. Increased chronic inflammatory cell content of lamina propria
4. Focal polymorph infiltration with crypt abscesses and edema
5. Vascular congestion
6. Mucin depletion of goblet cells

Resolving Phase

1. Reduction in vascular congestion
2. Gradual disappearance of polymorphs and crypt abscesses
3. Restoration of goblet cell population
4. Reactive epithelial hyperplasia and restoration of epithelial continuity
5. Declining population of lymphocytes and plasma cells

Colitis in Remission

1. Loss of parallelism, unequal separation and branching of crypts
2. Short tubules of varying length, separated from one another (mucosal atrophy)
3. Thickening of the muscularis mucosae
4. Paneth cell metaplasia

In the *active phase* of ulcerative colitis (Fig. 3a) there is mucosal inflammation of variable severity with an increase in the lymphocyte and plasma cell content of the lamina propria and polymorphonuclear infiltration which is usually focal and often in the form of crypt abscesses. It cannot be emphasized too strongly that the latter are not specific for ulcerative colitis, being seen in most inflammatory bowel disorders. The mucosal surface is irregular and covered with pus. Vascular congestion and hemorrhage are prominent. The epithelium shows a variable degree of destruction, especially of the superficial part of the crypts. This is accompanied by mucin depletion of the goblet cells and reactive hyperplasia of surviving epithelium. Mucin depletion is a very important sign of active disease [9] and objective methods of measuring it could be rewarding. More histochemical studies of mucosubstances in ulcerative colitis and other inflammatory bowel diseases should also be pursued.[10, 11]

Ulcerative colitis in an active phase can be graded subjectively into mild, moderate, or severe according to the severity of the mucosal destruction and other

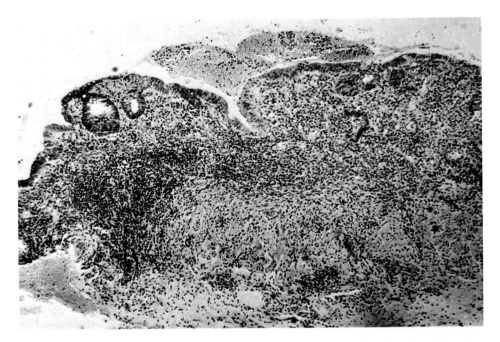

Fig. 4. Chronic ulcerative colitis in an active phase. There is mucosal atrophy with active inflammation. The thickened muscularis mucosae can be identified in the lower part of the photograph. Hematoxylin and eosin. × 93.

signs mentioned above. In mild cases the epithelial membrane can show mucin depletion but otherwise remains almost intact: at the other extreme in very severe attacks the entire mucous membrane consists only in a zone of inflammatory cells with a few surviving tubules and the muscularis mucosae is identifiable only as a line across which cells infiltrate into the submucosal layer (Fig. 4). In biopsies from very severe active ulcerative colitis it is even possible for the mucous membrane to be completely denuded of the epithelium. In such patients sigmoidoscopy can underestimate the severity of the disease.

The monitoring of patients by sequential rectal biopsy, e.g., once a week or once a fortnight, reveals the changes of ulcerative colitis in a *resolving phase* (Fig. 3B C). Among the first changes are a reduction in vascularity and gradual disappearance of polymorphs and crypt abscesses, but the increased content of plasma cells and lymphocytes is the last to decline. The restoration of the goblet cell population is among the earliest signs of resolution and is accompanied by reactive hyperplasia of the epithelium, especially at the base of the crypts, and restoration of epithelial continuity. Attempts to restore the normal architecture of the mucosa are accompanied by branching and irregularity of the epithelial tubules. In cases where there has been very severe mucosal loss, a single layer of columnar cells will cover an ulcerated area with differentiation into minitubules which grow in the direction of the muscularis mucosae, but usually fail to reach it. This leaves a permanent gap between the base of the crypts and the luminal side of the muscularis mucosae. This gap is an important sign of mucosal atrophy.

During the phase of resolution of an attack of colitis the inflammation, especially lymphocytes and plasma cells, may become patchy or focal, and this can give rise to difficulties in the differential diagnosı from Crohn's disease. The histopathologist will often examine rectal biopsies without much clinical information and he may receive a single sample at any stage of the inflammatory process. If he is uncertain about the diagnosis or the stage of colitis a further biopsy should be

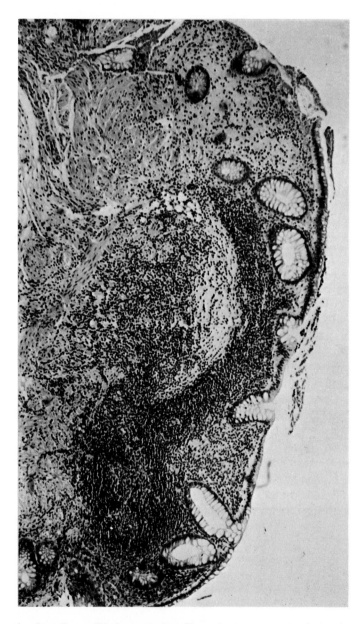

Fig. 5. Chronic ulcerative colitis in remission. There is severe mucosal atrophy with hyperplasia of lymphoid tissue, but no sign of active inflammation. The goblet cell population of the epithelium is normal. Note the thickening of the muscularis mucosae. Hematoxylin and eosin. × 100.

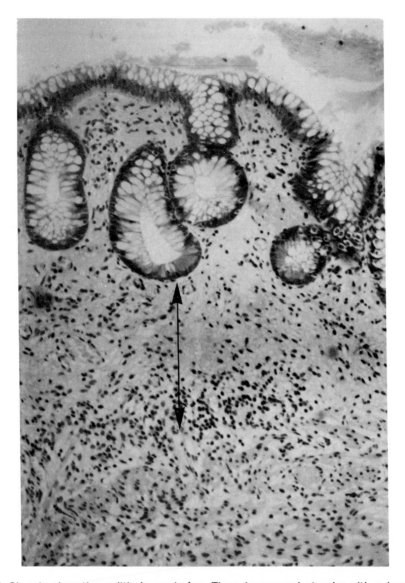

Fig. 6. Chronic ulcerative colitis in remission. There is mucosal atrophy with a large gap between the base of the crypts and the luminal side of the muscularis mucosae (arrows); there is also Paneth cell metaplasia at the base of the crypts. Hematoxylin and eosin. × 100.

requested for purposes of comparison. The time taken for an attack of colitis to resolve in response to treatment is quite variable and more research is required into the histology of sequential biopsies in order to gain experience regarding the microscopic changes in the different phases of the disease.

Rectal biopsies will sometimes be taken from patients with ulcerative colitis *in remission* (Fig. 3D; Figs. 5 and 6). Under these circumstances the sigmoido-scopic appearances can be quite normal. It does not follow that the rectal mucosa will be normal histologically. Sometimes it is possible for the pathologist to make a diagnosis of ulcerative colitis in remission when there is only a history of "colitis" and the patient has no symptoms. Such a diagnosis is valuable because it warns the physician or surgeon that the patient has had the disease, may have more attacks, and particularly may come into that group of mild and even symptomless colitics who are at risk from malignant change.

In ulcerative colitis in complete remission the inflammatory content of the rectal mucosa is within normal limits, epithelial continuity is restored, and the goblet cell population has returned to normal. However, there are nearly always some signs of *mucosal atrophy*. They may be minor, such as slight loss of parallelism, separation of the tubules, or branching of the crypts (Fig. 3C).[12] In patients with a long history of severe disease the atrophy can be very striking (Figs. 5 and 6). There is shortening of the crypts which fail to reach right down to the luminal surface of the muscularis mucosae leaving a characteristic gap. The muscularis mucosae itself is usually thickened with a tendency to splaying of its fibers.

Paneth cell metaplasia at the base of the crypts is a sign of a long history of colitis and is usually associated with some degree of atrophy (Fig. 6).

The presence of an increased number of lymphoid follicles in the mucosa is usually associated with a long history of colitis, but this is not always so. Some patients seem to have a particular capacity for forming lymphoid follicles and the mucous membrane may be packed with them, but the submucosal tissues are normal. This appearance is sometimes called "follicular proctitis" (Fig. 7) and probably represents a local immunologic response. It seems particularly sensitive to steroid therapy.

In some patients with long-standing chronic colitis there is a tendency for the mucosa to develop a villous structure. It may be that such patients are prone to malignant change but further study of this problem is required. In any case it is the degree of epithelial dysplasia which is more important in this context.

It is not always possible to classify rectal biopsy appearances into active colitis, resolving colitis, or colitis in remission with confidence. There are patients in whom the inflammation is a more continuous process of low grade activity in which the salient features of active disease are muted. Moreover, it would appear that attempts at resolution may be unsuccessful or incomplete and repeated biopsies then show the histology of colitis, held up as it were, in the resolving phase.

Histologic reports on most rectal biopsies should indicate the phase of the disease, an assessment of the severity of the attack, and whether there are signs of long-standing inflammation, such as mucosal atrophy and Paneth cell metaplasia. It is possible to see signs in one biopsy which show, for example, evidence of active disease superimposed on a mucosa which is atrophic (Fig. 4). This suggests that there have been previous attacks of colitis.

The introduction of colonoscopy and biopsy should make it possible for the sampling error inherent in rectal biopsy alone to be overcome. However, experience so far indicates that sequential rectal biopsies taken in conjunction with clinical and radiologic data usually give a reliable indication of the state of the patient.

Rectal biopsy has an important role in the management of the chronic colitic whose symptoms are mild but who, with increasing length of history, becomes

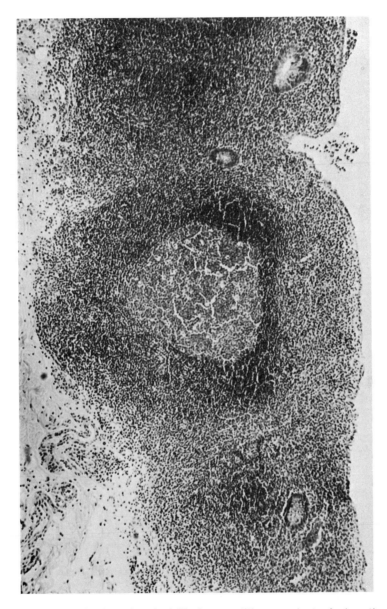

Fig. 7. Rectal biopsy showing chronic follicular proctitis, a variant of ulcerative colitis. Hematoxylin and eosin. $\times$ 100.

statistically at risk from malignant change.[13, 14] Such persons should be monitored by sequential biopsy about twice a year for evidence of epithelial changes which may indicate entry into a *precancerous phase*. The histologic criteria for a diagnosis of precancer in ulcerative colitis are insufficiently accurate at the present time. Histopathologists should have no difficulty in recognizing the more obvious signs of severe epithelial dysplasia or carcinoma-in-situ (Fig. 8),[15] but it is still

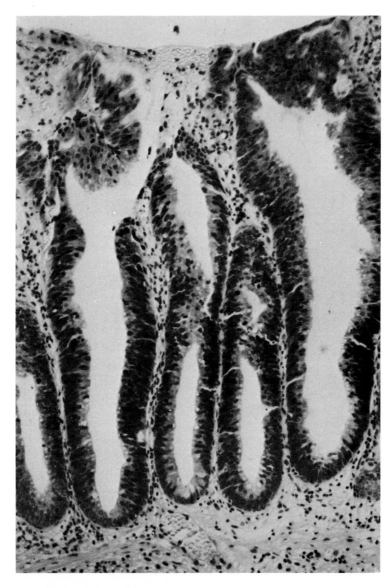

Fig. 8. Rectal biopsy from a patient with a very long clinical history of ulcerative colitis in remission. The appearances are those of carcinoma-in-situ. Hematoxylin and eosin. × 100.

difficult to assess the significance of minor changes. In the experience of the writer it is only possible to make a diagnosis of precancer in the absence of much inflammation because of the difficulty of distinguishing genuine dysplasia from reactive hyperplasia. Clearly much more research into the histologic and cytologic spectrum of the precancerous phase, as well as its extent and topographic distribution, is required. There is a sampling error in some patients and here again colonoscopy and biopsy will prove useful.

The signs of epithelial dysplasia are essentially the same as in other organs, e.g., the cervix. There is enlargement of nuclei which are pleomorphic, show hyperchromatism, and are often stratified with loss of polarity. The numbers of mitotic figures are increased and these are found at all levels of the mucous membrane, not only at the base of the crypts as in reactive hyperplasia. Goblet cell depletion may be marked, but in some cases there is an excess of mucin and this is usually accompanied by a tendency to a low villous type of growth pattern. The dysplasia usually involves the full thickness of the mucous membrane and can be graded into mild, moderate, and severe. The latter is virtually synonymous with carcinoma-in-situ.

Rectal biopsy in the chronic colitic is valuable in the detection of precancerous change. But it is also useful for the physician to know that the biopsy is not precancerous because this suggests that the patient, although statistically at risk from cancer, has no morphologic evidence of malignant change. Only a minority of patients who are statistically at risk actually get cancer. The pathologist can help to identify the *individual* who is at greatest risk. However, there is a sampling error inherent in rectal biopsy and, in theory at least, it is desirable for all total colitics with a history of symptoms for longer than ten years to have a colonoscopy and biopsy, especially if there is any suggestion of epithelial dysplasia in the rectal biopsy.

Crohn's Disease

Rectal biopsy is an important technique for the differential diagnosis of Crohn's disease from ulcerative colitis. The most useful sign is the detection of granulomas in the mucosa or submucosa (Fig. 9). These are small aggregates of epithelioid cell histiocytes, often including giant cells of the Langhans type, which can be missed unless they are looked for carefully in multiple or step sections of the biopsy. However, granulomas are not essential for the diagnosis of Crohn's disease. So-called *disproportionate inflammation* [16] in which there is much submucosal inflammation beneath an inflamed but intact mucous membrane is rather characteristic, especially when the main features of the inflammation are focal lymphocytic infiltration, edema, lymphangiectasia, and good preservation of the epithelium and its goblet cell population (Fig. 10). In other biopsies it is possible to indicate that the appearances are unlike ulcerative colitis because of the patchy nature of mucosal inflammation, which again is predominantly lymphocytic with a well-preserved epithelium and population of goblet cells. Although crypt abscesses are seen in Crohn's disease they are fewer than in ulcerative colitis. The writer has yet to see mucosal atrophy without inflammation in a biopsy from a patient with Crohn's disease.

In some patients with Crohn's disease of the colon and a clinically normal rectum, rectal biopsy may show no microscopic abnormality, but in others there is obvious edema of an otherwise normal rectal mucosa, perhaps with a little focal lymphocytic infiltration. Another feature of rectal biopsy histology which is suggestive of Crohn's disease is the presence of scattered ulcerating lymphoid follicles without any other mucosal abnormality.

Repeated biopsy at intervals over a period of a few weeks or longer provides opportunity for comparisons which can be very helpful in diagnosis. Generally

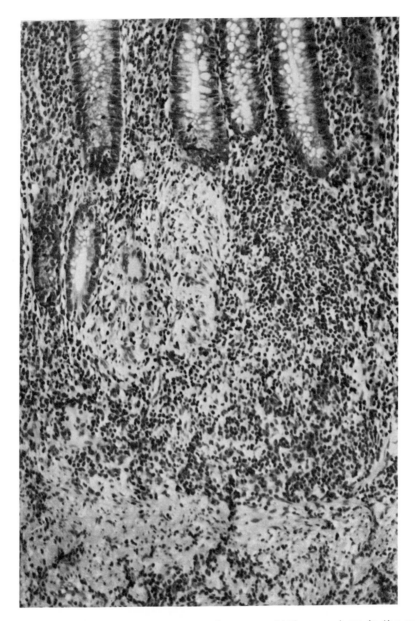

Fig. 9. Rectal biopsy in Crohn's disease showing a sarcoid-like granuloma in the mucous membrane. Hematoxylin and eosin. × 100.

speaking, ulcerative colitis is a disease in which rectal biopsy histology is likely to fluctuate considerably with or without treatment. In Crohn's disease, on the other hand, we are dealing with a persistent inflammation the quality of which changes little with time or in response to current therapy. However, the patchy nature of the condition will inevitably be reflected in samples taken from different parts of the rectum at the same or different moments in time. The most important sign-

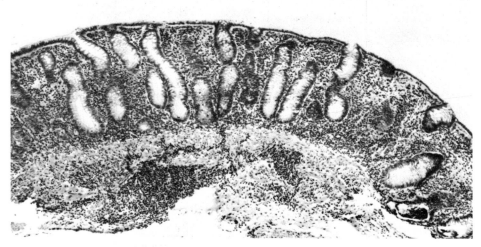

Fig. 10. Rectal biopsy from a patient with Crohn's disease showing mucosal and submucosal inflammation which is predominantly lymphocytic. Otherwise the epithelium and its goblet cell population are well preserved. Hematoxylin and eosin. × 83.

TABLE 2.   Some Signposts in the Biopsy Diagnosis of Ulcerative Colitis and Crohn's Disease

Ulcerative Colitis	*Crohn's Disease*
1. Primarily a mucosal inflammation	1. Mucosal or submucosal or both
2. Much submucosal disease only with severe mucosal inflammation or ulceration	2. Sometimes more submucosal than mucosal disease (disproportionate inflammation)
3. Granulomas absent	3. Granulomas may be present in mucosa or submucosa or both
4. Lymphocytic aggregates, if present, in otherwise abnormal mucosa only, and with germinal centers	4. Focal inflammation, predominantly lymphocytic, in an otherwise normal mucosa
5. Crypt abscesses commonly present in active phase	5. Crypt abscesses infrequent and fewer in number
6. Vascular congestion pronounced in active phase	6. Vascular congestion not a dominating feature
7. Submucosal lymphangiectasia not pronounced	7. Submucosal lymphangiectasia often pronounced
8. Mucin depletion in active phase	8. Goblet cell population usually well preserved
9. Mucosal atrophy	9. No mucosal atrophy
10. Paneth cell metaplasia sometimes present in chronic cases	10. Paneth cell metaplasia unusual
11. Thickening of muscularis mucosae	11. Thickening of muscularis mucosae not a usual feature
12. Epithelial dysplasia (precancer)	12. Epithelial dysplasia not seen

posts in the differential diagnosis of ulcerative colitis and Crohn's disease are summarized in Table 2.

All histopathologists continue to have difficulties in the interpretation of rectal biopsies in inflammatory bowel disease and equivocal reports are frequent. Further improvement in the quality of diagnosis will only come from improved technique, better collaboration between the endoscopist and the laboratory, and more experience in biopsy histology.

The Dysenteric Disorders

Ulcerative colitis and Crohn's disease are the most important in the differential diagnosis of inflammatory bowel disorders in the Western World. When examining rectal biopsies the histopathologist must, however, be alert for other conditions which may be easily confused with ulcerative colitis. The acute dysenteric disorders are an example and every biopsy should be consciously screened for *amoebic dysentery*. The *Entamoeba histolytica* is a large cell which is readily recognized, usually in the exudate covering the mucosa or adjacent to a mucosal erosion. The histology of the rectal biopsy appearances in acute intestinal amoebiasis has been described in detail and correlated with sigmoidoscopic appearances.[17, 18]

The histology of *shigellosis* shows certain differences from ulcerative colitis

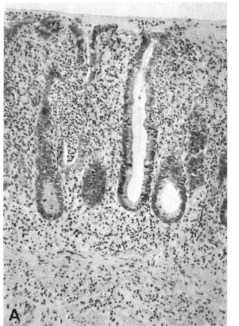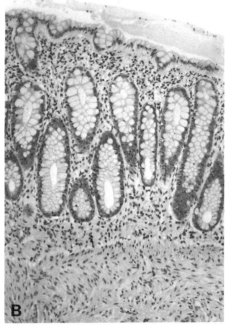

Fig. 11. A. Rectal biopsy from a patient with shigellosis. Most of the inflammatory cells are polymorphs and it is doubtful whether there is any increase in the chronic inflammatory cell population of the lamina propria. Hematoxylin and eosin. × 62. B. Rectal biopsy from the same patient with shigellosis after four days treatment with Neomycin. The mucosa is almost normal. Hematoxylin and eosin. × 62.

(Fig. 11A and B). In the former, a more diffuse polymorphonuclear infiltrate is characteristic, unlike the more focal distribution of these cells in active ulcerative colitis. According to the severity of the inflammation there is destruction of tissue with mucin depletion of the epithelial cells. However, the deeper layers of the mucosa are often spared any inflammation. Vascular congestion is not prominent and there is almost no increase in the plasma cell and lymphocyte population of the lamina propria. If the clinical situation also suggests an infective etiology a trial of antibiotic therapy will produce a dramatic response in the mucosal biopsy appearances, which will return to normal within a few days. This never happens in ulcerative colitis. In the writer's limited experience of *salmonella infections* the mucosal epithelium is well preserved, and there are scattered, rather small crypt abscesses but no increase in the lymphocyte and plasma cell content of the lamina propria. It would be helpful if pathologists could get more biopsies from patients with dysenteric colitis for purposes of comparison with the appearances of ulcerative colitis.

The Solitary Ulcer Syndrome

(Syns.: localized colitis cystica profunda; hamartomatous
           inverted polyp; the descending perineal syndrome)

This condition is often confused with ulcerative colitis and is probably commoner than was supposed at one time. It would appear that excessive straining at stool and abnormal habits of defecation can lead to internal prolapse of the rectal mucosa into the rectum or into the anal canal, where it becomes traumatized with subsequent development of a zonal proctitis which may proceed to a clinically characteristic lesion known as "solitary ulcer" of the rectum.[19] This is a poorly chosen name since the ulcers are not always solitary, nor is ulceration always present. This syndrome seems to be basically a proctitis, secondary to abnormal anorectal function. It is probably synonymous with the descending perineal syndrome.[20]

The rectal biopsy appearances are very characteristic (Fig. 12). Often there is very superficial and irregular mucosal ulceration with the formation of a surface exudate of mucus, fibrin, and pus cells. The crypts are hyperplastic but the most significant abnormality is seen in the lamina propria. This is obliterated by spindle-shaped cells, most of which are fibroblasts but others of which are smooth muscle fibers growing up between the crypts from the muscularis mucosae. The content of lymphocytes and plasma cells is reduced. There may be a tendency toward a villous surface configuration of the mucosa. The muscularis mucosae is thickened with splaying of its fibers. In very chronic cases epithelial tubules become misplaced into the submucosa and undergo cystic dilatation giving the appearances of so-called "localized colitis cystica profunda" [21, 22] or "hamartomatous inverted polyp." [23] In my opinion these are expressions which describe only one feature of the solitary ulcer syndrome which is not hamartomatous (as previously believed [19]), and the whole histologic spectrum is probably secondary to abnormal anorectal function. It is interesting and probably relevant that histologic changes identical with those seen in the solitary ulcer syndrome can also be found at the apex of an external rectal prolapse and on the surface mucosa of prolapsing hemorrhoids.

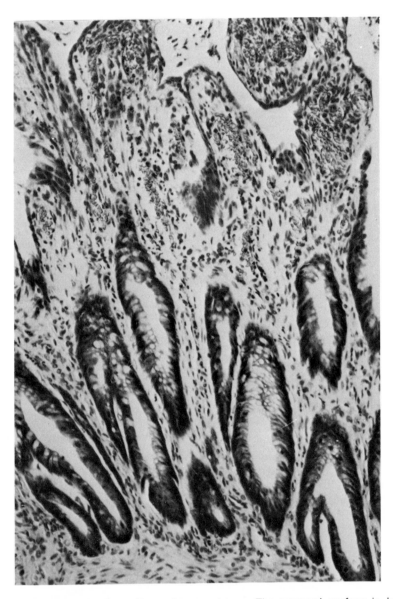

Fig. 12. Rectal biopsy in the solitary ulcer syndrome. The mucosal surface is irregular with attenuation of the covering epithelium and there is vascular congestion and poly-morphonuclear infiltration of the superficial mucosa. The crypts are hyperplastic. In between the crypts the lamina propria contains spindle cells, some of which are fibroblasts and others smooth muscle fibers derived from the muscularis mucosae. Hematoxylin and eosin. × 100.

Cathartic Colon

Another syndrome which can mimic ulcerative colitis is cathartic or purgative colon. Probably all of these patients have some degree of melanosis coli, but this may not be clinically obvious in the rectal segment. The presence of macrophages containing pseudomelanin in the lamina propria of a mucosal biopsy of the rectum should alert the histopathologist to the possibility that the patient also has the neurologic lesion of cathartic colon.[24] However, only a minority of persons with melanosis coli have the clinical and radiologic features of this syndrome. In cathartic colon the rectal mucosa can show some increase in its chronic inflammatory cell content which accounts for the endoscopic appearance of a proctitis. Other signs are thickening of the muscularis mucosae and an excess of submucosal adipose tissue.[25]

Ischaemic Disease of the Colon

Disorders of the mesenteric circulation, whether occlusive or nonocclusive, can produce mucosal changes in the rectum which mimic the symptoms of inflam-

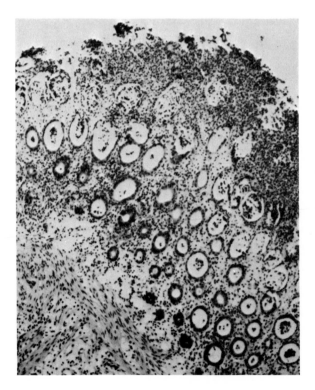

Fig. 13. Rectal biopsy in the membranous type of ischaemic enterocolitis. Hematoxylin and eosin. × 50.

matory bowel disease.[26] Whatever the mechanism of the ischaemic proctitis rectal biopsy has a useful role in diagnosis. Indeed, it is possible for the histopathologist to be the first to recognize acute ischaemic disease by the examination of a biopsy. The appearances are very different from ulcerative colitis.

Perhaps the most characteristic lesion is seen in so-called membranous or pseudomembranous colitis (Fig. 13). The changes can be diffuse or localized to give the "paint-spot" appearance observed macroscopically. The surface of the mucous membrane is covered by a membrane composed of mucin, pus, and red blood cells. The superficial part of the mucosa shows necrosis and the surviving crypts are distended, which gives a ballooning effect with atrophy and necrosis of the lining epithelium. These crypts are filled with mucin and cellular debris which appears to be bursting out to form a surface membrane. There is no infiltration by inflammatory cells but intravascular fibrin thrombi may be present. This type of ischaemic lesion can also be a manifestation of the intravascular coagulation syndrome.[27]

In some cases of ischaemic proctitis there is obvious necrosis of the mucosa without dilatation of the crypts and the formation of a surface membrane (Fig. 14).

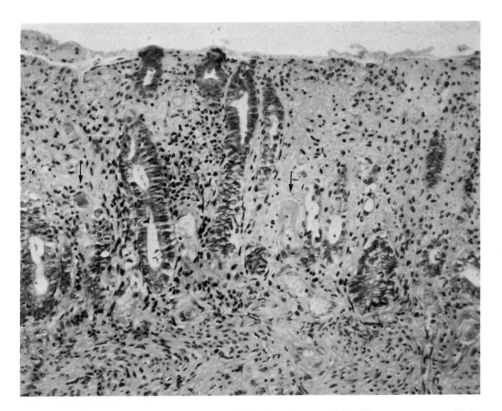

Fig. 14. Rectal biopsy from a patient with ischaemic proctitis. There are many fibrin thrombi present (arrows). Hematoxylin and eosin. $\times$ 100.

Intramucosal hemorrhage may be a feature and fibrinoid necrosis of the walls of blood vessels can be seen both in the mucous membrane and the submucosal layer. This is a secondary effect due to ischaemia following a slowing of the circulation, comparable to the appearance in ischaemic disease of the kidney, and probably the result of a similar mechanism.[28] A careful search of multiple sections of a biopsy, especially if there is much submucosal tissue present, may reveal evidence of atheromatous embolism.

References

1. Gabriel WB, Dukes CE, Bussey HJR: Biopsy of the rectum. Brit J Surg 38:401, 1951
2. Manson-Bahr P, Muggleton WJ: Rectal biopsy as an aid to the diagnosis of amoebic dysentery and allied diseases of the colon. Lancet 1:763, 1957
3. Truelove SC, Richards WCD: Biopsy studies in ulcerative colitis. Brit Med J 1:1315, 1956
4. Lumb G: Rectal biopsy in ulcerative colitis. Dis Colon Rectum 1:37, 1958
5. Lockhart-Mummery HE, Morson BC: Crohn's disease (regional enteritis) of the large intestine and its distinction from ulcerative colitis. Gut 1:87, 1960
6. Gear EV Jr, Dobbins WO: Rectal biopsy. A review of its diagnostic usefulness. Gastroenterology 55:522, 1968
7. Truelove SC, Horler AR, Richards WCD: Serial biopsy in ulcerative colitis. Brit Med J 2:1590, 1955
8. Dick AP, Lennard-Jones JE, Jones JH, et al: Technique for suction biopsy of the rectal mucosa. Gut 11:182, 1970
9. Morson BC: Pathology of ulcerative colitis. Proc R Soc Med 64:976, 1971
10. Hellstrom HR, Fisher ER: Estimation of mucosal mucin as an aid in the differentiation of Crohn's disease of the colon and chronic ulcerative colitis. Amer J Clin Path 48:259, 1967
11. Filipe MI, Dawson IMP: The diagnostic value of mucosubstances in rectal biopsies from patients with ulcerative colitis and Crohn's disease. Gut 11:229, 1970
12. Flick AL, Voegtlin KF, Rubin CE: Clinical experience with suction biopsy of the rectal mucosa. Gastroenterology 42:691, 1962
13. Morson BC, Pang LSC: Rectal biopsy as an aid to cancer control in ulcerative colitis. Gut 8:423, 1967
14. Hultén L, Kewenter J, Åhrén C: Precancer and carcinoma in ulcerative colitis. Scand J Gastroent 7:663, 1972
15. Evans DJ, Pollock DJ: In-situ and invasive carcinoma of the colon in patients with ulcerative colitis. Gut 13:566, 1972
16. Dyer NH, Stansfeld AG, Dawson AM: The value of rectal biopsy in the diagnosis of Crohn's disease. Scand J Gastroent 5:491, 1970
17. Prathap K, Gilman R: The histopathology of acute intestinal amoebiasis. Amer J Path 60:229, 1970
18. Gilman RH, Prathap K: Acute intestinal amoebiasis. Proctoscopic appearances with histopathological correlation. Ann Trop Med Parasitol 65:359, 1971
19. Madigan MR, Morson BC: Solitary ulcer of the rectum. Gut 10:871, 1969
20. Parks AG, Porter NH, Hardcastle J: The syndrome of the descending perineum. Proc R Soc Med 59:477, 1966
21. Wayte DB, Helwig EB: Colitis cystica profunda. Amer J Clin Path 48:159, 1967
22. Epstein SE, Ascari WQ, Ablow RC, Seaman WB, Lattes R: Colitis cystica profunda. Amer J Clin Path 45:186, 1966
23. Allen MS: Hamartomatous inverted polyps of the rectum. Cancer 19:257, 1954

BILIARY CIRRHOSIS

H. EDWARD MACMAHON

This is the story of biliary cirrhosis, its heritage, its birth, its adolescence, and its maturity. Traditions, customs, and habits and, at times, an unreasonable respect for the past have played no small part in much of our present-day nomenclature of disease and also in our knowledge, or lack of knowledge, of some of our more common diseases. The terms *cirrhosis* and *biliary cirrhosis* and the diseases they represent are such examples. First used by Laennec [1] in 1819 to describe the tawny yellow color of the liver of one of his patients, the term *cirrhosis,* though designating the least important characteristic of the disease he was describing, soon became universally adopted. In his description of the autopsy findings, there was "pleurésie chronique du côté gauche avec ascite, et maladie organique du fois." He described the liver as small, hidden, lightly nodular, and of a "grisejaunatre" color. When incised its surface was entirely composed of small, round-to-ovoid nodules varying in size from a millet to a hemp seed. He indicated that each nodule was separated from the others by a narrow interval containing what he believed to be normal liver parenchyma. He described the leathery consistency of the organ and considered the disease to be the commonest cause of ascites. Lastly, he believed that he was dealing with a scirrhous form of neoplasia in which the small nodules represented tumor tissue.

While it is clear to us today that Laennec was describing only one of a large group of diseases of the liver, a very common and important one that quickly acquired his name, this term soon became synonymous with scarring and sclerosis. Cirrhosis was being used, not only to include any form of scarring of the liver, but also to designate scarring of other organs, such as the pancreas, lungs, kidneys, and thyroid. One may still hear or see the expression *a cirrhotic lung,* but generally speaking the term *cirrhosis* today is exclusively used in reference to the liver.

Because this first use of the term *cirrhosis* by Laennec is so often associated with the first account of this disease, it is of some historic interest to point out that Mathew Baillie,[2] who wrote the first textbook of pathology in the English language (1795), gave a very good gross description of the same disease about 25 years earlier. In his book he referred to it as one of the most common, if not the most common, disease of the liver. He pointed out that it was much more common in men than women because of their drinking habits. He described the irregularity of the capsule and the uniform nodularity of the cut surface. He particularly stressed the hardness of the entire organ and indicated that while such a liver is usually of average size, it may be smaller than normal. As for color, it was often yellow due to bile retention. Lastly, he related the jaundiced color of the skin to the changes going on in the liver. In summing up his description, he said "this is the common appearance of what is generally called 'scirrhous liver.'" He did not use the term *cirrhosis*.

Prevailing Concepts Influence Contemporary Thinking

This unitarian concept of cirrhosis as a single disease of the liver, based purely on a gross examination of the organ, persisted for years. But with the development of histologic techniques and with the improvement in microscopy, it was only natural that pathologic histology should soon overtake gross anatomy as the basis for the classification and diagnosis of disease. This was particularly true of diseases of the liver and kidney. Soon other disciplines played an equally important role in the classification of the diseases of the liver. In tracing the steps through which our present classification has evolved, it is interesting to observe how basic discoveries have dominated the thinking of each period. For example, with the birth and almost explosive development of bacteriology in the latter half of the nineteenth century, every inflammatory reaction was considered to be bacterial in origin, and every form of fibrosis was regarded as the end stage of an inflammatory reaction. Indeed, many malformations were considered to be nothing more than the end stages of fetal infections.

Later, with the recognition of specific bacterial toxins, a new concept of humoral pathology developed. This seemed to be the answer to many unsolved problems, for what could not be explained by the actual presence of an organism was soon regarded as "toxic" in origin. This concept was soon extended to include a variety of chemical intoxications and also autointoxications which were so fashionable at the beginning of this century. Many years passed before the importance of viruses as a cause of liver disease was appreciated. Today there is probably no disease of the liver that has not been directly or indirectly ascribed to a virus.

As for the role of drugs in our own medicated society, quite apart from the use of alcohol or drug addiction, there is hardly a liver disease in which one or a combination of drugs has not in some way been incriminated. Also influencing our thinking today are the inherited enzyme deficiencies often manifesting themselves as "inborn errors of metabolism" which so often leave their fingerprint on the liver. This group includes one of the most recently detected of the enzyme deficiencies, namely, alpha-l-antitrypsin deficiency associated in certain patients with emphysema. But this listing is not all, for now we are confronted with the probability that some diseases of the liver may be nothing more than an expression of an inappropriate immunologic response on the part of the host, or an autoimmune reaction possibly to one's own mitochondria.

Each of these steps has left its mark. Each has made its own contribution, each in turn has enjoyed its own wave of enthusiasm, and each has temporarily influenced the thinking of each period. As the past so often reflects the probable course of the future, there can obviously be no stopping.

It is important for every pathologist to be aware of these changing concepts, for each represents an almost revolutionary advance in our thinking. It is important, too, to pursue vigorously the problems of etiology and pathogenesis, but it is equally important for the diagnostic pathologist to be very familiar with the histologic patterns of these diseases of the liver and to know the nature of each disease that has its own particular pattern. This is a prerequisite to accurate diagnosis. In respect to our knowledge of the histology of disease, nothing has contributed more than the day-to-day observations that are made at the autopsy table and at the surgical desk through the careful examination of biopsy material. Lastly, as important as either, is the necessity to have a good relationship between clinician and pathologist.

It is with this in mind, as I look back over nearly 50 years in the laboratory, that I need offer no apology for the contents of this paper, for it is concerned with the problem of diagnosis for the experienced and less experienced hospital pathologist. It is well to remember that it is the lesion itself, perfectly fixed and perfectly stained, that is our source of information. Our responsibility is to interpret this intelligently, for if one can establish an accurate diagnosis on the basis of a biopsy specimen, this may well prove to be the most meaningful piece of the puzzle in determining the ultimate care and prognosis of the patient.

The Mallory Era in America

Today almost every pathologist has his own definition of cirrhosis. Mallory, who in the first quarter of this century contributed so much to our knowledge of diseases of the liver, defined cirrhosis as "any sclerosed condition whether progressive or not in which destruction of liver cells is associated with real or apparent increase in connective tissue." In his classic paper of 1911 entitled "Cirrhosis of the Liver" [3] he described in detail what he regarded as five distinct types, the outcome of five separate and distinct diseases. That paper is not only a classic in description and interpretation, but is also unusual in that it includes 16 plates and drawings of excellent quality that are equal to any that may be found today.

His five types included (1) *toxic cirrhosis,* which he associated with some circulating toxin. Chloroform, for example, was frequently incriminated as the cause of this disease. His photomicrographs clearly show that this type would now be referred to as "postnecrotic cirrhosis."

His second type he called *infectious cirrhosis,* caused, he believed, by bacteria gaining entrance into the liver by way of the bile ducts. Here his photomicrographs and their legends are most helpful, for in this one type we find not one, as he had believed, but three separate entities including: (a) the actual presence of bacteria embedded in an inflammatory exudate within the cholangioles; (b) a classic example of what we now call congenital hepatic fibrosis with a superimposed infection and purulent inflammation; and (c) an example of long-standing uncomplicated extrahepatic cholestasis which we would now call "obstructive cirrhosis." At that time Mallory denied that bile stasis alone could lead to cirrhosis—a concept which probably relates to the prevailing influence that infection played in the thinking of that period. He did, however, concede that infection of the bile duct was commonly secondary to biliary obstruction, and in one of his plates there is an example of this combination.

His third type, *pigment cirrhosis,* had been recognized here and abroad for years. Histologically the keystone of this type was an excessive accumulation of hemosiderin in a scarred liver. In passing, it is of interest to recall that until his death in 1941 Mallory considered copper ingestion to be the most important factor in the etiology of this particular type of cirrhosis.

Syphilitic cirrhosis, caused by the actual presence in the liver of *Treponema pallidum,* was his fourth type. Here he divided this cirrhosis into those livers in which sclerosis was diffuse (congenital) and those in which scarring was focal, representing the disease of later life. One of his plates from a case of congenital syphilis shows masses of *Treponema* beautifully demonstrated within the space of Disse.

His last and fifth type, *alcoholic cirrhosis,* was the most important and the most common. Here we find Mallory's first description of what is now almost universally called "alcoholic hyalin," which has become such an important diagnostic sign. His plates show liver cells undergoing a peculiar form of degeneration before leukocytic infiltration. In all these five types he saw an inflammatory reaction, and to him cirrhosis was simply the late phase of a progressive or healed disease.

Before leaving that paper, it should be emphasized again that Mallory did not use the term *biliary cirrhosis.* This was purposeful for he found both the term and the literature confusing. He stressed the importance of ascending infections along the biliary passages ultimately leading to "infectious cirrhosis." He also admitted that infections of this type sometimes followed a preexisting obstruction, but he was unwilling to accept the terms *obstructive cirrhosis* or *obstructive biliary cirrhosis,* terms already in common use both here and abroad. He felt that in every case of cirrhosis in which an obstruction could be found along the course of the common duct, an underlying infection was always present.

The Spectrum of Cirrhosis Expands

Twenty years later, taking advantage of the annual Shattuck Lecture, which was delivered before the Massachusetts Medical Society, Mallory again discussed the subject of cirrhosis. The title of his lecture was "Cirrhosis of the Liver." [4] This was based on his own personal observations and investigations after 35 years as pathologist for the Boston City Hospital. He spoke of an analysis of all cases of cirrhosis which had come to postmortem examination. There were 550 cases, and these represented 5.88 percent of all autopsies. Again he stressed the point that cirrhosis of the liver was simply a late stage in the development of a dozen different diseases, and that to understand cirrhosis one must know the natural histories of the diseases from which it might arise. He emphasized here the importance of knowing the early stages of these diseases, for then the pattern of histology is often much more specific than at the end.

It must be remembered at this point that at the time of that lecture diagnostic needle biopsies of the liver were unknown, and surgical biopsies for diagnostic purposes were extremely uncommon. This meant that the autopsy was the only source of histologic material on which to base one's diagnosis and the only source of material on which to base a concept of what one believed to be the natural course of a disease of the liver. Today a needle biopsy taken during the early stage of a disease, or even a succession of biopsies, may not only be of great diagnostic importance but of inestimable value to the pathologist who is concerned with following the natural course of a disease. In Mallory's analysis of 550 livers showing cirrhosis, 104, or nearly 20 percent, were listed as unclassified. This was not only because he was very cautious, but rather because so many cases were seen in the late stage when, as he said, their specific identity may not be recognized.

Because some forms of cirrhosis were so uncommon and others so little known in this part of the world, he limited himself to seven types, not five as he had 20 years earlier. These seven now included *obstructive cirrhosis,* a type caused by the mechanical occlusion of either the hepatic or common bile ducts. This was best seen in infants with focal atresia of the common duct. The second type in his analysis was *colon bacillus cirrhosis,* a type which may occur alone or as a complication of obstruction. In the late or healed stages, because of the impossibility of distinguishing an obstructive from the colon bacillus type of cirrhosis, or a combination of the two, he admitted that this small group could be referred to a "biliary cirrhosis."

His third type he called *healed acute yellow atrophy.* This corresponded to the type he had classified earlier as "toxic." The extensive liver cell necrosis which was an essential component in the development of that disease was caused, he said, by a variety of toxins of bacterial origin, especially those derived from the streptococci and pneumococci and also by such chemicals as arsenic, phosphorus, chloroform, and carbon tetrachloride.

A fourth type was given the specific name of *streptococcus cirrhosis.*[5] On the basis of cases of streptococcal hepatitis showing massive liver cell necrosis and massive infection which he personally had seen, he believed that should a patient recover from such a disease, the healed stage could present a liver pattern which would be indistinguishable from that of "healed acute yellow atrophy." This concept is of some historic interest since it suggested the possibility of an infection as one factor in the etiology of "healed acute yellow atrophy," years before viruses were recognized as the most common cause of this disease. The fifth type was *syphilitic cirrhosis.* The sixth was *pigment cirrhosis,* and the seventh and last was *alcoholic cirrhosis.*

In comparing this list of seven types of cirrhosis with Mallory's original list of five, we find three terms that are common, namely, "alcoholic," "pigment," and "syphilitic" cirrhosis. The toxic cirrhosis of 1911 was now called "healed acute yellow atrophy." As for his original "infectious cirrhosis" caused by infections along the bile ducts, he became more specific and designated this type as "colon bacillus cirrhosis." [6] Of particular interest was his acceptance of a type of cirrhosis that could be initiated and developed by bile stasis alone. This acknowledgement was not based on a review of the literature but on work done in his own laboratory, first through a review of all cases of biliary obstruction from the files of the Boston City Hospital and Children's Hospital over a period of years,[7] and secondly by the experimental production of this type of cirrhosis under aseptic surgical conditions.[8] In this same lecture he also acknowledged for the first time the usefulness of the term biliary cirrhosis to designate the small group comprising (1) obstructive cirrhosis, (2) colon bacillus cirrhosis, and (3) combinations of the two. It must be admitted that this acceptance was rather late in coming to the Boston community, for these were terms that had been in general use in Europe and in other parts of this country for years.[9-16]

The Roessle Era in Germany

In Germany at about this time Roessle, who held the Virchow post of pathology at the University of Berlin, was the leading European authority on cirrhosis of the liver. His chapters covering the inflammatory diseases of the liver in Henke and Lubarsch (1930) are still considered as classics in this field. His concept of biliary cirrhosis [17] was based on the presence of a chronic interstitial inflammatory reaction in the portal areas arising in the bile ducts and cholangioles and also arising from a faulty elimination of bile.

With this as a basis he described three types of cirrhosis which could be included in this one category. First, *obstructive biliary cirrhosis;* second, a "cholangitic" type of infectious origin (cholangiohepatitis); and third, a *cholangiolotoxic* type (cholangiolohepatitis) arising in the terminal cholangioles. The last of these three was the most difficult to define. Among toxins that might initiate this reaction was manganese. Experimentally this chemical had been shown to produce a form of chronic interstitial inflammation within the portal areas. Today this third type has become one of the most common of all types of biliary cirrhosis, for it is related now, not only to viral infections and to many drugs in common use,[20] but also to such diagnostic and industrial hazards as beryllium [18] and thorotrast.[19] In brief, Roessle saw in the term *biliary cirrhosis* not one type of disease but at least three, differing in etiology yet having as a common denominator chronic interstitial hepatitis.

Concepts Versus Facts

In 1938 Thannhauser, a leading authority on diseases of intracellular lipid metabolism, and Magendantz [21] introduced the term *xanthomatous biliary cirrhosis* to designate what they believed to be a unique histologic pattern within the liver characterized by the accumulation of xanthoma cells and fibrous tissue in and about the walls of the intrahepatic bile ducts. The clinical syndrome that these investigators related solely to this type of biliary cirrhosis had been recognized for years. It was almost exclusively confined to female patients about 40 years of age. Addison and Gull,[22] as early as 1851, had given a full description of this symptom complex, but it was Thannhauser and Magendantz who first used the term *xanthomatous biliary cirrhosis* to designate not only the liver pattern which they considered to be specific, but also the complete clinical syndrome. Others years before had reported cases of this syndrome which was characterized by prolonged jaundice, a palpably enlarged liver, hypercholesterolemia, and xanthomatous changes over the body. They had used such terms as *cirrhosis*,[23, 24] *gall stone obstruction*,[25] *hypertrophic cirrhosis*,[26] and *hypertrophic biliary cirrhosis* [27, 28] to designate the changes within the liver, but none had referred to xanthomatous accumulations along the biliary tract. Thannhauser and Magendantz regarded this syndrome as an unusual manifestation of "familial hypercholesteremic xanthomatosis," which was also known as "essential xanthomatosis of the hypercholesteremic type." They presumed that in the course of this systemic disease cholesterol was deposited within the substance of the liver, thereby interfering with the flow of bile and causing jaundice and itching of the skin.

Because of this obvious lack of morphologic uniformity within the liver in patients showing this clinical syndrome, it was only natural that the introduction of a new term *xanthomatous biliary cirrhosis* should evoke considerable curiosity and interest. Fortunately the opportunity soon presented itself to study the histology of the liver in several patients in the Thannhauser clinic of the New England Medical Center. These patients were all females bewteen 40 and 50 years of age. Each was considered to show the classic signs of this syndrome. Utilizing both needle and surgical techniques, the investigators obtained an adequate amount of tissue to permit a thorough histologic examination.[29] None of these patients was seriously ill, yet each had had symptoms for months.

In all the sections that were representative of the earlier stages of the disease, there was a very distinct pattern, but in none was there a trace of xanthoma cells singly or in clusters. Instead, there was a chronic proliferative interstitial inflammatory reaction in each of the portal areas.[30, 31] There was also a marked infiltration with lymphoid cells. This inflammatory growth of tissue expanded each of the portal areas which joined to form perilobular rings of inflammatory granulation tissue. This reaction was most concentrated about the junction ducts at the margin of the portal areas and extended for a short distance into the periphery of the lobules. Liver cells lying in this peripheral zone showed regressive changes including a form of hyaline degeneration that was indistinguishable from that seen in "alcoholic cirrhosis." Some cells underwent necrosis in this area, just as mitotic activity in other areas indicated regeneration. The intertrabecular sinuses were collapsed, columns of liver cells were compressed, and bile canaliculi were blocked in some areas and distended in others; and most important there was a real or apparent loss of the intermediate collecting ducts from the portal areas. Bile canaliculi distended with bile would often end abruptly at the periphery of the lobule in a wall of fibrous tissue.

The Rebirth of an Old Disease

This particular pattern of biliary cirrhosis had features in common with the other types already referred to in this paper, but it also had distinctive characteristics. Because its etiology was obscure, because it seemed to differ from the obstructive and cholangitic types of biliary cirrhosis, because of its apparent close association with a particular syndrome, and especially because of the nature and location of the inflammatory reaction about the small bile ducts, the descriptive term *pericholangiolitic biliary cirrhosis* (pericholangiolohepatitis) was suggested. In any case there was no longer any justification for the use of the term *xanthomatous biliary cirrhosis* to designate this pattern of the liver.

After a period of 2 or 3 years, some of these patients on whom biopsies had been obtained came to autopsy with signs of severe parenchymatous dysfunction of the liver and evidence of portal hypertension. In each case the liver was large,

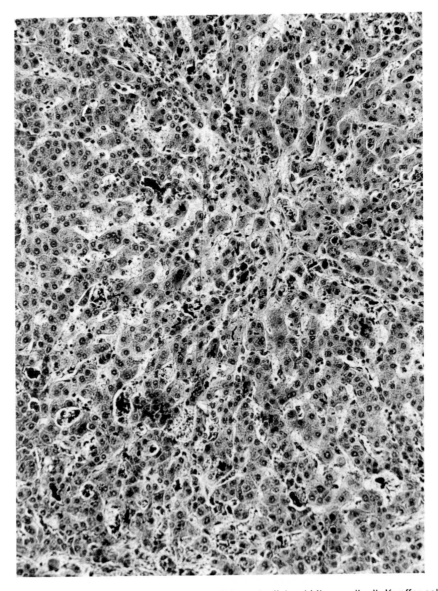

Fig. 1. Liver. Intense centrolobular bile stasis. Bile casts distend bile canaliculi. Kupffer cells, which are increased in size and number, are filled with inspissated bile. The pattern of the lobule is preserved. This section is from a severely jaundiced patient with obstruction of the common bile duct and early obstructive biliary cirrhosis ($\times$ 200).

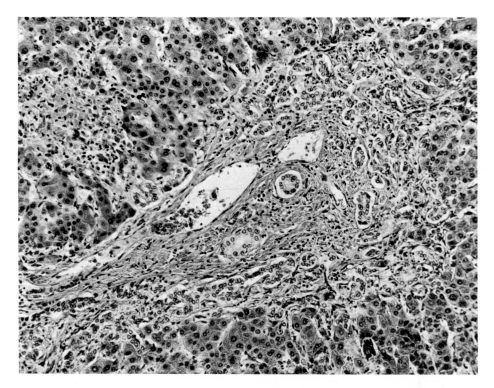

Fig. 2. Liver. Obstructive biliary cirrhosis of several weeks' duration. The portal area is enlarged as the result of a low-grade inflammatory reaction with an increase in tortuosity and number of distended cholangioles. A small area of necrotic liver cells infiltrated by histiocytes lies just to the left of the portal area. There is bile stasis in the canaliculi of the adjacent lobules ($\times$ 178).

heavy, firm, bile-stained, and coarsely fibrous. There was fragmentation of lobules, a complete loss of lobules, and the disease was obviously progressing. There were nodules of regenerated liver cells. There were areas of chronic progressive inflammation bordering residual lobules. There was bile stasis and a striking diminution of collecting bile ducts. In this late phase of fibrosis and nodular reconstruction, the pattern had little in common with the perilobular fibrosis so characteristic of the earlier phase of this disease. Seeing such a liver for the first time would tell little or nothing of the steps by which it had finally attained this distorted pattern.

Realizing that this disease could no longer be considered a variant of familial hypercholesterolemic xanthomatosis and realizing, too, that the concept of secondary xanthomatosis of the intrahepatic bile ducts could not be substantiated, Thannhauser offered the hypothesis that one was dealing here with a primary disease of the liver and that the clinical syndrome was apparently related to an excessive formation of cholesterol and lecithin by the liver together with an impaired excretion as the result of an obliteration and disappearance of cholangioles and collecting bile ducts. In brief, he now regarded pericholangiolitic biliary cirrhosis with its associated hypercholesterolemia and xanthomatosis as a specific disease of the liver.

Unfortunately Thannhauser suggested that the term *xanthomatous biliary cirrhosis* might be retained to designate the clinical syndrome.

This proved to be very confusing, and in 1950, just a year or two later, Ahrens et al.[32] in referring to the same disease coined a new term, *primary biliary cirrhosis* to designate this particular disease of the liver (pericholangiolitic biliary cirrhosis), and also to identify the complete clinical syndrome. This gained almost immediate

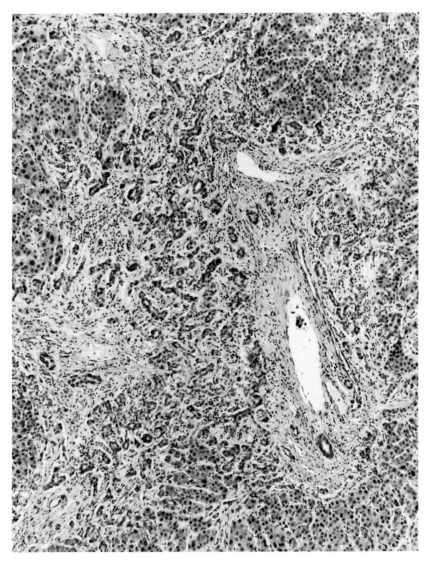

Fig. 3. Liver. Obstructive biliary cirrhosis. This section is from a patient with obstruction of the common bile duct of approximately 6 months' duration. All portal areas were involved, but the fibrosis was greatest along the course of the larger bile ducts. Here one sees a low-grade chronic interstitial inflammatory reaction. There is a minimal loss of liver cells together with an elongation and increase in the number of cholangioles. Lobules are well preserved but show extensive bile stasis ($\times$ 100).

general acceptance. Ahrens' paper was quickly followed by a succession of others that dealt with all aspects of this unusual disease.[33-47] For some, primary biliary cirrhosis was a specific histologic entity, though many felt that the clinical syndrome, partial or complete, might be found in association with other forms of liver disease. Still others felt that this particular form of cirrhosis was not always associated with the complete clinical syndrome.

If the reader has followed the sequence of events leading to the prevailing concept of biliary cirrhosis as of 1950, he will realize that it was not one but a category or group of diseases revolving about the bile duct system, having as a common denominator a chronic or healed interstitial inflammatory reaction more or less concentrated within the portal areas. It represented a comparatively mild group of diseases in which neither the liver cells nor the liver lobules, until the late stages, were seriously impaired. Included in this category were (1) obstructive biliary cirrhosis due to any factor or group of factors that might impede the flow of bile from the liver (Figs. 1–3); (2) cases of infectious biliary cirrhosis caused by bacteria, viruses, toxoplasma, and such parasites as flukes and roundworms (Figs. 4–7); (3) cases of toxic biliary cirrhosis, cholangiolitic or pericholangiolitic, which could be initiated by an ever-expanding list of drugs and chemicals, sometimes

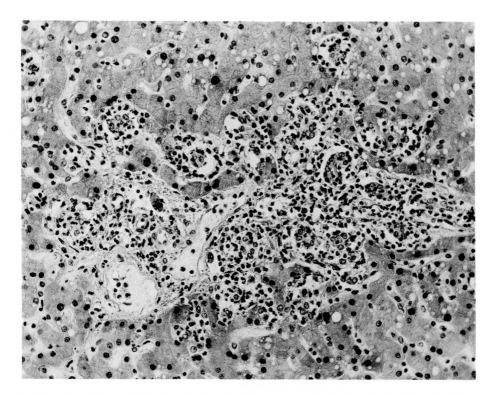

Fig. 4. Liver. The earliest stage in the development of cholangiolitic (infectious) biliary cirrhosis. Cholangioles contain polymorphonuclear leukocytes and bacteria. The interstitial tissue is infiltrated by an acute inflammatory cellular exudate which has already begun to spread into the bordering lobules. *E. coli* were grown in pure culture from this liver (× 168).

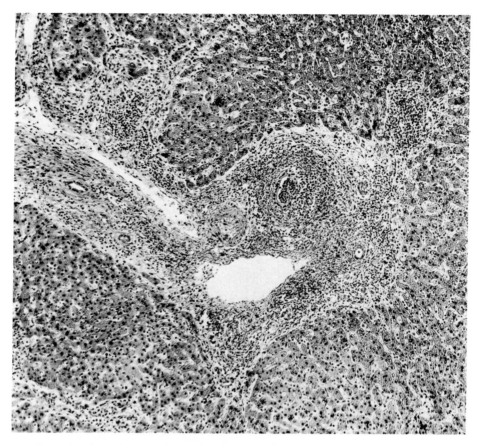

Fig. 5. Liver. Cholangitic and cholangiolitic (infectious) biliary cirrhosis. This is a very early lesion showing very little increase in fibrous tissue. One medium-sized bile duct and several cholangioles are distended with polymorphonuclear leukocytes. The surrounding interstitial tissue is edematous and richly infiltrated with the inflammatory cells. There is beginning proliferation of fibroblasts ($\times$ 100).

abetted by a state of hypersensitivity (Figs. 8–10); and (4) a specific type of questionable origin named, to distinguish it from the others, primary biliary cirrhosis. The last, also known as pericholangiolitic biliary cirrhosis, was the least common of the four (Figs. 11–15).

Acholangic Biliary Cirrhosis

The year 1952 introduced still another disease or deformity of the liver that, in the course of time, could lead to biliary cirrhosis.[48, 49] This was a congenital defect of varying degree, involving primarily the interlobular system of bile ducts which showed either a partial or complete lack of development (Figs. 16, 17). This condition is most commonly seen in infants and children who are jaundiced from

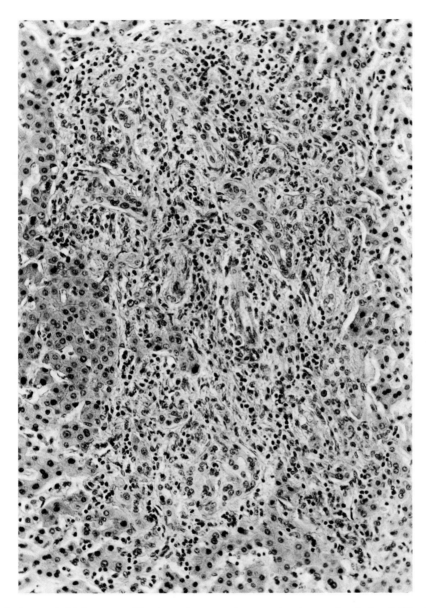

Fig. 6. Liver. A higher magnification of a portal area showing early cholangiolitic (infectious) biliary cirrhosis. The entire portal area fills most of the field. There is a marked proliferation of cholangioles, a mixed cellular inflammatory exudate. Hyperplasia of cholangioles is the most characteristic feature of this type of biliary cirrhosis. A similar picture was found in most of the portal areas throughout the liver ($\times$ 200).

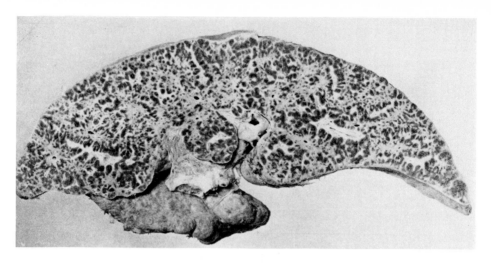

Fig. 7. Liver. Classical pattern of the gross picture of the healed stage of cholangitic and cholangiolitic (infectious) biliary cirrhosis. This liver was slightly enlarged, firm, finely nodular on the surface, and on section traversed by communicating bands of fibrous tissue. At this stage there can be a moderate elevation in portal venous pressure.

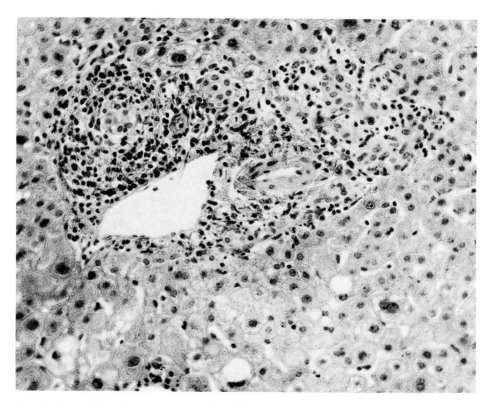

Fig. 8. Liver. "Toxic" cholangiohepatitis. This portal area is the site of a subacute inflammatory reaction centered in and about a small interlobular bile duct. The reaction is spreading into the periphery of the adjacent lobules. There is a small intralobular focus of inflammation at the base of this section. From a case of early Thorazine hepatitis (× 200).

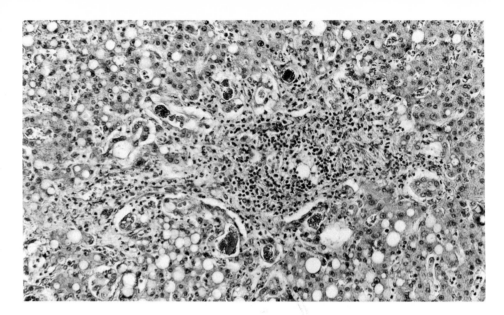

Fig. 9. Liver. An expanded portal area lies at the center of this field. Canals of Hering, leading up to the triad, are distended with casts of bile. There is no recognizable inter-lobular bile duct. The interstitial tissue is the seat of a chronic inflammatory reaction. The bordering liver cells are unusually rich in fat. From a case of early "toxic" biliary cirrhosis (chronic Thorazine intoxication) ($\times$ 100).

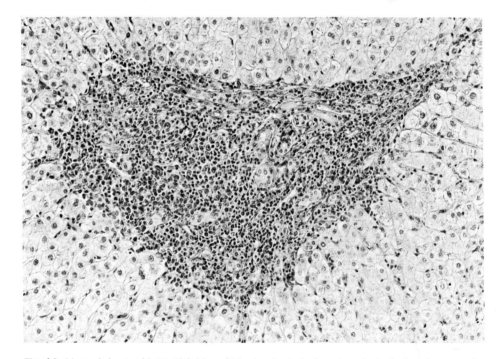

Fig. 10. Liver. A form of interstitial hepatitis dominated almost exclusively by plasma cells. The bordering liver lobules are remarkably well preserved. The veins, arteries, and bile ducts are almost completely obscured by this rich inflammatory infiltration. Early "toxic" biliary cirrhosis associated with drug addiction of undetermined type ($\times$ 100).

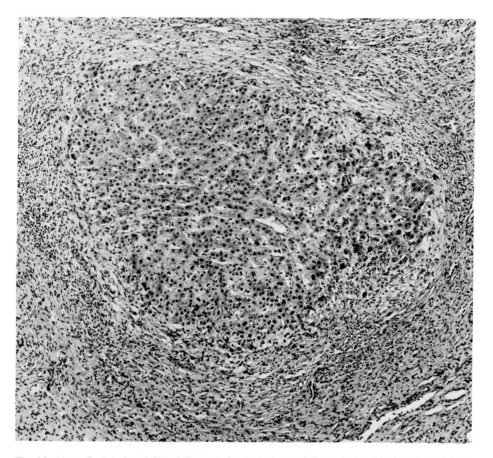

Fig. 11. Liver. Pericholangiolitic biliary cirrhosis (primary biliary cirrhosis). A solitary lobule, still largely intact with vein at the center. This lobule is incarcerated by a wall of inflammatory granulation and scar tissue. Bile ducts are greatly diminished, and many have disappeared. Bile stasis is most marked at the periphery of the lobule ($\times$ 100).

birth, but in lesser degree it may be found at any age. This anomaly may be seen in two or more members of the same family [51] and may also be found in association with such complex hereditary dysplasias as the Ellis–van Creveld syndrome. Some cases are associated with an extremely high level of serum cholesterol and with the most extreme form of cutaneous xanthomatosis. In its mildest form this anomaly may be responsible for transient and recurrent jaundice. Associated with this anomaly there may be a low-grade chronic interstitial inflammatory reaction that may dominate the histologic pattern.

Fibroxanthomatous Biliary Cirrhosis

Three years later, in 1955, still another disease that may lead to biliary cirrhosis was added to the list. Like acholangic biliary cirrhosis, this also is a disease

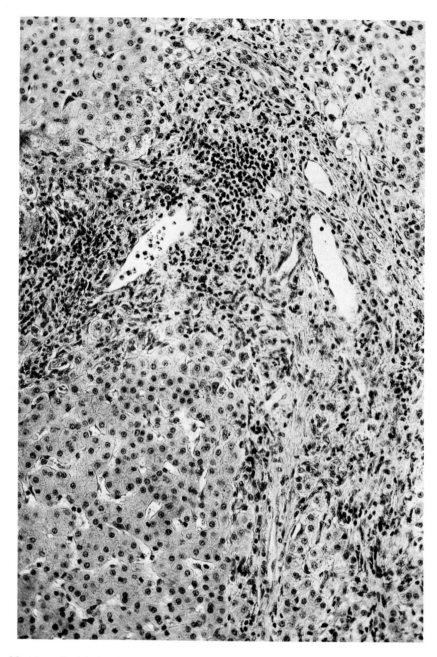

Fig. 12. Liver. Pericholangiolitic biliary cirrhosis (primary biliary cirrhosis). An early stage in the development of this type of biliary cirrhosis. This field includes portions of three lobules separated by a broad portal area that is the seat of a chronic interstitial inflammatory reaction in which there is a conspicuous depletion of bile ducts and cholangioles. Most of the inflammatory cells are lymphocytes ($\times$ 200).

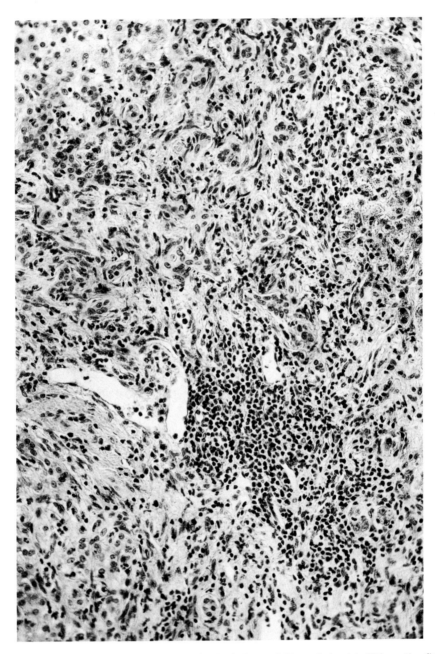

Fig. 13. Liver. Pericholangiolitic biliary cirrhosis (primary biliary cirrhosis). This entire field is occupied by an expanded portal area which is the seat of a chronic proliferative interstitial inflammatory reaction. There are many new vessels. There is a rich lymphocytic infiltration, and there is a conspicuous lack of bile ducts ($\times$ 200).

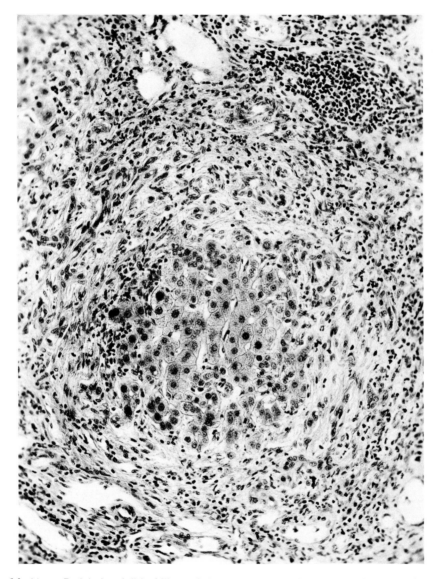

Fig. 14. Liver. Pericholangiolitic biliary cirrhosis (primary biliary cirrhosis). This field is from a more advanced stage of the disease showing the gradual erosion of the lobule as it becomes increasingly enveloped in fibrous tissue. Of particular interest is the conspicuous absence of bile ducts (× 200).

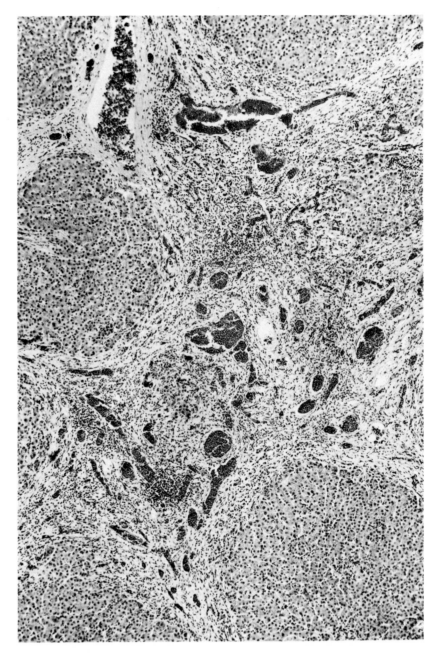

Fig. 15. Liver. Pericholangiolitic biliary cirrhosis (primary biliary cirrhosis). This section is from a patient who died of bleeding esophageal varices after a slow progressive down-hill course of 5 years. At this late stage there is nothing of a specific histologic nature that would enable one to offer a specific diagnosis of this particular type of biliary cirrhosis. Only with the aid of earlier biopsies was it possible to trace the steps leading to this final stage of the disease. As conspicuous as the absence of bile ducts is the un-usual distension of veins ($\times$ 100).

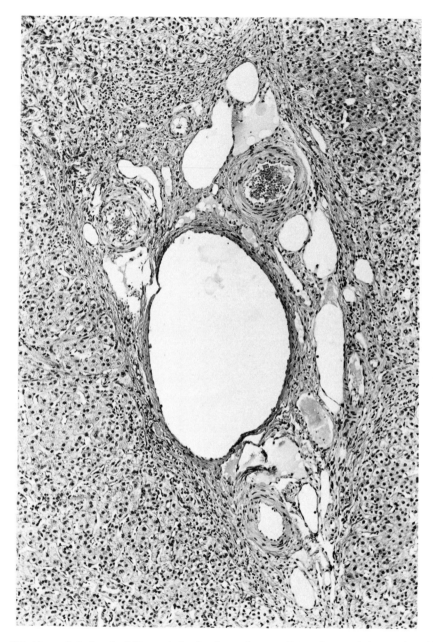

Fig. 16. Liver. Acholangic biliary cirrhosis. A random section of a portal area in which arteries, veins, and lymphatics are easily recognizable, but there is not a single bile duct. There is a minimal chronic interstitial inflammatory reaction throughout the entire portal area. Bordering liver cells and lobules are reasonably intact. This section is from a young boy who has been jaundiced since birth ($\times$ 100).

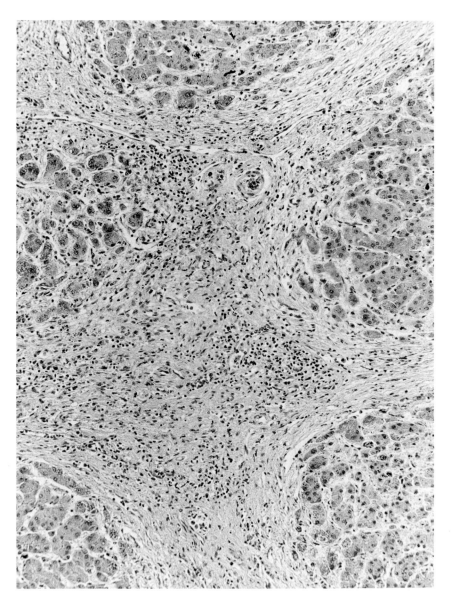

Fig. 17. Liver. A very late stage of acholangic biliary cirrhosis. This section is from a 17-year-old patient who had been jaundiced since birth. Here one finds wide paths of fibrous tissue devoid of bile ducts separating persistent lobules of liver cells. Earlier biopsies from this patient had shown the classic pattern of acholangic biliary cirrhosis. As the disease advances, its pattern becomes progressively nonspecific. Signs of portal hypertension dominated the clinical history ($\times$ 200).

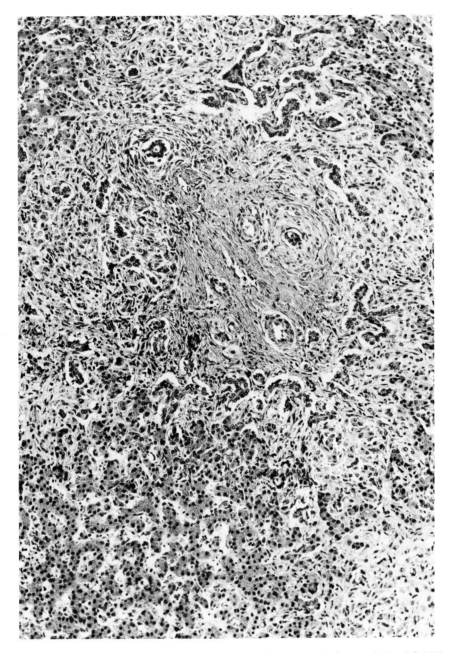

Fig. 18. Liver. Fibroxanthomatous biliary cirrhosis (a systemic form of Hand-Schüller-Christian disease). Most of this section is taken up by a single portal area from the liver of an infant. The interstitial tissue is greatly increased together with a rich accumulation of histiocytic cells (xanthoma cells) filled with lipids. The lesion involves particularly the walls of small interlobular bile ducts. This infant was moderately jaundiced. The cholesterol level was only slightly elevated, and the classic signs of primary biliary cirrhosis were absent ($\times$ 100).

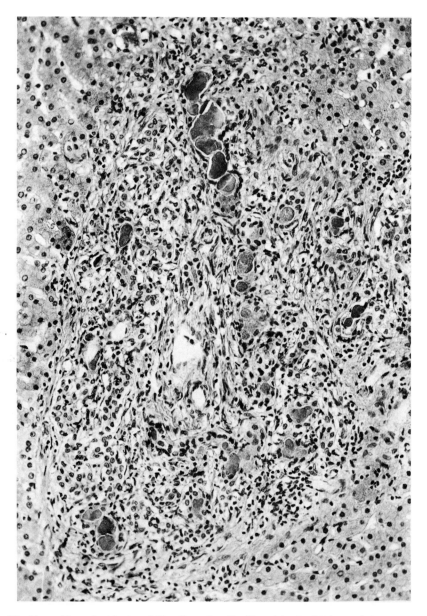

Fig. 19. Liver. Mucoviscidosis of the liver (cystic fibrosis). A single portal area, greatly enlarged, showing maximal distention of marginal cholangioles and small collecting ducts by thick inspissated bile-tinged mucus. The rest of this portal area is the seat of a low-grade chronic interstitial inflammatory reaction. The bordering liver parenchyma is reasonably intact (× 100).

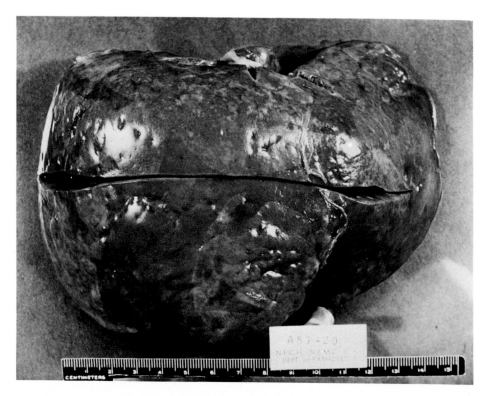

Fig. 20. Liver. Mucoviscidosis (cystic fibrosis). Entire liver showing the smooth, but pitted, mottled surface characteristic of this type of biliary cirrhosis.

of infancy and childhood. Here one is dealing with a systemic form of the Hand-Schüller-Christian syndrome (normal cholesterolemic xanthomatosis) in which every portal area within the infant's liver is involved by a rich deposition of cholesterol in histiocytes, and a definite proliferation of fibrous tissue. In this process, portal areas are enlarged. These gradually spread from the triads into the peripheral zones of the adjacent lobules (Fig. 18). Associated with this disease, which would appear to originate in the walls of the interlobular bile ducts, is a mild chronic interstitial inflammatory reaction.[50] To designate this form of biliary cirrhosis, the simple descriptive term of *fibroxanthomatous biliary cirrhosis of infancy* is suggested. This type of liver disease must be clearly distinguished from any of the others so far described.

Cystic Fibrosis as a Cause of Biliary Cirrhosis

Three years later, in 1958, another disease was added to this expanding group that could terminate as biliary cirrhosis. This was cystic fibrosis, a disease also

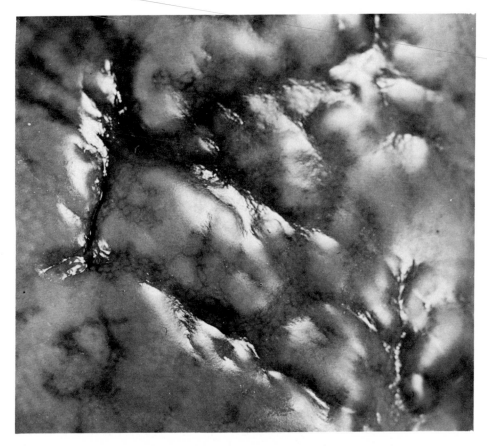

Fig. 21. Liver. Mucoviscidosis (cystic fibrosis). Observe the coarse wrinkling of the capsular surface though the capsule itself is smooth and glistening.

known as mucoviscidosis. This condition may be seen in infancy and childhood. The liver is regular in size and shape. The capsule is smooth but deeply wrinkled. Characteristic of this type of biliary cirrhosis is an accumulation and retention of mucus, sometimes bile-tinged, within distended intrahepatic bile ducts. Cholangioles become elongated and increased in number as the whole portal area becomes the site of a low-grade chronic interstitial inflammatory reaction (Figs. 19–21). In this reaction there is an infiltration of lymphocytes, histiocytes, eosinophiles, and occasionally multinucleated giant cells. This pattern is unique.[52]

Carcinomatous Biliary Cirrhosis

In that same year, 1958, a type of biliary cirrhosis was described that was secondary to a diffuse lymphatic dissemination of tumor cells throughout the portal areas of the liver (Fig. 22). This spread led to a secondary low-grade chronic interstitial inflammatory reaction within the portal areas and to a moderate degree of bile stasis. The dissemination of tumor cells was not associated with an obstruction to any part of the extrahepatic biliary tract. Grossly the liver was slightly enlarged, bile-stained, firm, finely nodular, and diffusely scarred (Figs. 23, 24). The clinical signs, symptoms, and laboratory findings of this disease of the liver can mimic those of uncomplicated long-standing extrahepatic biliary obstruction. The disease can be readily overlooked clinically. At autopsy, unless malignancy is suspected, the true nature of the disease within the liver can be completely overlooked. The liver is neither greatly enlarged nor coarsely nodular, and its shape is retained.[52]

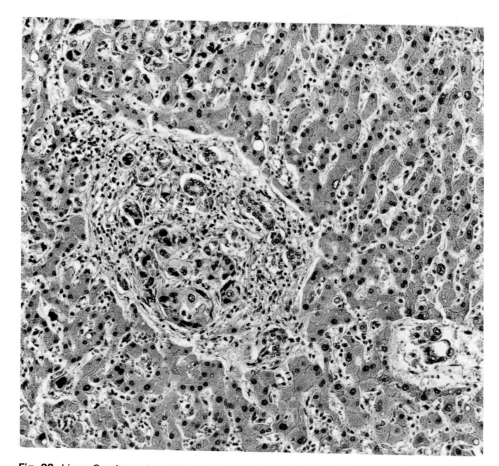

Fig. 22. Liver. Carcinomatous biliary cirrhosis. A single portal area lies at the center of the field. All lymphatics are blocked and distended by tumor cells. There is a low-grade chronic inflammatory reaction throughout the interstitial tissue with edema, cellular infiltration, and beginning proliferation of fibrous tissue. There is moderate bile stasis within the bordering lobules (× 200).

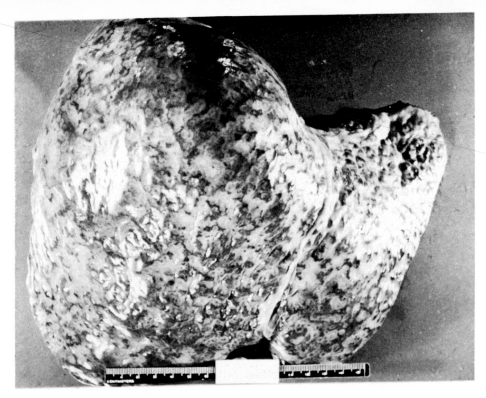

Fig. 23. Liver. Carcinomatous biliary cirrhosis. The size and shape of the liver are retained. The surface is wrinkled and mottled gray and green. The right and left lobes may be easily distinguished. Note the absence of coarse lobation so commonly seen in extensive metastatic liver disease.

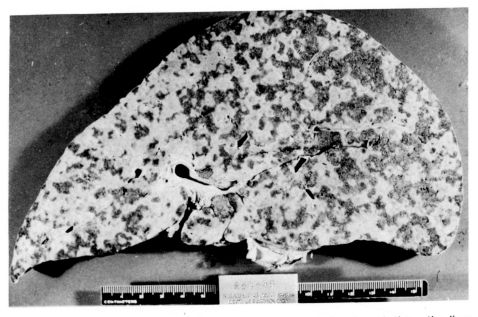

Fig. 24. Liver. Carcinomatous biliary cirrhosis. This cross section through the entire liver clearly reveals the communicating trabeculae of fibrous tissue isolating islands of bile-stained liver cells. Small and medium-sized vessels and bile ducts are compressed.

Biliary Cirrhosis—a Group or Category of Diseases

Once again it might be helpful to pause, to gather together this growing list of diseases that must be taken into consideration when one refers to biliary cirrhosis as a group. Actually, an awareness of these is in a sense a prerequisite to establishing a definitive histologic diagnosis—for one never diagnoses beyond one's realm of thought. This list now includes obstructive biliary cirrhosis, cholangitic biliary cirrhosis (infectious), toxic biliary cirrhosis, which as pointed out earlier is being seen more commonly year after year, primary biliary cirrhosis, acholangic biliary cirrhosis, fibroxanthomatous biliary cirrhosis of infancy, biliary cirrhosis associated with mucoviscidosis, and last, carcinomatous biliary cirrhosis. At this point one might ask if the term *biliary cirrhosis,* including such a variety of diseases differing

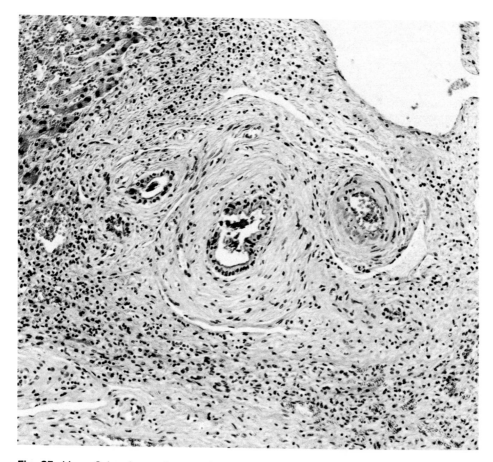

Fig. 25. Liver. Scleroderma (progressive systemic sclerosis). A section from a patient in which this disease was largely confined to the liver, gastrointestinal tract, pancreas, and mesentery. The large and medium-sized arteries were particularly damaged. Here, there is a profuse proliferative inflammatory reaction throughout the portal areas associated with a moderate infiltration of lymphocytes and plasma cells ($\times$ 100).

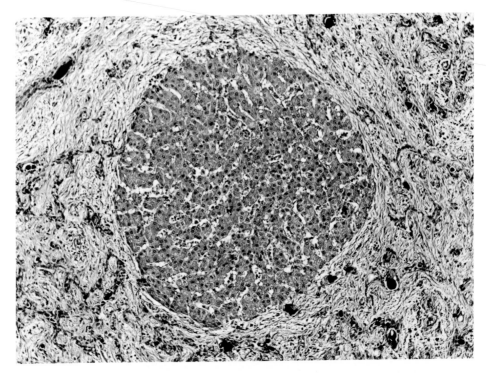

Fig. 26. Liver. Progressive obliterative biliary cirrhosis (a variant of obstructive biliary cirrhosis). This section from the liver of an infant 8 months of age who experienced a progressively downhill course from birth. An island of residual liver parenchyma is becoming progressively incarcerated in fibrous tissue. Casts of inspissated bile can still be seen in compressed degenerating bile ducts (× 100).

in etiology and pathogenesis, serves any useful purpose. The answer would appear to be yes, for as long as the term *cirrhosis* is to be used in a general way to designate the sclerotic state of the liver, it is useful to have such a term as *biliary cirrhosis* to separate this from other large groups of liver disease. Such a classification based on morphology alone must not eliminate other ways of identifying and classifying diseases of the liver, but until we have one that is better, the present histologic classification should be retained.

Scleroderma as a Cause of Biliary Cirrhosis

No sooner had these eight distinct types of biliary cirrhosis been assembled than another and another and still another had to be added to this list. To consider the first of these, there is the large and expanding family of diseases loosely referred to as "the collagen diseases." One of these is "systemic scleroderma," also known as progressive systemic sclerosis. This is a disease that may involve many organs of the body. In the liver it may involve branches of the hepatic artery and the connective tissue of the portal area leading to extensive sclerosis of these triads and constriction of the bile ducts.[53] The liver may be of average size or slightly enlarged, but this type of biliary cirrhosis may be easily overlooked in the gross examination.

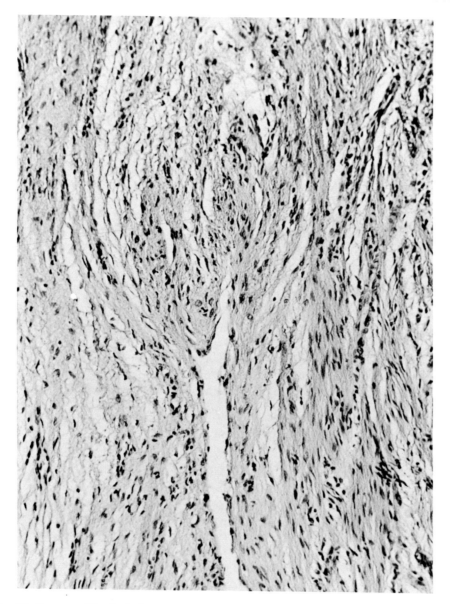

Fig. 27. Common bile duct. Progressive obliterative biliary cirrhosis (a variant of obstructive biliary cirrhosis). This field was selected to show the gradual destruction and obliteration of the common bile duct ($\times$ 100).

Histologically, if one is aware, it may be recognized at once. This increase in hyalinized connective tissue can reduce the caliber of arteries to a mere fraction of the normal and can transform the connective tissue of the portal areas into dense collagen. This sclerosis can constrict bile ducts causing intrahepatic cholestasis. Along with these changes there is an infiltration of lymphocytes, histiocytes, and plasma cells (Fig. 25). In one case in which the vessels were very badly narrowed, the patient developed massive necrosis of the liver following a transitory circulatory collapse.

A Variant of Biliary Cirrhosis

Another disease, not a new one but one that has attained considerable prominence, has been described as "a variant of obstructive cirrhosis." [54] Seen in infancy, the lesion is dominated by an excessive growth of fibrous tissue involving not only the extrahepatic biliary tract but also the intrahepatic bile ducts as well (Figs. 26, 27). As this fibrosis progresses, large and small bile ducts become sclerosed and eliminated. With this progressive growth of fibrous tissue, there is a corresponding destruction of liver cells. This disease may progress for months. It terminates fatally, and in the light of our present knowledge it offers no surgical or medical cure. Grossly the liver is larger than normal and deeply bile-stained, and when it is sectioned, there is a progressive degree of scarring fanning out from the hilus. This type of biliary cirrhosis must be clearly distinguished from the simple obstructive type in which all the changes in the liver are secondary and dependent upon some form of extrahepatic obstruction. The term *biliary atresia* has been suggested for this type of biliary cirrhosis, but this is quite inadequate since atresia, which literally means occlusion of a natural channel, may be confined to a single segment of the extrahepatic biliary tree. Because bile ducts within the liver gradually disappear in this disease, one must clearly distinguish this type from the acholangic type already described. Because the etiology of this sclerosing disease remains obscure, because it is unique, and because it is only found within the first year, the descriptive term *progressive obliterative biliary cirrhosis of infancy* is suggested.

Sarcoidosis

Now the list has grown to 10, and still this is not the end of the story, for no report of this type would be complete without referring to that nebulous disease of man—sarcoidosis. This may turn up in any part of the body, and the liver is not exempt.[55] When it strikes the liver, it may be confined to the portal areas. Characteristic of this disease histologically is a granulomatous type of inflammation that in the past has often been mistaken for tuberculosis (Fig. 28). When this disease involves the liver, the clinical signs may be negligible, and in the gross examination the disease can be easily overlooked. It may turn up as a totally unsuspected finding in a needle biopsy specimen. Its importance lies in recognizing it when found, for this may be the first indication of an otherwise unsuspected case.

Galactosemia

A metabolic disease of infancy that must now be included in this group is one associated with an inability on the part of an infant to handle galactose normally. This is due to an enzyme defect responsible for the conversion of galactose to utilizable glucose. In addition to the excessive accumulation of fat in the liver, which

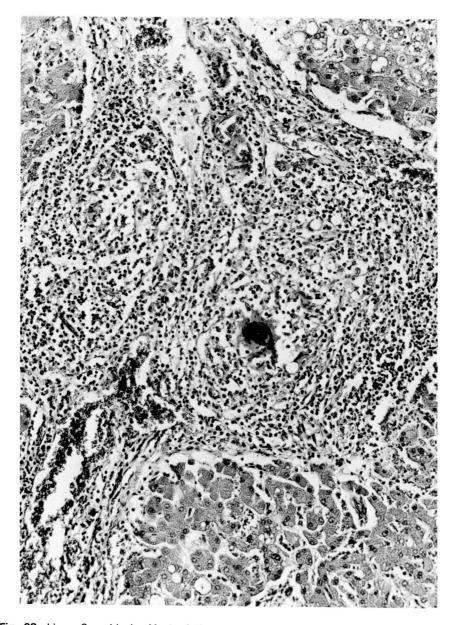

Fig. 28. Liver. Sarcoidosis. Most of the portal areas of this liver were enlarged by a chronic granulomatous interstitial inflammatory reaction. In this field a solitary multi-nucleated giant cell lies at the center of a single granuloma. This patient had extensive sarcoidosis of the mediastinal nodes. There is a rich lymphocytic histiocytic and fibrous tissue proliferation ($\times$ 100).

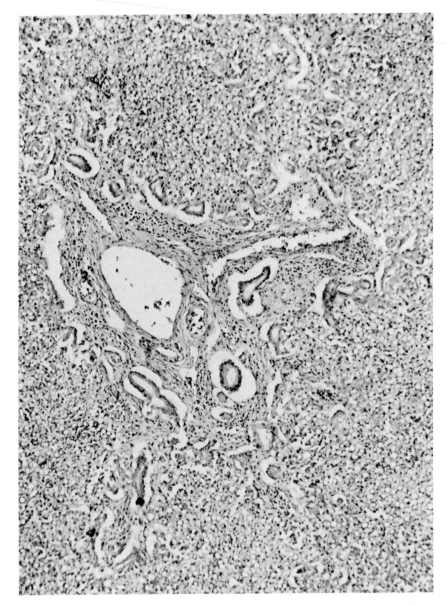

Fig. 29. Liver. Galactosemia. A random section from a somewhat enlarged liver of an infant with congenital galactosemia. The portal area is larger than normal. There is an apparent or real increase in the canals of Hering. The stroma is increased and there is a light lymphocytic infiltration. The bordering liver cells are rich in neutral fat ($\times$ 100).

is responsible for the enlargement of this organ, there may be a distinct increase in the number of cholangioles bordering the portal triad, an increase in connective tissue within the portal triad, and an infiltration of inflammatory cells (Fig. 29). While the sum total of these histologic changes is minimal, this disease should be included in this group since once again it is only through an awareness of this entity as a very mild form of biliary cirrhosis that a meaningful histologic diagnosis can be made.[56]

Alpha-I Antitrypsin Deficiency

Each year will undoubtedly bring out new diseases together with the rediscovery of old ones that properly belong to this expanding category. One of the most recent to be added to this group is an unusual type of biliary cirrhosis that may be found in certain emphysematous patients who have inherited a deficiency of

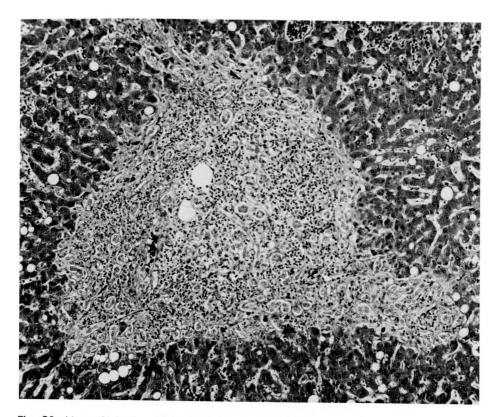

Fig. 30. Liver. Alpha-1 antitrypsin deficiency. This pattern was found in portal areas throughout the liver. It resembles most closely cholangiolitic biliary cirrhosis (infectious biliary cirrhosis). In this liver the small and large bile ducts contain no leukocytes. There is a symmetric chronic interstitial inflammatory reaction dominated by a striking increase in the number of cholangioles. There is no significant bile stasis ($\times$ 90). (Courtesy of G. J. Gherardi of Framingham Union Hospital.)

alpha-1 antitrypsin in their serum.[57, 58] The concentration of this substance is controlled by alleles of a pair of codominant genes that produce variants of the normal trypsin molecule. Of practical importance in a clinical sense is the fact that the livers of patients showing this defect may have two significant variations from the normal. The first is a chronic interstitial inflammatory reaction that histologically is almost indistinguishable from the pattern of cholangiolitic biliary cirrhosis (Fig. 30). The second variant lies in the presence of a homogeneous eosin-staining cytoplasmic globule that may be found within the liver cells. This could be mistaken for "alcoholic hyalin" but is said to be a nonlipid glycoprotein that stains positively by PAS.

This new entity brings the list of diseases that today may be included in the category of biliary cirrhosis to 13 in all. It may be recalled that Mallory only 32 years ago, in speaking of all forms of cirrhosis in general, said there must be at least a dozen different types. In this report it has been possible to describe and to demonstrate at least 13 types belonging to a single group, and of course there will be others.

Diseases That May Mimic Biliary Cirrhosis

If a chronic or healed interstitial inflammatory reaction throughout the portal areas of the liver is to be the accepted hallmark of biliary cirrhosis, and this seems a reasonable basis upon which to base the histologic diagnosis, then it is necessary to consider briefly other diseases that also involve the liver which could be confused with the histologic pattern of the diseases already described.

Congenital Hepatic Fibrosis

The first of these is congenital hepatic fibrosis, a developmental anomaly of the liver, but one that is not infrequently complicated by infection (Figs. 31–34). This anomaly may be found incidentally in the course of an autopsy on a patient of any age, for it may be entirely devoid of any clinical signs and symptoms.[59, 60] At one time this anomaly was thought to be the end stage of a chronic inflammatory reaction, had this been true, it would have been included in the aforementioned category of biliary cirrhoses. It can easily be mistaken for metastases from a distant tumor by an unsuspecting surgeon in the course of an exploratory laparotomy, or by a pathologist in the course of a routine autopsy. This anomaly, though the term *congenital hepatic fibrosis* is of relative recent vintage, is not a recent discovery since it has been described among developmental anomalies of the liver for years. It is characterized by an excess of large communicating bile ducts coursing along the portal triads. These are engulfed or surrounded by an increase in fibrous tissue that becomes increasingly collagenous with age. In earlier descriptions it was often related to cystic diseases of the kidney, including medullary cystic disease, and to other anomalies within the liver, such as congenital cysts or peliosis of the capillaries. This anomaly may be limited to a very small portion of the liver and could be easily overlooked. One of its most interesting features is that it is sometimes associated with a very important defect in the portal system of veins, apparently dating

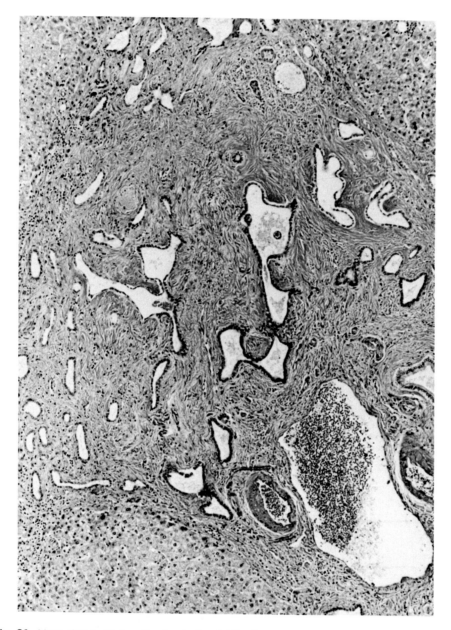

Fig. 31. Liver. Congenital cystic dysplasia of bile ducts (congenital hepatic fibrosis). This histologic pattern was repeated many times throughout the liver. It was an incidental finding in the liver of a 73-year-old male patient. There were no recognizable clinical signs or symptoms. As one grows older this type of congenital malformation, characterized by an overgrowth of bile ducts and connective tissue along the portal areas, becomes increasingly collagenous. A vein and artery are included in this field ($\times$ 100).

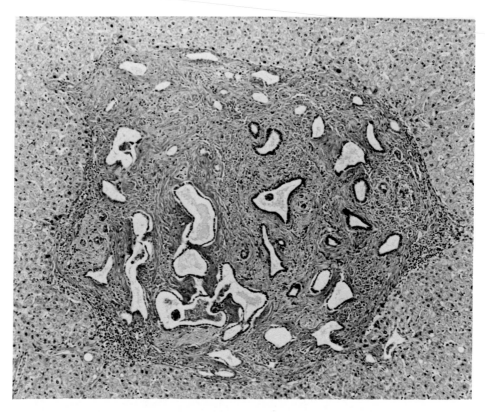

Fig. 32. Liver. Congenital cystic dysplasia of bile ducts with partial agenesis of portal veins (congenital hepatic fibrosis). Section from the liver of a 33-year-old male patient who had experienced recurrent attacks of esophageal bleeding. He had esophageal varices, portal hypertension, and an enlarged spleen without any evidence of liver cell dysfunction. In this section there is an overgrowth of anomalous bile ducts and a conspicuous absence of portal veins ($\times$ 90).

back to the early transformation of the vitelline circulation into the permanent system of portal veins. In the latter case many of the portal triads will be found to have no branches of the portal vein. Associated with this is the fact that such patients, usually young adults, may experience recurrent bleeding from esophageal varices without showing any other sign, symptom, or laboratory finding of a liver disease. Since this anomaly can lead to portal hypertension, it must be recognized, for it is amenable to surgical therapy. A disease with which this anomaly has at times been confused is "pipe-stem cirrhosis," a very late stage of infectious biliary cirrhosis that may develop in the course of schistosomiasis.

Systemic Mast-Cell Disease

This is a relatively rare disease whose pattern in the liver may be confused with that of biliary cirrhosis. In this there is an accentuation of all portal areas,

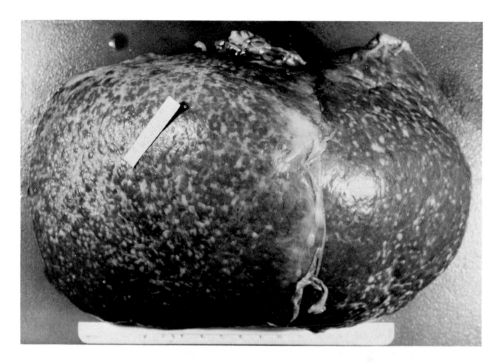

Fig. 33. Liver. Congenital cystic dysplasia of bile ducts (congenital hepatic fibrosis). This liver is mottled and slightly enlarged, but the shape is retained. It is from a 63-year-old male patient operated on for carcinoma of the sigmoid. At the time of operation the gray nodules throughout the liver were erroneously considered to be multiple metastases. Histologically there was not a trace of tumor in the liver. This anomaly had been present since birth.

which are richly infiltrated with mast cells and which show in addition a low-grade chronic interstitial inflammatory reaction (Fig. 35).

Pigment Cirrhosis

Cases of pigment cirrhosis have been known to masquerade clinically under the guise of primary biliary cirrhosis. Histologically, however, the very presence of hemosiderin in the liver cells, which is so easily recognizable with the use of appropriate stains, sets this disease aside as a distinct category in its own right. Nevertheless, when one examines sections showing the early stage of pigment cirrhosis, one is at once aware of the fact that this form of cirrhosis begins by a widening of the portal triads at the expense of the liver cells at the periphery of the lobule. In other words, were the pigment not present, the patterns would be that of biliary cirrhosis (Fig. 36).

Hodgkin's Disease, Letterer-Siwe Disease, and the Leukemias

Hodgkin's disease, when it is diffusely scattered throughout the portal areas of the liver (Fig. 37), cases of reticuloendotheliosis of the Letterer-Siwe type which

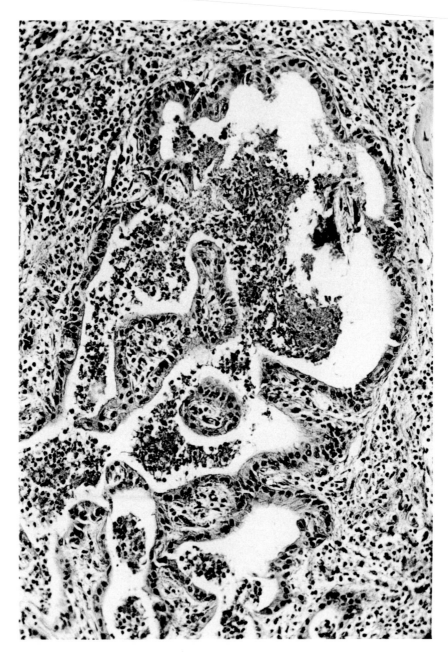

Fig. 34. Liver. Cystic dysplasia of bile ducts (congenital hepatic fibrosis) complicated by bacterial infection. The surrounding interstitial tissue is the site of a chronic inflammatory reaction. Such lesions were once regarded as simply infectious in origin, pathologists being unaware of the underlying basic anomaly. This type of anomaly is unusually susceptible to secondary bacterial infection ($\times$ 200).

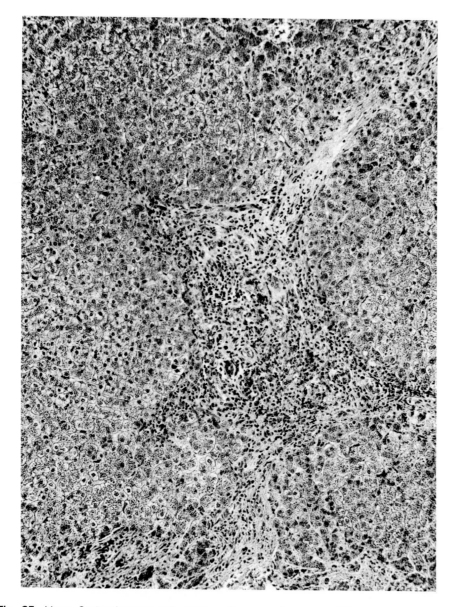

Fig. 35. Liver. Systemic mast-cell disease. Every portal area within this liver was accentuated by an unusual infiltration of mast cells. There was an increase in the size of the portal areas. The liver was slightly larger than normal, but the shape was retained. On gross examination the portal areas stood out unusually well. The spleen was considerably enlarged and showed a striking increase in mast cells involving particularly the follicles ($\times$ 100).

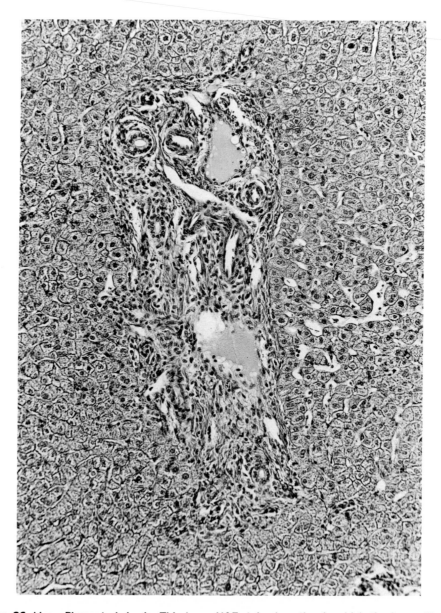

Fig. 36. Liver. Pigment cirrhosis. This is an H&E-stained section in which the hemosiderin is scarcely visible. At this stage in the development of uncomplicated pigment cirrhosis, the pattern is one of biliary cirrhosis with a chronic interstitial inflammatory reaction extending out from every portal area. There is minimal bile stasis. The most striking feature of this disease, namely, the accumulation of hemosiderin, is not visible in this section (× 90).

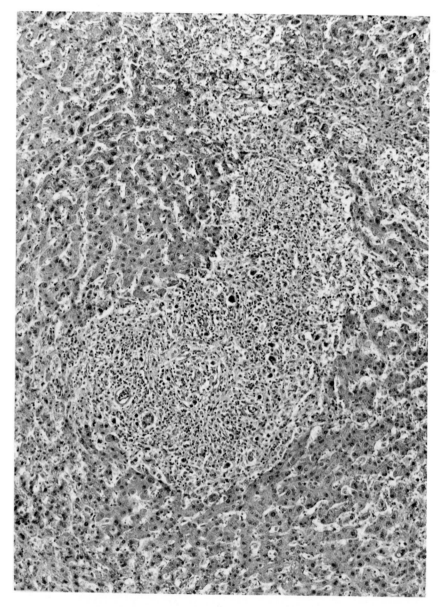

Fig. 37. Liver. Hodgkin's disease. Every portal area throughout the liver was considerably enlarged as the result of a proliferation of cells including classic Sternberg-Reed giant cells. The whole pattern mimics that of biliary cirrhosis. In this section the portal vein, hepatic artery, and bile duct are obscured by this neoplastic type of granulation tissue. There is moderate bile stasis in the adjacent lobules (× 100).

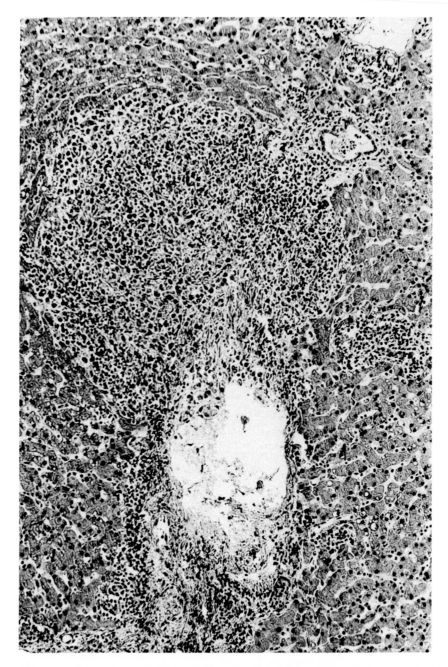

Fig. 38. Liver. Systemic reticuloendotheliosis (Letterer-Siwe disease). In this field the tumor is extending out in an asymmetric fashion from the portal areas, progressively encroaching upon the bordering liver parenchyma. This pattern throughout the portal areas of the liver can mimic both grossly and histologically that of a chronic interstitial inflammatory reaction so characteristic of biliary cirrhosis ($\times$ 100).

may also involve every portal area (Fig. 38), and some of the leukemias, particularly chronic lymphocytic, monocytic, and eosinophilic leukemia, can very closely mimic biliary cirrhosis. In each of these diseases the portal areas may become very accentuated, not only by the presence of the neoplastic cells, but also by the presence of proliferating connective tissue that may be associated with these diseases. This increase in connective tissue may stand out very clearly when, as the result of therapy, the leukemic cells have disappeared leaving only a fibrous tissue background.

Discussion

This portion, because of the limitation of space and time, will be very brief since this paper is primarily concerned with the morphology of a number of diseases which comprise, or may be confused with, what one considers to be a category or group of biliary cirrhoses. It has been necessary to exclude detailed histologic descriptions of most of these diseases, let alone their etiology, pathogenesis, clinical significance, therapy, and prognosis. These all lie beyond the primary scope of this paper which was to share with others, especially the younger pathologists of today, some of the observations and experiences that I have had in the laboratory and at the autopsy table over a period of almost 50 years.

It has not been possible to include all or even the majority of references bearing on this particular subject, for the growth of the literature bearing on biliary cirrhosis seems inexhaustible. Instead, I have relied very heavily on my own personal observations and many times have referred to papers written in earlier years. It was my good fortune to have been able to spend some time with Dr. Mallory at the Boston City Hospital, with Dr. Roessle at the Charité in Berlin, and with Dr. Thannhauser at the New England Medical Center. To each of these men I owe a debt which can never be fully repaid.

Summary

Biliary cirrhosis is described as a category of diseases involving the liver, having as its hallmark a chronic inflammatory reaction of varying intensity throughout the interstitial tissue of the portal areas. In this paper an attempt has been made to discuss some of the problems related to the recognition and acceptance of the term *biliary cirrhosis*. At one time it was used to indicate a single disease associated with uncomplicated biliary obstruction. Today, at least to the pathologist, this term designates an expanding spectrum of histologic patterns, some new and some old, which must be recognized by the hospital pathologist. Because this group of diseases is sometimes confused with others involving the liver, a few of the latter have been briefly included with the hope that a recognition of these may be helpful to others.

References

1. Laennec, R. T. H. De l'auscultation médiate. Paris, J. A. Brosson et J. S. Chaudé. 1819, Vol. 1.
2. Baillie, M. The Morbid Anatomy of Some of the Most Important Parts of the

Human Body, 1st ed. Albany, Barber and Southwick, for Thomas Spencer, 1795.

3. Mallory, F. B. Cirrhosis of the liver. Five different types from which it may arise. Johns Hopkins Med J 22:1, 1911.

4. Mallory, F. B. Cirrhosis of the liver. N Engl J Med 206:1231, 1932.

5. MacMahon, H. E., and Mallory, F. B. Streptococcus hepatitis. Am J Pathol 7:299, 1931.

6. MacMahon, H. E. Infectious cirrhosis. Am J Pathol 7:77, 1931.

7. MacMahon, H. E., and Mallory, F. B. Obstructive cirrhosis. Am J. Pathol 5:645, 1929.

8. MacMahon, H. E., Lawrence, J. S., and Maddock, S. J. Experimental obstructive cirrhosis. Am J Pathol 5:631, 1929.

9. Wyss, O. Zür Aetiologie des Stauungsicterus. Virchows Arch [Pathol Anat] 36:454, 1866.

10. Mayer, H. Über Veränderungen des Leberparenchyms bei dauerendem Verschluss des Ductus choledochus. Med Jahr (Wien) 133, 1872.

11. Charcot, J. M., and Gombault, A. Note sur les altérations du foie consecutives à la ligature du canal cholédoque. Arch Physiol Norm Pathol 3:272, 1876.

12. Hanot, V. Sur une forme de cirrhose hypertrophique du foie. Thèse de Paris, 1876.

13. Legg, J. W. Congenital deficiency of the common bile duct, the cystic and hepatic ducts ending in a blind sac; cirrhosis of the liver. Trans Pathol Soc Lond 27:178, 1876.

14. Heinecke, H. Zür Kenntnis der biliaren Leberzirrhose. Beitr Pathol 22:259, 1897.

15. Nicati, W., and Richard, A. Recherches sur la cirrhose biliare du lapin domestique. Arch Physiol Norm Pathol 7:501, 1880.

16. MacCallum, G. A. A Textbook of Pathology, 2nd ed. Philadelphia, Saunders, 1922, pp. 330–334.

17. Roessle, R. Handbuch der Speziellen Pathologischen Anatomie und Histologie. Henke-Lubarsch. New York, Springer. 5 (No. 1):429, 1930.

18. MacMahon, H. E., and Olken, H. G. Chronic pulmonary beryllosis in workers using fluorescent powder containing beryllium. Arch Ind Hyg Occup Med 1:1, 1949.

19. MacMahon, H. E., Murphy, A. S., and Bates, M. I. Endothelial cell sarcoma of liver following thorotrast injection. Am J Pathol 23:585, 1947.

20. Waitzkin, L., and MacMahon, H. E. Hepatic injury found during chronic chlorpromazine therapy. Ann Intern Med 56:220. 1962.

21. Thannhauser, S. J., and Magendantz, H. The different clinical groups of xanthomatous diseases; a clinical physiological study of 22 cases. Ann Intern Med 11:1662, 1938.

22. Addison, T., and Gull, W. On a certain affection of the skin, vitiligoidea (a) plana; (b) tuberosa, with remarks. Guys Hosp Rep 7:265, 1851.

23. Murchison, C. The lesions found in the liver and skin in a fatal case vitiligoidea associated with chronic jaundice and enlargement of the liver. Trans Pathol Soc Lond 20:187, 1869.

24. Fagge, C. H. Diseases, etc., of the skin. General xanthelasma or vitiligoidea. Trans Pathol Soc Lond 24:242, 1873.

25. Pye-Smith, P. H. Xanthelasma (vitiligoidea plana) of skin, peritoneum and mucus membrane, associated with jaundice. Autopsy. Trans Pathol Soc Lond 24:250, 1873.

26. Futcher, T. B. Xanthelasma and chronic jaundice. Am J Med Sci 130:939, 1905.

27. Pinkus, F., and Pick, L. Zür Struktur und Genese der symptomatischen Xanthome. Deutsch Med Wochenschr 34:1426, 1908.

28. Dyke, S. C. Case of hypercholesteremic splenomegaly associated with xanthomatosis and biliary cirrhosis. J Pathol 31:173, 1928.

29. MacMahon, H. E. The examination of needle biopsy specimens. Gastroenterology 56:426, 1969.
30. MacMahon, H. E. Biliary xanthomatosis. Am J Pathol 24:527, 1948.
31. MacMahon, H. E., and Thannhauser, S. J. Xanthomatous biliary cirrhosis (a clinical syndrome). Ann Intern Med 30:121, 1949.
32. Ahrens, E. H., Jr., Payne, M. A., Kunkel, H. G., Eisenmenger, W. J., and Blondheim, S. H. Primary biliary cirrhosis. Medicine (Baltimore) 29:299, 1950.
33. Shay, H., and Harris, C. Changing concepts of xanthomatous biliary cirrhosis. Am J Med Sci 223:286, 1952.
34. Jesserer, H., and Wewalka, F. Über einen Fall von sogennanter primärer biliärer Zirrhose. Wien Z Inn Med 10:427, 1952.
35. Haubrich, W. S., and Sancetta, S. M. Spontaneous recovery from hepatobiliary disease with xanthomatosis. Gastroenterology 26:658, 1954.
36. MacMahon, H. E. Liver patterns in biliary hypercholesteremic xanthomatosis. Mt Sinai J Med NY 24:1024, 1957.
37. Hartmann G. So-called xanthomatous biliary cirrhosis and chronic pseudo-xanthomatous pericholangitis. Frank Zeitschr Pathol 68:55, 1957.
38. MacMahon, H. E. Diagnostic patterns in intra-hepatic cholestatic jaundice. Gastroenterology 34:1033, 1958.
39. Cameron, R. Some problems in biliary cirrhosis. Br Med J 1:535, 1958.
40. Hamilton, J. D. The pathology of primary biliary cirrhosis. Lab Invest 8:701, 1959.
41. Rubin, S. Schaffner, F., and Popper, H. Chronic non-suppurative destructive cholangitis. Am J Pathol 46:387, 1965.
42. Williams, G. E. G. Pericholangiolitic biliary cirrhosis. J Pathol 89:23, 1965.
43. Popper, H. Primary biliary cirrhosis (non-suppurative cholangitis, chronic destructive). Proceedings of 33rd Seminar of the American Society of Clinical Pathologists. 1967, p. 15.
44. Wessler, S., and Avioli, L. A. Primary biliary cirrhosis. JAMA 206:1285, 1968.
45. Foulk, W. T., and Baggenstoss, A. H. Biliary cirrhosis. In Schiff, L., ed. Diseases of the Liver, 3rd ed. Philadelphia, Lippincott, 1969, p. 739.
46. Doniach, D., Walker, J. G., Roitt, I. M., and Berg, P. Autoallergic hepatitis. N Engl J Med 282:86, 1970.
47. Popper, H. The pathology of viral hepatitis. Proceedings of Canadian Hepatic Foundation Symposium on Viral Hepatitis. Can Med Assoc J 106:447, 1972.
48. Ahrens, E. H., Jr., Harris, R., and MacMahon, H. E. Atresia of the intrahepatic bile ducts. Pediatrics 8:628, 1951.
49. MacMahon, H. E., and Thannhauser, S. J. Congenital dysplasia of the intra-lobular bile ducts with extensive skin xanthomata: congenital acholangic biliary cirrhosis. Gastroenterology 21:488, 1952.
50. MacMahon, H. E. Biliary cirrhosis; Differential features of five types. Lab Invest 4:243, 1955.
51. Gherardi, G. J., and MacMahon, H. E. Hypoplasia of terminal bile ducts: Occurrence in two jaundiced male siblings. Am J Dis Child 120:151, 1970.
52. MacMahon H. E. Biliary cirrhosis. Arch Intern Med 102:841, 1958.
53. MacMahon, H. E. Systemic scleroderma and massive infarction of intestine and liver. Surg Gynecol Obstet 134:10, 1972.
54. MacMahon, H. E. A variant of obstructive biliary cirrhosis. Am J Pathol 60:371, 1970.
55. Klatskin, G., and Yesner, R. Hepatic manifestations of sarcoidosis and other granulomatous diseases. A study based on histological examination of tissue obtained by needle biopsy of the liver. Yale J Biol Med 23:207, 1950.
56. Smetana, H. F. and Olen, E. Hereditary galactose disease. Am J Clin Pathol 38:3, 1962.

57. Gherardi, G. J. Alpha-1—antitrypsin deficiency and its effect on the liver. Hum Pathol 2:173, 1971.
58. Lieberman, J., Mittman, C., and Gordon, H. W. Alpha-1 antitrypsin in the livers of patients with emphysema. Science 175:63, 1972.
59. MacMahon, H. E. Congenital anomalies of the liver. Am J Pathol 5:499, 1929.
60. Kerr, D. N. S., Harrison, C. V., Sherlock, S., and Walker, R. M. Congenital hepatic fibrosis. Q J Med 30:91, 1961.

RADIATION INJURY WITH PARTICULAR REFERENCE TO THOROTRAST

GIUSEPPE GRAMPA

Thorotrast, widely used as a contrast medium in X-ray diagnosis during the years 1930-45, was practically discarded after 1945 since harmful late effects from its use were noted.

It may be estimated from data on Thorotrast manufacture and from epidemiologic studies[14,40,154,165] that more than 50,000 patients have been injected with Thorotrast, mainly for arteriography, but also for hepatolienography,[168] retrograde pyelography, mammography, hysterosalpingography, and paranasal sinus cavity visualization. From 3,000 to 4,000 Thorotrast-bearing men are still living in West Germany.[180]

It is astonishing, in retrospect, how a potentially harmful contrast medium has been employed for years in spite of reiterated warnings, such as the recommendation of the American Medical Association, Council of Pharmacy and Chemistry, in 1932.[29] Thorotrast-induced lesions constitute, by now, a well-defined chapter of human and experimental pathology.

A discussion on the dosimetry and toxicity of Thorotrast held in Vienna in October, 1965,[80] jointly by I.A.E.A. and by W.H.O., and a conference on distribution, retention, and late effects of thorium dioxide, sponsored by the New York Academy of Sciences in April, 1966,[162] summarized the bulk of knowledge collected in this field from all over the world.

Injected into the blood vessels, Thorotrast* is retained mostly in the reticuloendothelial system (R.E.S.) and therefore in the organs where reticulo-

Work done in part under contract 343/RB of the International Atomic Energy Agency in Vienna, Austria.

*Thorotrast is a 25 percent colloidal thorium dioxide suspension in aqueous solution of dextrin.[162,185]

333

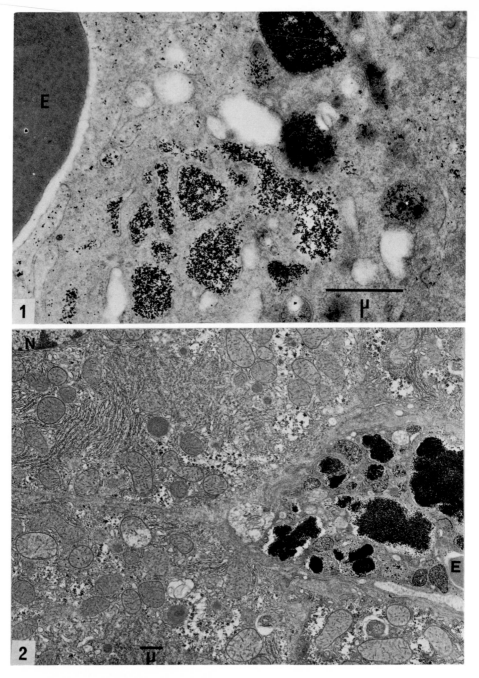

Fig. 1. Thorium dioxide granules in the cytoplasm of a Kupffer cell, 1 hour after injection. E=erythrocyte. Rat liver, X19,800.

Fig. 2. Large thorium dioxide aggregates of differing densities in the cytoplasm of a Kupffer cell, 3 months after injection. No Thorotrast is seen in two adjacent liver parenchymal cells. E=erythrocyte. Rat liver, X6,570. (Adapted from Grampa. 1965. Atti Soc. Ital. Path., 9:717-720.)

endothelial cells are more numerous, such as spleen, lymph nodes, bone marrow, and liver.[61,199] Dextrin, which is added to thorium dioxide for stabilizing the colloidal suspension, is rapidly removed by blood amylase.[10] Thorium dioxide particles, before being phagocytosed by histiocytic cells, are coated with proteins, mostly fibrin. Histiocytes absorb Thorotrast rapidly by a process of pinocytosis, as shown with electron microscopic observations. Thorotrast particles appear as very electron dense, remarkably uniform granules measuring approximately 70 Å in diameter, usually grouped in small aggregates. Within a few minutes after injection, thorium dioxide particles are seen in cytoplasmic canaliculi and in membrane-bound osmiophilic organelles of lysosome type (Fig. 1).

In the liver, thorium dioxide is mainly observed in Kupffer cells; hepatocytes do also absorb Thorotrast, especially if it is injected in large doses. Thorotrast deposits are recognizable grossly as fine whitish reticulum or thick bands of whitish chalky color.

By optic microscopic observations, thorium dioxide is seen as grayish granules measuring 0.5 to 3 μ in diameter. Single granules form masses of greater diameter with lapse of time.

Enlarged histiocytes loaded with Thorotrast project into the lumen of sinusoids, and eventually disintegrate: subsequent phagocytosis of Thorotrast particles by other histiocytes leads to a pattern of Thorotrast distribution that changes from diffuse to focal with time[167]; in later observations dense aggregates are seen mainly in portal spaces (Fig. 2). Thorotrast redistribution in the R.E.S. may be followed by changes in X-ray pictures taken at different time intervals.

Fibrosis

The late lesion most frequently observed after Thorotrast injection is fibrosis, both local, due to Thorotrast extravasation at the site of injection, and diffuse, in the organs where Thorotrast is deposited (liver, spleen, lymph nodes, and bone marrow).

The external surface of the liver has a coarse nodular appearance, due to the retraction of the fibrotic areas around Thorotrast deposits (Fig. 3). Histologically, foci of necrosis are frequently observed in association with fibrosis; the most common lesion, however, is atrophy of the hepatocytes, in the immediate neighborhood of Thorotrast deposits and in the centrolobular areas; rupture of the trabeculae and of the reticular fibers produces a pattern of "pseudolobulation" (Fig. 4), defined as "Thorotrast cirrhosis" by some authors, even if Thorotrast by itself does not cause the parenchymal distortion, which is the main feature of liver cirrhosis.

In the spleen, as the liver, Thorotrast distribution changes from diffuse to focal with time. The spleen capsule is thickened and smooth, due to connective tissue proliferation (Fig. 5).

In histologic sections, large deposits of Thorotrast are observed near the splenic trabeculae, and around follicular arteries, extensive fibrosis being accompanied by progressive parenchymal necrosis and atrophy (Fig. 6). In long-standing cases, the spleen is much reduced in volume and composed of bands of hyaline

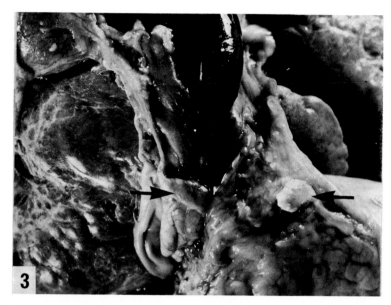

Fig. 3. Thorotrast fibrosis of the liver and massive Thorotrast deposition in lymph node (arrows). (Female patient 76 years old; femoral arteriography at age 55.) (From Grampa and Tommasini Degna. 1958. Rec. Progr. Med., 26:290-318.)

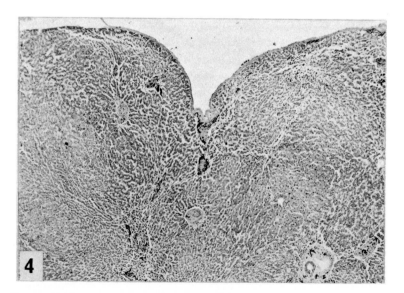

Fig. 4. Thorotrast fibrosis of the liver: slight changes of the lobular pattern in the subcapsular zone. Increased connective tissue and thorium dioxide deposits in the portal spaces. (Same patient as in Fig. 3.) H&E. X25. (From Grampa and Tommasini Degna. 1958. Rec. Progr. Med., 26:290-318.)

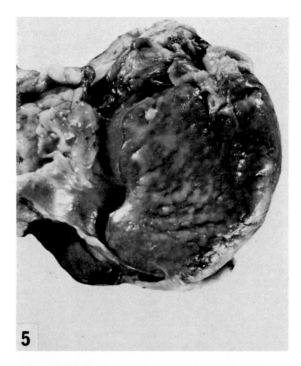

Fig. 5. Thorotrast fibrosis of the spleen: whitish thickened areas of the capsule correspond to thorotrast deposition. (Same patient as in Fig. 3.)

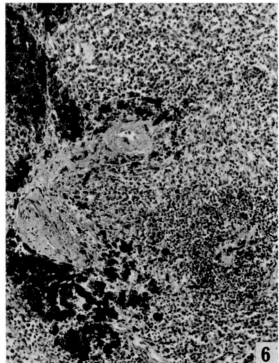

Fig. 6. Fibrosis of the spleen with massive Thorotrast deposits along splenic trabeculae and around splenic arteries. (Same patient as in Fig. 3.) H&E. X120.

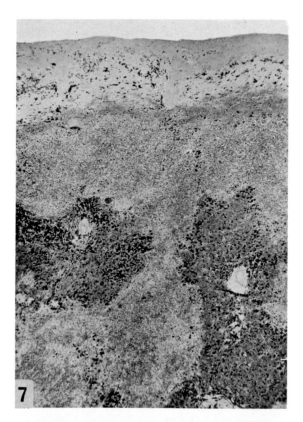

Fig. 7. Thorotrast fibrosis of the spleen: large Thorotrast aggregates in the thickened capsule and in hemorrhagic zones around the central follicular arteries. (Same patient as in Fig. 9.) H&E. X25. (From Grampa and Tommasini Degna. 1958. Acta Genet., 8:65-78.)

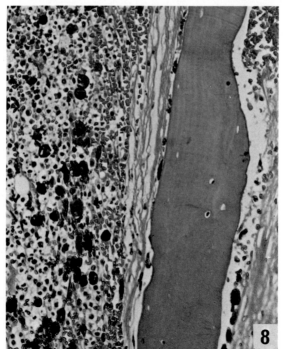

Fig. 8. Thorotrast deposition in the bone marrow: slight fibrosis close to a bone trabecula. (Same patient as in Fig. 3.) H&E. X220.

fibrous tissue around Thorotrast deposits, with great reduction of splenic parenchyma (Fig. 7).

Very similar pictures may be observed in the hilar lymph nodes of the liver,
which also show, as a result, complete replacement of lymphatic parenchyma
by Thorotrast and fibrous tissue (Fig. 3).

Bone marrow usually does not disclose pathologic changes on gross examination.[52] Histologically, thorium dioxide aggregates are seen both free and in
reticular cells, more numerous in proximity to bone than in the central portion
of marrow spaces. Bone trabeculae, frequently surrounded by slight fibrosis,
are not appreciably modified (Fig. 8).

Thorotrastomas

A distinctive form of fibrosis is produced by extravascularly deposited
thorium dioxide. It is estimated that in at least 3 percent of angiographies there
has been extravascular leakage.[14]

The local formation of fibrous tissue around Thorotrast deposits is called
thorotrastoma, or Thorotrast granuloma. Most cases of thorotrastoma are
located in the cervical region, as cerebral angiography is by far the most frequent
diagnostic procedure involved. The granulomas are very hard, partly calcified,
and adherent to the contiguous structures. On cut section they are chalky white,

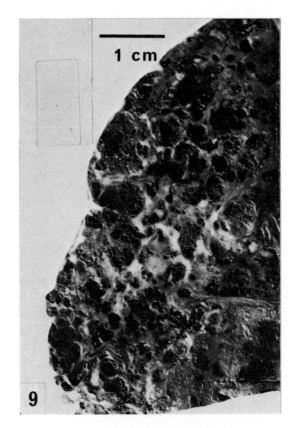

Fig. 9. Liver hemangioendothelioma. Cut surface shows dark
hemorrhagic nodules surrounded by whitish twigs of thorotrast. (Male patient 61 years
old; hepatolienography with 75
ml Thorotrast at age 32. (From
Grampa and Tommasini Degna.
1958. Rec. Progr. Med., 26:290-
318.)

sometimes with softening zones. Large areas of softening are likely the result of ischemia from radiation-induced obliteration of the blood supply.

Histologically, the granuloma is composed of very dense, hyalinized connective tissue, in which Thorotrast may be found both free and in the cytoplasm of histiocytes (Fig. 9). Paravascular granulomas have been recorded also near the portal vein, femoral arteries, and the aorta; in addition thorotrastomas have been observed in the renal pelvis following retrograde pyelography,[153] as well as in joint spaces, peritoneum, liver, and brain,[48] following intracavitary injection.

Malignant Tumors

Development of malignant tumors constitutes the most severe damage induced by Thorotrast.[62,101] Criteria generally accepted in order to ascribe a tumor to Thorotrast are as follows: thorium dioxide granules should be found in the immediate vicinity of the tumor, the latency period should be sufficiently long, and the radiation dose should be sufficiently high.[30,31]

The number of malignances in subjects injected with Thorotrast is steadily increasing as foreseen.[8,62,154,181] Approximately 200 pathologically confirmed cases are by now reported in the literature. Over half of these are tumors located in the liver, namely 31 cases of hepatocellular carcinomas (mean latency 23 years), 47 cases of cholangiocellular carcinomas and carcinomas of extra-hepatic biliary system (mean latency 21 years), and 46 cases of sarcomas (mean latency 22 years).

In addition to single case reports, three relatively large series of liver tumors in Thorotrast patients have been investigated by Silva da Horta[152] (12 hemangio-endotheliomas, 1 reticulum cell sarcoma, 1 cholangiocarcinoma, and 1 carcinoma of common hepatic duct), by Dahlgren[31] (1 hemangioendothelioma, 4 adeno-carcinomas, 3 liver cell carcinomas, and 2 undifferentiated carcinomas), and by Takahashi et al.[164,197] (5 cases of hepatomas, 17 of cholangiocarcinomas, 5 of hemangioendotheliomas).

The amount of Thorotrast injected in patients developing malignant tumors of the liver is usually large (in excess of 30 ml) and a definite correlation between the amount of contrast medium and the development of hepatic tumors has been pointed out.[14]

The increased frequency of cholangiocarcinomas and hemangioendotheliomas in Thorotrast-treated subjects appears statistically significant, as compared with the distribution of causes of death in the autopsied Japanese population.[164]

Hemangioendotheliomas deserve special mention for their striking frequency in Thorotrast-treated patients (over one-third of the cases) as compared with their very low incidence among liver tumors as a whole (around 1 percent). The external surface of the liver is irregular, due to the bulging of reddish and bluish nodules of different size; whitish strands are seen in the depressed grooves between nodules. On cut section an irregular lobular pattern is produced by white lines encircling hemorrhagic nodules scattered throughout the hepatic parenchyma (Fig. 10).

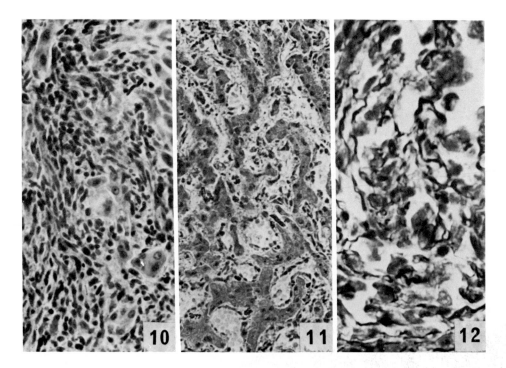

Fig. 10. Liver hemangioendothelioma. Solid masses of elongated tumor cells compress remnants of hepatic cords. (Same patient as in Fig. 9.) H&E. X30. (Adapted from Grampa and Tommasini Degna. 1958. Rec. Progr. Med., 26:290-318.)

Fig. 11. Liver hemangioendothelioma. Kupffer cell proliferation dissociates liver trabeculae. (Same patient as in Fig. 9.) H&E. X180.

Fig. 12. Liver hemangioendothelioma. Net of reticulin fibers in close connection with neoplastic cells. (Same patient as in Fig. 9.) Gomori reticulum stain. X800.

Histologically, nodules composed of spindle cells replace the cords of hepatocytes. Some nodules are mainly solid (Fig. 11), others show tiny clefts or well-formed vascular spaces. The initial tumor change appears as Kupffer cell proliferation in the sinuses, with preserved trabecular pattern of the liver parenchyma (Fig. 12). Transitional forms from the solid to the angiomatous type are often recognizable. Reticulum stain reveals a delicate network of reticulin fibers in the tumor tissue (Fig. 13). In the vascular spaces foci of myeloid cells may be observed. Thick bands of fibrous connective tissue surround large aggregates of thorium dioxide.

The causative effect of Thorotrast in liver tumors is supported by experimental work, in which liver tumors both of hemangioendotheliomatous and carcinomatous type were obtained in several animal species, viz., mice,[68,148] rats,[60] and rabbits,[84,85,163] after Thorotrast administration (Fig. 14).

A second group of malignant tumors develops after local deposition of Thorotrast used for visualization of body cavities and tubular structures. Thirty-one cases of kidney tumors, namely 23 carcinomas of the renal pelvis (mean latency 25 years), 6 carcinomas of the renal parenchyma (mean latency 21 years), and 2 sarcomas of the renal pelvis (mean latency 23 years) are reported after ret-

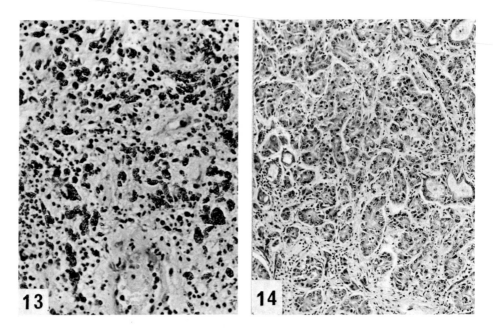

Fig. 13. Cervical thorotrastoma. Numerous thorium dioxide aggregates surrounded by granulation tissue. H&E. X180.

Fig. 14. Cholangiocellular carcinoma in a rat treated with Thorotrast 23 months before death. H&E. X200.

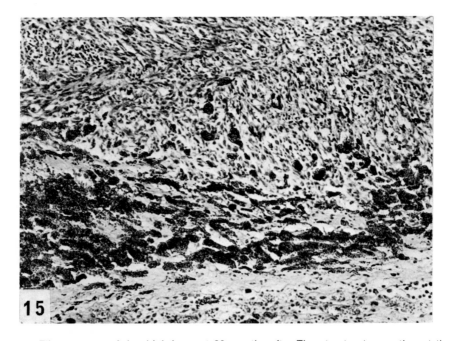

Fig. 15. Fibrosarcoma of the thigh in a rat 20 months after Thorotrast extravasation at the site of intravenous injection. H&E. X180.

rograde pyelography. A clear cell kidney carcinoma was observed[50] after arteriography.

In addition, 6 cases of carcinomas of maxillary sinuses, 4 spindle cell sarcomas in the lateral cervical region or other site of Thorotrast extravasation, and 12 cases following more uncommon procedures, such as urethrography and hysterosalpingography, have been described.

Spindle cell sarcomas have been obtained by several authors[15,64,116,128,136,145,146,192,193] in experimental animals (mouse, rat, guinea pig, hamster), usually by subcutaneous injection (Fig. 15). It is to be pointed out that tumors of this type were the first to be related to Thorotrast and led to the subsequent rich surge of studies on Thorotrast cancerogenesis.[79]

To complete the variety of tumors in patients injected with Thorotrast, approximately 50 cases of leukemias and other hematologic disorders (myeloid aplasia, erythremia, purpura) must be considered. Leukemias are usually of myeloid type, develop after a long latent period, and show a rather acute course.[1]

References of pathologically confirmed Thorotrast tumors are listed below.*

In many cases the relationship between Thorotrast and tumor is debatable especially when the organ involved is frequently affected by spontaneous tumors or the latency period is short.

Chromosomal Damage

In peripheral granulocytes of people treated with Thorotrast, chromosomal aberrations (deletions, dicentric and ring chromosomes) and polyploid cells have been observed.[45,82]

Statistical data show a significant correlation between frequency of chromosomal breaks and radiation dose.

Tumors of liver
Sarcomas: 7,17,20,24,25,40,42,46,49,51,64,71,73,88,100,103,111,113,118,132,143,149,151,152,155,160, 164,166,171,178,180,182,188,196.

Carcinomas: a) Hepatocellular carcinomas: 9,31,33,40,43,46,47,49,52,54,96,98,107,110,115,157,164, 169,173,179,183,187; b) Cholangiocellular carcinomas: 5,6,17,30,43,46,67,91,97,99,108,121,123,138,158, 159,164,180,188; c) Carcinomas of gall bladder and bile ducts: 6,9,54,55,71,72,73,99,131,188.

Tumors developed after local deposition of Thorotrast: Carcinomas of renal pelvis: 3,16,18,21,34, 37,44,49,70,77,94,95,124,129,130,147,170,172-175,184. Sarcomas of renal pelvis: 75,190.

Clear cell carcinomas of the kidney: 37,50,81,172,176. Carcinomas of maxillary sinuses after sinusography: 22,42,66,74,90,102.

Tumors after perivascular extravasation: a) spindle cell sarcomas: 30,89,93,126; b) chondrosarcoma: 140; c) squamous cell carcinoma of the skin: 92.

Tumors after other procedures:
Salpingography: Peritoneal hemangioendothelioma: a) 26, and mesothelioma: 27; b) Ovary carcinoma: 144.

Mammography: Carcinomas of the breast: 4,19.

Dacryocystography: Carcinoma of the eyelid: 137.

Urethrography: Squamous cell carcinoma of the urethea: 32.

Cecal fistulography: Peritoneal spindle cell sarcoma: 141.

Urinary bladder fistulography: Seminal vesicle carcinomas: 57.

Leukemia and other hematologic diseases: 1,12,13,17,35,41,43,55,56,65,83,112,114,117,125,127, 135,142,154,156,188.

Reports on tumors of lung, (2,17,40,69,76,120,134,154,177); stomach, (40,150); intestinal tract, (22, 40); pancreas, (17,40,150,186); larynx, (154); uterus, (40); bone, (195); and on Hodgkin's disease, (176); mycosis fungoides, (191); Kaposi's sarcoma, (198); and meningioma, (194) may also be listed.

Pathogenesis

Although the pathogenesis of Thorotrast-induced lesions is still under discussion, their close resemblance to lesions induced by other radioactive substances and by X rays (parenchymal necrosis, fibrosis, occurrence of malignant tumors, and leukemias after a long latent period, also chromosomal aberrations) points to Thorotrast radioactivity as the main factor.[36, 53, 161]

On the other hand, tissue reactions induced by Thorotrast are not different from those of other fibrogenetic substances. Radiation could therefore reinforce a nonspecific foreign body tissue reaction; fibrosis may, in part, be related also to the property of thorium dioxide to become bound to serum albumins. However, while several mechanisms are discussed, no conclusive evidence supporting a nonradioactive basis for the carcinogenic effects of Thorotrast has been obtained.[11]

Thorotrast Radioactivity and Dosimetric Information

Thorium (^{232}Th) is the first of a family of 11 radioactive isotopes, mostly alpha-emitters, with a very different half-life.

A scheme of ^{232}Th decay series is given in Table 1. Thorotrast radioactivity is easily demonstrated in tissue sections by autoradiographic technique (Fig. 16). Dosimetry refers to the measurement of the energy absorbed from the Thorotrast radiation per unit mass of tissue (radiation dose) and is expressed in rads. Over

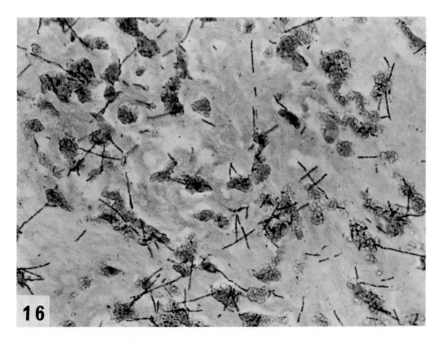

Fig. 16.   Liver hemangioendothelioma. Histoautoradiography showing numerous alpha tracks departing from Thorotrast aggregates. (Same patient as in Fig. 9.) H&E. X500.

TABLE 1. Decay Scheme for [232]**Th**

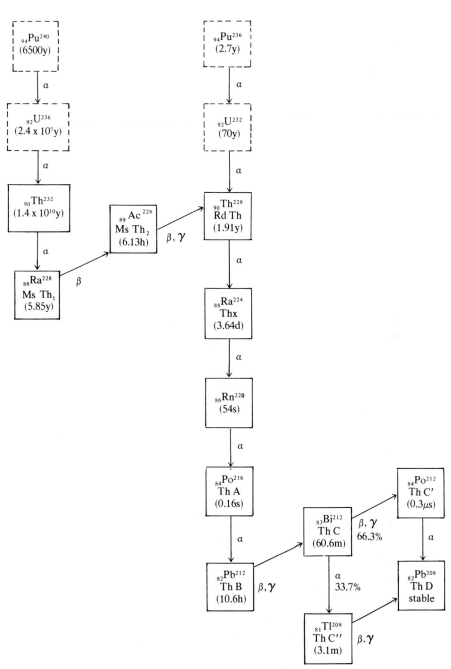

(Modified from Cohn et al. Ann. N.Y. Acad. Sci., 145:608–622, 1967.)

90 percent of the radiation energy is associated with alpha particles: this accounts for the fact that doses contributed by beta and gamma rays are usually ignored.[36]

Many techniques, including alpha and gamma spectrometry, autoradiography, radiography, and light and electron microscopy have been applied in order to estimate the doses to various organs from the several components of the Thorotrast complex.[28,36,78,109,122,133]

Dosimetric determinations constitute a complex problem, because radiation delivered to tissues depends on many factors, some hardly estimable, such as the way of administration, the range of equilibrium between single isotopes, the amount of alpha particles self-absorbed into thorium dioxide aggregates, the increased volume of aggregates with time, and the steady process of redistribution of the aggregates in the organs.[29,36]

The distribution of chemical ^{232}Th among the various organs of the body probably accurately reflects the distribution of the colloidal particles of thorium dioxide contained in Thorotrast, since thorium dioxide is extremely stable and insoluble in body fluids. The knowledge of its precise distribution in men among the various portions of the R.E.S. (liver, spleen, red bone marrow, and lymphatic system) and between them and other organs, is far from accurate.

Parr,[122] gathering together some available measurements, calculated the following values: liver 70 percent, spleen 17 percent, red bone marrow 8 percent, lung 0.8 percent, skeleton 0.6 percent, heart 0.05 percent, and kidney 0.1 percent.

Such figures should be cautiously applied to a particular Thorotrast case, as wide departures from these average values are often found.

Although reliable data on lymph nodes are rare, their ^{232}Th concentration may exceed that of the liver by at least a factor of 10, so that in some cases a significant proportion of the whole radiation burden is confined to the lymph nodes. Also, perivascular deposits may exceed 50 percent of the total body radioactivity.

The wide variations in Thorotrast uptake by the different parts of the R.E.S. from patient to patient can probably be related to the different pathologic conditions, including endocrine imbalance, by which the patients were affected[59]; values with differences of 50 percent should be regarded as satisfactory, due to the number of factors involved.[104]

Quantitative information on the uniformity of distribution in a single organ are scanty. For the liver, differences by a factor of two were reported between peripheral and central parts, the former containing the higher concentration.

On the microscopic scale, the inhomogeneities in distribution are even greater and the difference between the minimum and the maximum radiation rates has been estimated as having a ratio of 50 or 100.[133] With these limitations, it has been calculated that in 20 years, after injection of 20 ml of Thorotrast, 500 to 540 rads are delivered to the spleen and 1,200 to 1,400 rads to the liver.[86,138,139]

For the same Thorotrast dose and time interval, Kaul[87] estimates 10 rads to the bone and 220 rads to the bone marrow. In accordance with the low dose to the skeleton is the fact that few cases of bone tumor induced by Thorotrast have been reported so far.[195]

According to Marinelli,[106] doses received by bone marrow and lung are in the range of those received by people submitted to X-ray therapy for cervical arthrosis. In bone tissue and in the kidney, radiation doses are more or less uniform, approximately 1 to 5 rads per year, relatively close to those that the International Commission for Radiation Protection considers permissible for the whole human working life.

Conclusions

The effect of radiation from a radioactive substance, such as thorium dioxide, deposited in the body is not completely identical to that of an external radiation source.

Thorotrast use, as regrettable for the adverse effects mentioned as it may be, constitutes a radiobiologic experiment of very high interest, since Thorotrast patients offer a unique opportunity for an appraisal of the effects of long-standing alpha radiation in man.[28,105] Investigations are in progress in different countries, with the aim of performing radioactivity tests, blood examinations, morphologic, autoradiographic, and radiochemical studies on tissues and statistical evaluation on the frequency of malformation in descendants of patients treated with Thorotrast.

It is highly desirable that through international institutions such as W.H.O. and I.A.E.A., data may be evaluated with uniform criteria in order to provide definite results on the largest possible number of cases.

Dosimetric studies are important for comparison with other forms of radiation at the level of practical radiation protection.

Knowledge in this field of pathology and information acquired in the study of Thorotrast cases will give a valuable contribution to problems related to the use of nuclear energy in contemporary civilization.

References

1. Abbatt, J. D. Leukemia and other fatal blood dyscrasias in thorium dioxide patients. Ann. N.Y. Acad. Sci., 145:767–775, 1967.
2. Abrahamson, L., O'Connor, M. H., and Abrahamson, M. L. Bilateral alveolar lung carcinoma associated with injection of Thorotrast. Irish J. Med. Sci., 293:229–235, 1950.
3. Alken, C. E., Roucayrol, J. C., Oberhausen, E., Taupitz, A., and Überberg, H. Zur Frage der Carcinoma-Entstehung nach Pyelographie mit Thorotrast. Urol. Int. 10:137–156, 1960.
4. Austoni, B. Epitelioma mammario maschile in sede di mastite cronica da Thorotrast. Chirurgia (Milano), 5:145–152, 1950.
5. Baserga, R., Yokoo, H., and Henegar, G. C. Thorotrast-induced cancer in man. Cancer, 13:1021, 1960.
6. Batzenschlager, A., Keiling, R., and Kuntzmann, F. Cancer des voies biliaires sur thorotrastose du foie. Ann. Anat. Path., 6:457, 1961.
7. ——— Reville, P., and Weill-Bousson, M. Sarcome endothélial angioplastique caverneux du foie et thorotrastose hépatique. Bull. Ass. Franc. Etude Cancer, 48:347–364, 1961.
8. ——— Dorner, M., and Weill-Bousson, M. La pathologie tumorale du Thorotrast chez l'homme. Oncologia, 16:28–63, 1963.

9. ———— Weill-Bousson, M., and Mandard, A. M. Cancers hépatiques et biliaires par thorotrastose hépato-ganglionnaire. Arch. Anat. Path., 15:295–300, 1967.

10. Bell, E. The origin and nature of granules found in macrophages of the white mouse following intravenous injection of Thorotrast. J. Cell. Physiol., 42:36, 1953.

11. Bensted, J. P. M. Experimental studies in mice on the late effects of radioactive and nonradioactive contrast media. Ann. N.Y. Acad. Sci., 145:728–737, 1967.

12. Bernard, J., Boiron, M., Guérin, R. A., Gérard-Marchant, R., Ripault, J., Moulias, R., and Delaporte, P. Leucémie aiguë à promyélocytes survenue 17 ans après une artériographie carotidienne au thorotrast. Presse Med., 74:487–491, 1966.

13. Birkner, R. Die Spätschäden des Thorotrasts, beurteilt nach dem ältesten, bisher bekannten Thorotrastschädensfall. Strahlentherapie., 78:587–608, 1949.

14. Blomberg, R., Larsson, L. E., Lindell, B., and Lindgren, E. Late effects of Thorotrast in cerebral angiography. Ann. N.Y. Acad. Sci., 145:853–858, 1967.

15. Bogliolo, L. Sopra i blastomi sperimentali da ossido di torio. Patologica, 30:422, 1938.

16. Bömke, F. Thorotrastschäden der Nieren. Zbl. Path., 95:464–468, 1956.

17. Boyd, J. T., Langlands, A. O., and Maccabe, J. J. Long-term hazards of Thorotrast. Brit. Med. J. No. 5604, 2:517–521, 1968.

18. Brauman, H., Gepts, W., Gompel, C., and Stuckens, M. Sequelles tardives d'une pyelographie au thorotrast. Acta Clin. Belg., 21:326–337, 1966.

19. Brody, H., and Cullen, M. Carcinoma of the breast seventeen years after mammography with thorotrast. Surgery, 42:600–606, 1957.

20. Brozman, M., and Simko, M. Haemangioendothelioma of the liver after thorotrast. Bratisl. Lek. Listy, 38:638, 1958.

21. Bücheler, E. Doppelseitige Nieren-Thorotrastose mit maligner Neubildung einer Niere. Fortschr. Röentgenstr., 104:361–367, 1966.

22. Buda, J. A., Conley, J. J., and Rankow, R. Carcinoma of the maxillary sinus following thorotrast instillation. Amer. J. Surg., 106:868, 1963.

23. Budin, E., and Gershon-Cohen, J. The danger of cancer from thorotrast as a diagnostic medium Amer. J. Roentgen., 75:1188–1193, 1956.

24. Buschmann, O., and Hünig, R. Thorotrastose. Med. Klin., 61:14–18, 1966.

25. Caroli, J., Etévé, J., Platteborse, R., and Fallot, P. Thorotrast et hémangioréticulome malin du foie. Rev. Med. Chir. Mal. Foie, 31:53–68, 1956.

26. Casper, J. Peritoneal haemangioendotheliomatosis after salpingography with thorotrast. Ann. N.Y. Acad. Sci., 145:798–805, 1967.

27. Cattel, R. B., and Kahn, F. Thorotrast and carcinogenesis: report of one case. J.A. M.A., 174:413–415, 1960.

28. Cohn, S. H., Gusmano, E. A., and Robertson, J. S. Calculation of radiation dose from thorotrast using whole-body gamma-ray spectral data. Ann. N.Y. Acad. Sci., 145:608–622, 1967.

29. Council on Pharmacy and Chemistry. Thorotrast (preliminary report). J.A.M.A., 99: 2183–2185, 1932.

30. Dahlgren, S. Thorotrast tumours. A review of the literature and report of two cases. Acta Path. Microbiol. Scand., 53:147–161, 1961.

31. ———— Late effects of thorium dioxide on the liver of patients in Sweden. Ann. N.Y. Acad. Sci., 145:718–723, 1967.

32. ———— Effects of locally deposited colloidal thorium dioxide. Ann. N.Y. Acad. Sci., 145:786–790, 1967.

33. Di Gennaro, A., and Bassi, M. Un caso di cirrosi epatica e di mesotelioma peritoneale insorti dopo 18 anni da un'iniezione di Toriofanina. Riforma Medica, 73:244–251, 1959.

34. Drefke, F. Spätschäden, insbesondere Tumorbildungen, nach retrograde Pyelographie mit Thorotrast und ihre Problematik. Med. Diss. Halle, 1962.

35. Duane, G. W. Aplastic anaemia 14 years following administration of Thorotrast. Amer. J. Med., 23:499, 1957.

36. Dudley, R. A. A survey of radiation dosimetry in thorium dioxide cases. Ann. N.Y. Acad. Sci., 145:595–607, 1967.

37. Dunant. J., and Rutishauser, G. Thorotrast-Tumoren der Niere. Drei weitere Fälle. Schweiz. Med. Wschr., 96:1156–1160, 1966.
38. Edmondson, H. A. Tumors of the liver and intrahepatic bile ducts. Atlas of Tumor Pathol., Sec. VII, Fasc. 25, Washington, A.F.I.P., 1958, pp 80–86.
39. Ellis, P. A. A case of thorium-induced cholangioma. Brit. J. Surg., 51:74–76, 1964.
40. Faber, M. Thorium dioxide patients in Denmark. Ann. N. Y. Acad. Sci., 145:843–848, 1967.
41. ――――― and Johansen, C. Leukemia and other hematological diseases after thorotrast. Ann. N.Y. Acad. Sci., 145:755–758, 1967.
42. Fabrikant, I. J., Dickson, R. J., and Fetter, B. F. Mechanisms of radiation carcinogenesis at the clinical level. Brit. J. Cancer, 18:459–477, 1964.
43. Federlin, K., and Scior, H. Spätschäden und Tumorentwicklung nach Thorotrast Injection. Frankf. Z. Path., 68:225, 1957.
44. Feine, U., and Leonhardt, J. Nierenbeckencarcinom nach Thorotrast-Pyelographie. Krebsforsch.. 64:323–327. 1961.
45. Fisher, P., Golob, E., Kunze-Mühl, E., and Müllner, T. Chromosomal aberrations in thorium dioxide patients. Ann. N.Y. Acad. Sci., 145:759–766, 1967.
46. Fitzgerald, P. J. Personal communication.
47. Forbes, I. J., Geddes, R. A., and Wood, N. M. Thorotrast induced hepatoma with dysimmunoglobulinaemia. Med. J. Aust., 55(1):762–765, 1968.
48. Freeman, W. Thorium granulomas in the brain. Report of 4 cases following prefrontal lobotomy. Ideggyog. Szle, 21:26–34, 1968.
49. Freese, P., and Kemnitz, P. Beitrag zur Entstehung bösartiger Geschwülste nach Thorotrast. Zbl. Path., 105:161–169, 1964.
50. Friedrich, W. Hypernephroides Karcinom nach Thorotrastanwendung und eosinophiles Adenom der Hypophyse. Z. Krebsforsch., 63:456, 1960.
51. Fruhling, L., Gros, Ch. M., and Batzenschlager, A. Sarcome endothélial angioplastique généralisé chez un malade ayant subi 12 ans auparavant une injection intra-artérielle et para-artérielle de thorotrast. Bull. Ass. Franc. Cancer, 42:559–563, 1955.
52. ――――― Gros, Ch. M., Batzenschlager, A., and Dorner, M. La maladie du Thorotrast. Ann. Med., 57:297–350; 409–486, 1956.
53. ――――― and Batzenschlager, A. Lésions dues à l'action ionisante par injection de thorotrast chez l'homme. Conference Int. sur l'influence des conditions de vie et de travail sur la santé, Cannes, 1957. Comptes Rendus, 533–539, 1957.
54. Gardner, D. L., and Ogilvie, R. F. The late results of injection of thorotrast: Two cases of neoplastic disease following contrast angiography. J. Path. Bact., 78:133–144, 1959.
55. Gaus, H., Gülzow, M., and Meyer-Hofmann, G. Spätschäden nach Thorotrastanwendung. Klin. Wschr., 44:32–39, 1966.
56. Gebauer, A., and Hinecker, R. Iatrogene und gewerbliche Radium und Thoriumschäden. Strahlentherapie, 98:558–569, 1955.
57. Gelzer, J., and Scheidegger, S. Samenblasenkarzinom (14 Jahre nach Kontrast Darstellung einer Harnfistel mit Thorotrast). Oncologia, 12:27–33, 1959.
58. Grampa, G. Osservazioni al microscopio elettronico sulla distribuzione del Thorotrast nel fegato di ratto. Atti Soc. Ital. Pat., 9:717–720, 1965.
59. ――――― Reticuloendothelial system stimulation by estrogens and Thorium dioxide retention in rat liver. Int. Symposium on atherosclerosis and R.E.S., Villa Olmo, Sept. 8–10, 1966. New York, Plenum Publishing Corporation, 1967, pp. 214–220.
60. ――――― Liver distribution of colloidal Thorium dioxide and development of liver epithelial tumors in rats. Ann. N.Y. Acad. Sci., 145:738–747, 1967.
61. ――――― and Cefis, F. Le cellule di Kupffer dopo iniezione di Thorotrast. Atti X Congr. Naz. Soc. Ital. Path., 843–847, 1967.
62. ――――― and Tommasini Degna, A. Lesioni da Thorotrast in patologia umana. Rec. Progr. Med., 26:290–318, 1958.
63. ――――― and Tommasini Degna, A. Hemangioendothelioma of the liver following intravenous injection of Thorotrast. Acta Genet., 8:65–78, 1958.

64. ——— Grigolato, P. G., and Lange A. Fibrosarcomi da Thorotrast nel ratto. Atti X Congr. Naz. Soc. Ital. Pat., Roma, 1969.

65. Grebe, S. F. Beitrag zur Frage der Thorotrastspätschädigung Eine myeloische Leukämie nach diagnostischer Thorotrastapplikation. Strahlentherapie., 94:311–319, 1954.

66. Gros, Ch. M., Fruhling, L., and Keiling, R. Injection de thorotrast dans le sinus maxillaire. 15 ans aprés: Apposition d'un épitheliome malpighien. Bull. Ass. Franc. Etude Cancer, 42:556–558, 1955.

67. Grossiord, A., Rougrayrol, J. C., Duperrat, B., Ceccaldi, P. F., and Meeus-Bith, L. Adenocancer du foie avec cirrhose 21 ans apres une arteriographie au thorotrast. Sem. Hop. Paris, 32:184–193, 1956.

68. Guimaraes, J. P., and Lamerton, L. F. Further experimental observations on the late effects of thorotrast administration. Brit. J. Cancer, 10:527–532, 1956.

69. Hackenthal, P. Beitrag zu den morphologischen Veränderungen durch Thorotrastablagerungen. Zbl. Path., 94:352–359, 1956.

70. Hartig, W., and Neideck, J. Contribution to the problem of thorotrast damage after retrograde pyelography. Z. Urol., 56:249–268, 1963.

71. Hassler, O., Boström, K., and Dahlbäck, L.-O. Thorotrast tumors. Report of 3 cases and a microradiological study of the deposition of thorotrast in man. Acta Path. Microbiol. Scand., 61:13–20, 1964.

72. Heitmann, W. Carcinom der Gellengangs und der Leber nach Thorotrast-Injektion. Chirurg., 25:223–225, 1954.

73. Hieronymi, G. Kritische Untersuchung sogenannter Thorotrast-tumoren nebst Mitteilung zweier Fälle. Zbl. Path., 97:513–523, 1958.

74. Hofer, O. Kieferöhlencarzinom durch radiumhaltiges Kontrastmittel hervogerufen. Deutsch. Zahnaerztl. Z., 7:736, 1952.

75. Holl, H., and Kammerer, V. Nierensarkom nach retrograder Pyelographie mit Thorotrast-Kasuistischer Beitrag. Med. Welt, 12:712–715, 1967.

76. Holthusen, W. Carcinomentstehung nach Thorotrast. Quoted by Batzenschlager et al., 1963.[8]

77. Hubmann, R., and Hoer, P. W. Nierenbecken Carcinome nach retrograder Pyelographie mit Thorotrast. Urologe, 3:227, 1964.

78. Hursch, J. B. Loss of thorium daughter by thorium dioxide patients. Ann. N.Y. Acad. Sci., 145:634–641, 1967.

79. I.A.E.A. Bibliography on Thorotrast. Vienna, 1964; Suppl. 1965.

80. ——— 106: The Dosimetry and Toxicity of Thorotrast. Vienna, 1968.

81. Jakob, H., and Schostock, P. Früh-und Spätfolgen nach Thorotrastanwendung. Langenbecks Arch. Klin. Chir., 285:341–352, 1957.

82. Janower, M. L., Sidel, V. W., Baker, W. H., Fitzpatrick, D.E.P., Guarino, F.I., and Plynn, M. J. Late clinical and laboratory manifestations of Thorotrast administration in cerebral arteriography. A follow-up of thirty patients. New Eng. J. Med., 279:186–189, 1968.

83. Jedlica, V., Hermanska, Z., and Kubat K. Idiopathic myelofibrosis with terminal effusion of reticular cells in the peripheral blood. The presence of phagocytosed thorotrast in the histological examination of the organs. Acta Med. Scand., 169:479, 1961.

84. Johansen, C. A disseminated, transmissible, reticuloendothelial sarcoma in rabbits provoked by intravenously deposited thorium. Acta Path. Microbiol. Scand., 105: 92, 1955.

85. ——— Tumors in rabbits after injection of various amounts of thorium dioxide. Ann. N.Y. Acad. Sci., 145:724–727, 1967.

86. Kaul, A. Dose in liver and spleen after injection of Thorotrast into blood. In The Dosimetry and Toxicity of Thorotrast. Vienna, I.A.E.A., 1968, pp. 30–43.

87. ——— Dose in skeleton and bone marrow following Thorotrast injection into blood. In The Dosimetry and Toxicity of Thorotrast. Vienna, I.A.E.A., 1968, pp. 69–78.

88. Kemnitz, P. Multizentrische angioplastische Retikuloendotheliomatose der Leber nach Thorotrast-Arteriographie. Zbl. Path., 106:189–197, 1964.

89. ———— and Vinz, H. Uber ein durch paravasale Injection von Thorotrast am Applicationort entstendenes Sarkom. Zbl. Path., 106:502–511, 1964.
90. Kligerman, M., Lattes, R., and Rankow, R. Carcinoma of the maxillary sinus following thorotrast instillation. Cancer, 13:967, 1960.
91. Kohoutek, J., and Novak, D. Cholangiogenni Karcinoma jater po thorotrastu. Ces'k. Rentegen., 14:110, 1960.
92. Kolár, J., and Vrabec, R. Ein ungewöhnlicher Thorotrast-Spätschäden. Med. Klin., 61:2070–2071, 1966.
93. Krick, W., and Heck, G. Spindelzellsarkom im Abdomen nach Thorotrast. Med. Klin. 57:1899, 1962.
94. Krückemeyer, K. Entwicklung eines Nierencarcinoms nach Thorotrast-Pyelographie. Urologe, 2:73, 1963.
95. ———— Lessmann, H., and Pudwitz, K. Nierenkarzinom als Thorotrastschäden. Fortschr. Roentgenstr., 93:313–321, 1960.
96. Kuisk, K., Sanchez. J. S., and Mizuno, N. S. Colloidal thorium dioxide (Th) in radiology with emphasis on hepatic cancerogenesis. A case report of occluded carotid and jugular vessel and a case of hepatoma, 27 and 33 years after its administration. Amer. J. Roentgen., 99:463–475, 1966.
97. Larson, B. A case of post-angiography Thorotrast deposition and primary squamous cell carcinoma of the liver. Acta Path. Microbiol. Scand., 58:389, 1963.
98. Lauche, A. (quoted by Hieronymi) Path. Anat. Demonstr. Med. Ges., 2:11, 1955.
99. Levy Kahn, H. Two cases of carcinoma after thorotrast administration. Ann. N.Y. Acad. Sci., 145: 700–717, 1967.
100. Looney, W. B. An investigation of the late clinical findings following thorotrast (thorium dioxide) administration. Amer. J. Roentgen., 83:163–185, 1960.
101. ———— and Colodzin, M. Late follow-up studies after internal deposition of radioactive materials. J.A.M.A., 160:1–3, 1956.
102. ———— Hursch, J. B., Colodzin, M., and Stedman, L. T. Tumor induction in man following thorotrast (thorium dioxide) administration. Acta Uniocontra Cancrum, 16: 435–447, 1960.
103. Lüdin, M. Jr. Hämangio-endotheliomatose von Leber und Milz bei Thorotrastspeicherung. Schweiz. Path., 16:987, 1953.
104. Marinelli, L. D. Dosimetry in relation to epidemiology: Its applications in radiogenic leukemias and bronchial carcinoma (Thorotrast). Radiological Physic Division Annual Report, Argonne Nat. Lab. July, 1966 to June, 1967, pp. 37–41.
105. ———— Problemi inerenti alla determinazione delle dosi massime di radiazioni ammissibili per l'uomo. Atti Accad. Med. Lombard, 22:167–177, 1967.
106. ———— The doses from Thorotrast and migrated descendants: status, prospects, and implications. The dosimetry and toxicity of Thorotrast. Vienna, I.A.E.A., pp. 86–99, 1968.
107. Matthes, T. Thorotrastschäden und Krebsgefahr. Arch. Geschwulstforsch., 6:162–182. 1954.
108. ———— Zur Frage der Entstehung eines Carcinoms auf dem Boden einer Thorotrast-Narbenleber. Strahlentherapie., 99:94–106, 1956.
109. May, H., Marinelli, L. D., and Corcoran, J. B. In vivo counting of thorium dioxide patients: special techniques and preliminary results. Ann. N.Y. Acad. Sci., 145:623–633, 1967.
110. McKay, J. S., and Ross, R. C. Hepatoma induced by thorium dioxide (Th). Canad. Med. Ass. J., 94:1298–1303, 1966.
111. McMahon, E., Murphy, A. S., and Bates, M. J. Endothelial-cell sarcoma of liver following Thorotrast injections. Amer. J. Path., 23:585, 1947.
112. Meesen, H. Leukämie nach Thorium X. Deutsch. Med. Wschr., 5:169, 1955.
113. Möbius, C., and Lembcke, K. Thorotrasttumoren der Leber. Zbl. Path., 105:41–56, 1963.

114. Moeschlin, S., Marti, H. R., and Germann, W. Tödliche Panmyelopathie durch Thorotrast (Thoriumdioxyd). Schweiz. Med. Wschr., 83:1061, 1953.

115. Morgan, A., Jayne, W., and Marrack, D. Primary liver cell carcinoma 24 years after intravenous injection of Thorotrast. J. Clin. Path., 11:7–18, 1958.

116. Mori, T., Sakai T., Okamoto, T., Nozue, Y., Ishida, T., Umeda, M., and Tamura, N. Preliminary report on a spindle-cell sarcoma in the Syrian hamster produced by Thorotrast. Gann, 57:431–433, 1966.

117. Netousek, M., Bores, J., and Dvorak, K. Chronic myelosis following the use of Thorotrast. Blood, 12:391, 1957.

118. Nettleship, A., and Fink, W. J. Neoplasms of the liver following injection of Thorotrast. Amer. J. Clin. Path., 35:422–426, 1961.

119. Nielsen, G. Thorotrastspätschäden. (Vereinigung Pathologischer Anatomen, Hamburgs, 27 Jan. 1956). Zel. Allg. Path., 95:159, 1956.

120. ———— and Kracht, J. Zur Cancerogenese nach diagnostischer Thorotrastanwendung. Frank. Zschr. Path., 68:661, 1958.

121. Okinaka, S., Nakao, K., Ibayashi, H., Nakaidzumi, M., Kakehi, H., and Sugimura, T. A case report on the development of biliary tract cancer eleven years after the injection of Thorotrast. Amer. J. Roentgen., 78:812, 1957.

122. Parr, R. M. Information on Thorotrast dosimetry supplied by the radiochemical analyses of tissue specimens. Ann. N.Y. Acad. Sci., 145:644–653, 1967.

123. Person, D. A., Sargent, T., and Isaac, E. Thorotrast induced carcinoma of the liver. A case report including results of whole body counting. Arch. Surg., 88:503–510, 1964.

124. Pfeifer, K. Plattenepithelkarzinom der Niere mit sarkomartigen Anteilen nach Thorotrast-Pyelographie. Zbl. Path. Anat., 107:556–565, 1965.

125. Pijpers, P. M. Acute monocytaire leukemia, 13 jaar na carotis arteriografie met thorotrast. Nederl. T. Geneesk., 112:799–802, 1968.

126. Plenge, K., and Krückemeyer, K. Über ein Sarkom am Ort der Thorotrast Injection. Zbl. Path. 92:255–260, 1954.

127. Porton, W. M., and Revers, F. E. Monoblasten-leukemie bij een patiente met thorotrastose. Nederl. T. Geneesk., 112:797–798, 1968.

128. Prussia, G. Contributo allo studio dei tumori sperimentali da Thorotrast. Sperimentale, 90:522, 1936.

129. Rijnders, W. P., Donker, P. J., Ten Berg, J. A., and Ybema, H. J. Renal tumor after pyelography with Thorotrast. Nederl. T. Geneesk., 105:1657, 1961.

130. ———— Ybema, H. J., Donker, P. J., and Ten Berg, J. A. Renal changes following retrograde pyelography using Thorotrast. Arch. Chir. Neerl. 15:157–173, 1963.

131. Roberts, J. C., and Carlson, K. E. Hepatic duct carcinoma seventeen years after injection of thorium dioxide. Arch. Path., 62:1–7, 1956.

132. Rosenbaum, F. J. Lebersakom nach Thorotrast. Deutsch Med. Wschr., 84:428–433, 1959.

133. Rotblat, J., and Ward, G. B. Analysis of the radioactive content of tissues by alphatrack autoradiography. Phys. Med. Biol., 1:57–70, 1956.

134. Roth, F. Thorotrast Karzinom der Bronchien. Zbl. Path. 96:417, 1957.

135. Rotter, W. Uber Gewebschäden durch Thorotrast unter besonderer Berücksichtigung der Gefässveranderungen und aplasticher Knochenmarkreactionen. Beitr. Path. Anat., 111:144–157, 1951.

136. Roussy, G., Oberling, C., and Guérin, M. Action cancérigène du dioxyde de Thorium chez le rat blanc. Bull. Acad. Med., 35:809–816, 1934.

137. Rudolphi, H. Spätentwicklung eines Unterlid-Karzinoms nach Thoriumoxydinjektion. Beitr. Path. Anat., 111:158–164, 1950.

138. Rundo, J. Considerations of the limits of radiation dosage from Thorotrast. Brit. J. Radiol., 28:615–619, 1955.

139. ———— The determination of the distribution of internally deposited Thorium by means of studies with a realistic phantom. Acta Radiol., 47:65–77, 1957.

140. Schajowicz, F., Defilippi-Novoa, C. A., and Firpo, C. A. Chondrosarcoma of the axilla induced by Thorotrast. Boll. Soc. Argent. Ortop. Traum., 30:199–210, 1965.

141. Scheibe, G. Malignes intraperitoneales Thorotrastom beim Menschen. Zbl. Chir., 80: 588–592, 1955.
142. Schmidt, W., Schulte, A., and Lapp, H. Klinischer und pathologisch-anatomischer Beitrag zur Frage der Schädigung durch Thorotrast (Panmyelopathie nach Thorotrast Injektion vor 10 Jahren). Strahlentherapie, 81:93–102, 1950.
143. Schreiner, L. Uber Thorotrastschäden mit Entstehung eines sarkomatösen Hämangio-endothelioms der Leber. Z. Krebsforsch., 64:169–175, 1961.
144. Schwenzer, A. W., and Federlin, K. Salpingographie mit Thorotrast vor 23 Jahren und Enstehung eines Ovarialkarzinoms. Geburtsh. Frauenheilk., 17:225–236, 1957.
145. Selbie, F. R. Experimental production of sarcoma with Thorotrast. Lancet, 2:847, 1936.
146. ———— Tumors in rats and mice following injection of Thorotrast. Brit. J. Exp. Path., 19:100, 1938.
147. Seynsche, O. Thorotrastschädigung der Niere. Zbl Path., 103:161–162, 1962.
148. Shibata, H. Experimental study on the development of tumors induced by Thorotrast. Nippon Acta Radiol., 16:1336–1347, 1966.
149. Silva da Horta, J. Lebersarkom einer Frau, 3 Jahre und 2 Monate nach Thorotrast-injektion. Chirurg., 24:218–223, 1953.
150. ———— As formas anatomo-clinicas resultantes da acçao do thorotraste. In: Colectanea de Trabalhos Médicos de Discípulos de Pulido Valente, Lisbon, Livraria Luso-Espanhola, 1954, pp. 17–44.
151. ———— Late lesions in man caused by colloidal thorium dioxide (Thorotrast); new case of sarcoma of liver 22 years after injection. Arch. Path., 62:403–418, 1956.
152. ———— Late effects of Thorotrast on the liver and spleen and their efferent lymph nodes. Ann. N.Y. Acad. Sci., 145:676–699, 1967.
153. ———— Effects of colloidal thorium dioxide extravasates in the subcutaneous tissues of the cervical region in man. Ann. N.Y. Acad. Sci., 145:776–785, 1967.
154. ———— and Cayolla da Motta, L. Follow-up study of thorium dioxide patients in Portugal. Ann. N.Y. Acad. Sci., 145:830–842, 1967.
155. Smolinski, E., and Huth, J. H. Akute Abdomen als Folge eines Thorotrastschädens. Arch. Geschwulstforsch., 7:283–290, 1966.
156. Spier, J., Cluff, L. E., and Urry, W. D. Aplastic anemia following administration of Thorotrast. J. Lab. Clin. Med., 32:147, 1947.
157. Sposito, M., and Petroni, V. A. Epatoma insorto dopo 26 anni dalla epatografia con Thorotrast. Epatologia, 7:159, 1961.
158. Stemmermann, G. Adenocarcinoma of the intrahepatic biliary tree following Thorotrast. Amer. J. Clin. Path., 34:446, 1960.
159. Suckow, E., Henegar, G. C., and Baserga, R. Tumors of the liver following administration of Thorotrast. Amer. J. Path., 38:663, 1961.
160. Swarm, R. L. Quoted by Looney, 1960.[100]
161. ———— The neoplasms of the liver following the deposition of thorium dioxide. In: The Dosimetry and Toxicity of Thorotrast. Vienna, I.A.E.A., 1968, pp. 117–120.
162. ———— Conference Chairman: Distribution, Retention and Late Effects of Thorium Dioxide. Ann. N.Y. Acad. Sci., 145:523–858, 1967.
163. ———— Miller, E., and Michelitch, H. J. Malignant vascular tumors in rabbits injected intravenously with colloidal Thorium Dioxide. Path. Microbiol., 25:27–44, 1962.
164. Takahashi, S., Kitabatake, T., Yamagata, S., Miyakawa, T., Masuyama, M., Mori, T., Tanaka, T., Hibino, S., Miyakawa, M., Kaneda, H., Okajima, S., Komiyama, H., Adachi, T., Koga, Y., Hashizume, T., and Hashimoto, Y. Statistical study on Thorotrast-induced cancer of the liver. Tohoku J. Exp. Med., 87:144–154, 1965.
165. Telles, N. C. Follow-up of thorium dioxide patients in the United States. Ann. N.Y. Acad. Sci., 145:674–675, 1967.
166. Tesluk, H., and Nordin, W. A. Hemangioendothelioma of liver following thorium dioxide administration. Arch. Path., 60:493, 1955.
167. Tessmer, C. F., and Chang, J. P. Thorotrast localization by light and electron microscopy. Ann. N.Y. Acad. Sci., 145:545–575, 1967.

168. Thomas, F. S., Henry, G. W., and Kaplan, H. S. Hepatolienography: Past, present and future. Radiology, 57:669, 1951.

169. Ueshima, M. An autopsy case of carcinoma of the bile duct with metastasis to the skin (Japanese). J. Jap. Soc. Intern. Med., 53:1194–1198, 1964.

170. Van Lancker-Delvigne, M. A., and Smoliar, V. Renal lesions produced by Thorotrast. Rev. Belge Path., 31:271–279, 1965.

171. Vellenga, L. R. Een geval van hemangiosarcoom van de lever, 25 jaar na injectic van Thorotrast voor cerebrale angiografie. J. Belge Radiol., 45:682, 1962.

172. Verhaak, R. Nierafwijkingen na pyelographie met Thorotrast. Tilburg, Holland, H. Bergmans, 1958. Quoted by Batzenschlager, Dorner, and Weill-Bousson, 1963.

173. ———— Zu einem Fall von Karzinom in einer Thorotrastleber. Fortschr. Rontgenstr., 101:539–543, 1964.

174. ———— Tumor induction in a Thorotrast kidney. Oncologia, 19:20–32, 1965.

175. ———— The Thorotrast kidney. J. Belg. Radiol., 48:711, 1965. Quoted by Brauman et al., 1966.

176. Verner, J. V., and Smith, A. Hodgkin's disease following administration of Thorotrast. Southern Med. J., 56:524–528, 1963.

177. Vögtlin, J., and Minder, W. Über Thorotrastschäden nach Bronchographie, retrograder Pyelographie, Salpingographie und Arteriographie. Radiol. Clin., 21:96–115, 1952.

178. Wald, A. M. and Richter M. Quoted by Looney et al., 1960.[102]

179. Walko, R., and Fodor, I. Retikuläre Leber, totale Milz und ausgedehnte Mesenterial-drüsenverkalkungen, bei Lebercirrhose. Fortschr. Rontgenstr., 99:712–716, 1963.

180. Wegener, K., and Zahnert, R. Bericht über pathologisch-anatomische und quantitative Untersuchungen an 9 Fallen menschlicher Thorotrastose. Virchows Arch. (Path. Anat.), 351:316–332, 1970.

181. Wenz, W. Thorotrasttumoren nach intraoperativer Cholangiographie. Ein Beitrag zur diagnostischen Bedeutung der Zöliakographie beim Gallengangskarzinom. Fortschr. Roentgenstr., 102:570–575, 1965.

182. ———— and Ott, G. Aktuelle Thorotrastprobleme: Ein Lebersarkom mit intraperito-nealer Blutung. Strahlentherapie., 127:464–469, 1965.

183. Wertheman, A. Über Spätschäden verschiedener Organe durch Thorotrast und auto-radiographisher Nachweis desselben. Path. Microbiol., 22:350–362, 1959.

184. Weyeneth, R. Spätschäden nach Pyelographie mit Thorotrast. Z. Urol., 9:513–542, 1958.

185. Wiedemann, O. Manufacture of Thorotrast. In The Dosimetry and Toxicity of Thoro-trast. Vienna, I.A.E.A., 1968, pp. 1–4.

186. Wuketich, S., and Mark, T. Doppelcarcinom nach Thorotrast-Arteriographie. Z. Krebsforsch., 62:95–108, 1957.

187. Zastrow, R., and Roloff, W. Late effects of Thorotrast. Clinical studies. Z. Ges. Inn. Med., 20:365–374, 1965.

188. Zak et al., 1956. Quoted by Kohoutek and Novak, 1960.[91]

189. Zeitlhofer, J., and Speiser, P. Hämangioendotheliomatose beim Kaninchen nach ex-perimenteller Thorotrast-verabreichung. Z. Krebsforsch., 60:161–168, 1954.

190. Zollinger, H. U. Ein Spindelzellsarkom der Niere, 16 Jahre nach Thorotrast Pyelogra-phie. Schweiz. Med. Wschr., 52:1266–1268, 1949.

191. Hundeiker, M., Berger, H., and Petres, J. Mycosis fungoides nach Thorotrastanwen-dung mit Entwicklung zur Reticulumzellsarkomatose. Arch. Klin. Exp. Derm., 232:56–65, 1968.

192. Ikeda, M. Experimental studies on sarcoma formation with thorium dioxide sol (thoro-trast). Fukuota Acta Med., 52:481–493, 1961.

193. Kharlampovich, S. I., Podsosov, S. P., and Svinogeeva, T. P. The transplantable rat sarcoma T-1 induced by thorium dioxide sol. Vop. Onkol., 14:98, 1968.

194. Kyle, R. H., Oler, A., Lasser, E. C., and Rosomoff, H. I. Meningioma induced by thorium dioxide. New Engl. J. Med., 268:80–82, 1963.

195. Matzen, P., and Giuliani, K. Peteosthor und Tumorgenese. Zbl. Chir., 87:881–886, 1962.

196. Mignot, J., Barge, J., and Lozac'Hmeur, M. T. Les tumeurs provoquées par le thoro-trast. Apropos d'un sarcome à localisations multiples. Arch. Anat. Path., 16:294–304, 1969.
197. Mori, T., Sakai, T., Nozue, Y., Okamoto, T., Tanaka, T., and Tsuya, A. Malignancy and other injuries following Thorotrast administration: follow-up study of 147 cases in Japan. Strahlentherapie, 134:229–254, 1967.
198. Perkins, H. T., Verner, J. V., Yoneyama, T., and Estes, E. H. Unusual clinico-pathologi-cal syndromes with Kaposi's visceral and related sarcomata. Report of three cases, one associated with thorium dioxide administration. A.M.A. Arch. Int. Med., 105: 733–744, 1960.
199. Simmons, D. J., Cummins, H., and Nirdlinger, E. Observations on the deposition of thorotrast in rat tissues. Amer. J. Roentgen., 103:902–918, 1968.

Addendum

Since 1971, studies on biologic effects of Thorotrast have been pursued, both in man and in experimental animals; the proceedings of a meeting held in 1973 at the Finsen Institute [1] contain much of these recent contributions. Liver tumors, both carcinoma (hepatocellular and cholangiocarcinomas) and sarcoma (heman-gioendotheliomas) type, have been reported in Syrian hamsters [2] and rats,[3] the latter species associated with lung tumors.[4]

Patients injected with Thorotrast are currently under intensive investigation in countries where its use has been widespread, namely West Germany,[5–7] Portugal,[8–10] Denmark,[11] England,[12, 13] Japan,[2] and the United States.[14] A total of about 5,000 patients have been traced and autopsy records of many of the deceased are available, while living patients are under periodic medical and labor-atory examinations, including liver function tests. The data from the different series show the liver to be the most damaged organ. In fact, the liver is a fre-quent seat of cirrhosis (6.6 percent of cases versus 2.7 percent in a control group).[5] It is of interest that the number of cases appear to be increasing with time, as this could support the possibility of a dependency of the cirrhosis on Thoro-trast.[11]

Even more striking is the number of malignant liver tumors, which are steadily increasing as time passes. Out of a total of 456 malignant tumors discovered in Thorotrast patients (including leukemias and other fatal blood disorders) 249 (54.6 percent) proved to be malignant liver tumors. Concerning the histologic type, among 129 histologically confirmed cases, 49 (30.21 percent) were heman-gioendotheliomas and the remaining were hepatocellular and cholangiocarcino-mas. The relevance of these figures stands out if compared with autopsy series from general hospitals. In the latter, primary liver tumors account for about 4 percent of all malignant tumors,[15] and the incidence of hemangioendotheliomas, among primary liver tumors, is exceedingly low (0.2 percent).[16]

The carcinogenic effect of Thorotrast on malignant liver tumors, and on hemangioendotheliomas in particular, is, therefore, unquestionable. Radiation certainly remains the most important factor in the mechanism of this effect.

The latency period and the rate of appearance are practically the same in different series, with reported mean values of 22 to 26 years. Hemangioendotheliomas develop after a latency period of at least 15 years.[11]

A number of investigations on the role of nonradioactive properties of Thorotrast [17] led to controversial results: in fact, tumor induction with nonradioactive components of Thorotrast, like dextrine, or with nonradioactive substances physically comparable to Thorotrast, like Zirconotrast, either failed or was not confirmed by other experiments. No liver tumor has been obtained with injection of chemically inert substances like India ink.[3] On the other hand, the importance of radiation is further supported by the observation that using ^{230}Th enriched Thorotrast (with an alpha activity from 7 to 49 times that of commercial Thorotrast), hemangioendotheliomas appear in rabbits at shorter intervals than in animals injected with commercial Thorotrast.[18]

The amount of Thorotrast deposited in the different organs is difficult to assess, due to the process of its redistribution. According to Kaul [19] the liver would account, in a "standard Thorotrast patient," for 59 percent of the injected quantity.

It is well known that patients who receive Thorotrast in high doses develop liver tumors more frequently than patients injected with low doses,[20] but the calculation of the radiation doses delivered to the liver is a problem of great complexity. The large number of radionuclides involved in the ^{232}Th decay series, their inhomogeneous distribution in several different physical phases, and the self-absorption of radiations in Thorotrast aggregates, which reduces the tissue doses by a factor in the range of 0.65,[19] are among the most important items to be considered. However, "best estimates" for dose-rate calculations in patients with long-term Thorotrast burdens have been published; for the liver, after injection of 40 ml of Thorotrast and an exposure time of 30 years, an average dose of 930 rads may be assumed.[6]

Further follow-up studies of Thorotrast patients (some patients are now living 40 years after the administration) are important for gathering optimal and useful radiobiologic data. This painstaking effort is well deserved, as Thorotrast patients represent a unique and irreplaceable potential source of information on the long-term effects of chronic radiations in man.

References

1. Faber M (ed): Proceedings of the Third International Meeting on the Toxicity of Thorotrast, Finsen Institute, Copenhagen, April 1973. Danish Atomic Energy Commission—Riso Report No. 294, Copenhagen, 1973
2. Mori T, Okamoto T, Umeda M, et al: Thorotrast-induced spindle cell sarcoma and hepatic cholangiocarcinoma in Syrian hamsters. In Faber M (note 1), pp 267–80
3. Grampa G, Di Ferrante ER, Marzo A, Sardini D: Liver tumors induced by Thorotrast in rats: morphological, alpha spectrometric, and biochemical correlations. (Abstract)—10th International Cancer Congress, Houston, 1970
4. Grampa G: Lung tumors in rats after Thorium-dioxide administration. 5th International Congress Radiation Research, Seattle, July 1974

5. Van Kaick G, Scheer KE: Actual status of the German Thorotrast study. In Faber M (note 1), pp 157–62
6. Van Kaick G, Muth H, Lorenz D, Kaul A: Malignancies in German Thorotrast patients and estimated tissue dose. Meeting on Biological Effects of Injected ^{224}Ra (ThX) and Thorotrast, July 1974
7. Wesch H, Kampmann H, Wegener K: Assessment of organ distribution of Thorium by neutron-activation-analysis. In Faber M (note 1), pp 52–60
8. Da Silva Horta J, Cayolla L, Tavares MH: Epidemiological follow-up studies of the Portuguese Thorotrast series (up-dated results). In Faber M (note 1), pp 193–211
9. Da Silva Horta J, Cristina ML, Baptista AS: Liver ultrastructural findings in patients injected with Thorotrast. In Faber M (note 1), pp 219–32
10. Da Silva Horta J: Tumours developed in people injected with Thorium dioxide (Thorotrast) (Portuguese experience). In Faber M (note 1), pp 233–47
11. Faber M: Follow-up of Danish Thorotrast cases. In Faber M (note 1), pp 137–47
12. Boyd JT, Langlands AO, Maccabe JJ: Long-term hazards of Thorotrast. Br Med J 2:517, 1968
13. Buckton KE, Langlands AO: The Edinburgh Thorotrast series. Report of a cytogenetic study. In Faber M (note 1), pp 114–25
14. Janower ML, Miettinem OS, Flynn MJ: Effects of long-term Thorotrast exposure. Radiology 103:13, 1972
15. Giordano A, Grampa G, Riviera L: Modificazione della frequenza dei tumori maligni al tavolo anatomico: rilievi comparativi tra i quinquenni 1926–1930 e 1956–1960. Simposio sulla Statistica nelle Ricerche sui Tumori, Roma, October 1963. Ann Stat Series VIII, 14:719, 1964
16. Mori R, Nozue Y, Miyazi T, Takahashi S: Thorotrast injury in Japan. In Faber M (note 1), pp 175–92
17. Riedel W, Muller B, Kaul A: Non-radiation effects of Thorotrast and other colloidal substances. In Faber M (note 1), pp 281–93
18. Faber M: The effect of Thorotrast enriched with Th^{230}. In Faber M (note 1), pp 294–302
19. Kaul A: Mean organ dose rates in man following intravascular injection of Thorotrast. In Faber M (note 1), pp 40–51
20. Faber M: Dose effect relations in hepatic carcinogenesis. In Faber M (note 1), pp 308–16

PRIMARY CARCINOMA OF THE LIVER AS A PATHOLOGIST'S PROBLEM*

JOHN HIGGINSON

DONALD J. SVOBODA

An understanding of the biology of primary carcinoma of the liver is of interest to the pathologist for several reasons. First, the frequency in man of this carcinoma shows marked geographic variations which are almost certainly of environmental origin. Second, since experimental hepatic tumors can be induced easily and tend to be relatively homogeneous, they lend themselves readily to comparative studies from both morphologic and biochemical viewpoints. Thus, failure to gain meaningful information from such comparative investigations could cast considerable doubt on the possible value of animal experimentation in identifying etiologic and environmental factors in man. Third, the production of experimental hepatomas is frequently regarded as an important index of the oncogenic potential of new chemical substances, whether synthetic or natural, not only for the liver but also for other organs. The correct evaluation of substances of potential carcinogenic significance, such as aflatoxin, is of significance from both health and socioeconomic viewpoints.

Although there have been several recent reviews on primary liver cancer,[4, 10, 64] we believe it is useful to reconsider the subject with a view toward integrating laboratory investigations and field studies with respect to the most pertinent trends in both areas of endeavour.

The present paper is largely confined to analyzing the problem of liver carcinoma based on recent studies in experimental and human hepatocarcinogenesis, with special reference to morphogenic pathways. Accordingly, no attempt will be made to cover the vast literature on the biochemical aspects of the problem except where pertinent to the discussion. This does not imply that the authors are unaware that meaningful cancer prevention will require a full understanding of the mechanisms

---

* The following abbreviations are used in this paper: FAA, acetylaminofluorene; DEN, diethylnitrosamine; DMN, dimethylnitrosamine; DNA, deoxyribose nucleic acid; ER, endoplasmic reticulum; DAB, dimethylaminoazobenzene; CCl₄, carbon tetrachloride; MCA, 20-methylcholanthrene; DAST, 4-dimethyl-aminostilbene.

of action of individual carcinogens, but rather that they recognize a *de facto* situation in which critical analysis of the overall biologic picture in man and animals may give leads to possible causative factors. Emphasis is placed on experimental observations, since these may suggest related approaches in the study of human liver cancer. There has often been a surprising failure to correlate between experimental and field studies, especially in areas where liver cancer is common, although changes in the human liver can be studied readily by biopsy.

Human Liver Carcinoma

Geographical Pathology

Recent epidemiologic studies have been directed largely to systematizing earlier work. During the last decade there has been a considerable increase in the availability of accurate morbidity data on hepatic cancer, which is partly summarized in Figure 1. Liver cancer is uncommon in North America, Western Europe, the USSR, and Australia, where no significant sex or racial differences are noted. With a few exceptions, liver cancer appears to be rare in Central and South America and in the Caribbean area. Most areas of Africa and parts of South East Asia, however, show a high frequency, especially in males. There is little evidence that there is a true increase of liver cancer in Japan or in the Indian subcontinent, with the possible exception of Kerala.[16, 28, 86] The highest incidence is in Bantu males in Mozambique where, in the younger age-groups, the rate is approximately 500 times that of the United States. In the older age-group, the rate is closer to that observed in North America. It is considered unlikely that this levelling off of incidence in Southern Africa is a cohort effect.

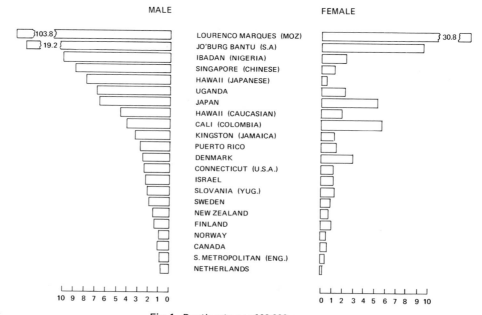

Fig. 1. Death rate per 100,000 per year.

Histopathologic Aspects

The classification and pathologic characteristics of liver cancer have been adequately covered elsewhere.[4, 10, 18, 30, 64, 92] In brief, carcinomas are broadly classified as hepatocellular (liver cell type, Fig. 2) or cholangiocellular (bile duct type), and occasionally mixtures of the two. Hepatocellular carcinomas show a wide range of morphologic patterns[18] usually described as trabecular, atypical or anaplastic, and acinar.[29] The last have sometimes been misclassified as cholangiocellular tumors (Fig. 4). Bile production is regarded as pathognomonic for liver cell carcinoma. In the neoplastic cells, the glycogen content tends to be low, and cytoplasmic hyaline occlusions may be found.[65]

The increase in liver cancer in Africa and Asia is due essentially to an increase in hepatocellular tumors.[28] Steiner,[91] moreover, found no essential morphologic difference between tumors in areas of high (Africa) and low incidence (United States). It would thus appear justifiable to regard the two cell types as representing distinct biologic entities in man. In South East Asia, however, an unusual adenocarcinoma sometimes associated with hepatocellular carcinoma may be found with parasitic infestation[33] (Fig. 3).

The rare embryonal carcinoma (hepatoblastoma) of children may be only epithelial or it may also contain mesenchymal elements. The epithelial element is composed for the most part of embryonal liver cells or better differentiated fetal liver cells.[35] No geographic variations are shown but it has been described in association with various congenital anomalies.[22]

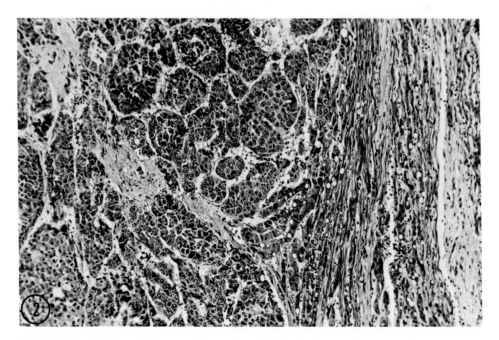

Fig. 2. Typical hepatocellular carcinoma in African Bantu showing trabecular pattern of relatively normal looking liver cells. H&E. X120; reduced 15%.

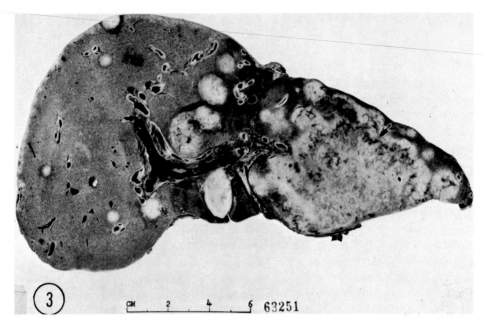

Fig. 3. Primary adenocarcinoma arising in the liver in association with **Clonorchis sinensis** in a Chinese patient from Hong Kong. (Courtesy of Prof. J. B. Gibson.)

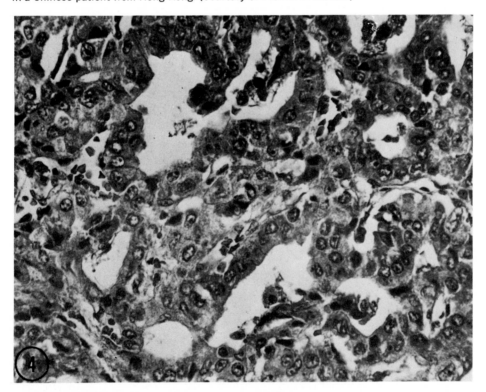

Fig. 4. Primary hepatocellular carcinoma in a 52-year-old white male. Much of the tumor consists of acini lined by elongated cells (adenohepatoma). H&E. X290.

Liver Cancer in Animals

Most spontaneous and induced liver tumors have been described in many animal species. It is of course not possible to determine in many cases whether so-called "spontaneous" tumors merely represent a situation in which the inducing agent has not yet been identified. Further, many animals in earlier studies were fed on stock diets, possibly contaminated with aflatoxin, organic long-acting pesticides, or other possible hepatocarcinogens.

Domestic and Nonlaboratory Animals

While spontaneous primary liver carcinoma has been reported in many species, including cattle, fish, and birds, the overall incidence would appear to be relatively low, and geographic variations correlating with those seen in man in the same regions have not been reported.[13] The relatively low frequency reported among domestic animals in countries of high incidence of human cancer may be of some importance as negative evidence when considering the possible role of naturally occurring carcinogens in man, such as the senecio alkaloids, to which it would be anticipated that both animals and man would be exposed.[9]

Laboratory Animals

Spontaneous liver cell tumors occur in mice, rats, and hamsters[108] but appear rare in higher species. In rodents the frequency of spontaneous tumors shows a considerable genetic influence.[108]

Experimental Tumors

Carcinoma of the liver has been produced by several agents which show significant variation in hepatocarcinogenic potentiality in different strains. While the majority of studies have been done in mice and rats,[108] tumors have also been produced in hamsters,[103] guinea pigs,[14] fish,[2, 36, 89] dogs, mastomys, ducks,[11] and nonhuman primates.[38]

Histopathology

The histopathology of experimental tumors has been extensively discussed.[92] In general, most carcinogens cause hepatocellular tumors, but some also produce adenocarcinomas. Cytologically and histologically, hepatocellular carcinomas in man show close similarities to those induced in experimental animals (Figs. 4 and 5). In contrast, cholangiocarcinomas in man tend to arise in noncirrhotic livers, while with certain carcinogens, notably the azo dyes, in rats such tumors tend to arise in association with foci of cholangiofibrosis, a lesion very rare in man.

Different chemical carcinogens tend to produce tumors of various histologic patterns ranging from well-differentiated hepatomas seen with aflatoxin to the anaplastic and mixed patterns with 3′-Me-DAB.[92] Chemically induced tumors produced by a carcinogen in the liver of a single animal show both chromosomal[66] and immunologic individuality.[39, 73] Experimental hepatoblastomas appear to be very rare.

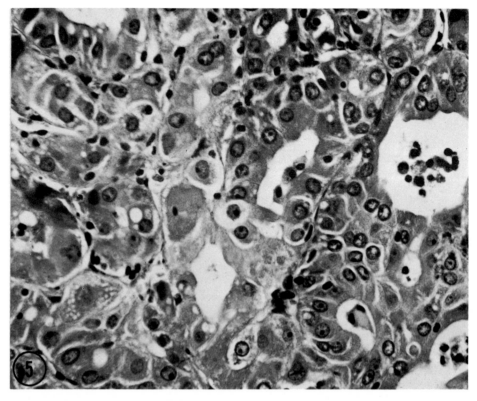

Fig. 5. Primary hepatocellular carcinoma induced in the liver of a male rat by feeding 1 ppm of aflatoxin B_1 in the diet for 33 weeks. Like the human hepatoma in Figure 4, this tumor, in some areas, is composed of acinar structures. H&E. X290.

Pathogenesis of Primary Liver Carcinoma

Cirrhosis

MAN. In man, a high proportion of liver cell carcinomas arise in cirrhotic livers. Nodular hyperplasia with cirrhosis alone, however, is not a sufficient stimulus for neoplasia. In general, the proportion of cirrhotic livers showing malignant change tends to correlate with the frequency of the disease, especially in the younger age groups.[28] Unfortunately, due to semantic variations in classification, it is unknown whether carcinoma arises with equal frequency in the same morphologic type of cirrhosis in countries of high and low incidence, much less whether such cirrhoses have similar etiologic backgrounds. The latter hypothesis would appear unlikely because liver cell carcinoma definitely appears in some cirrhotic livers due to excess alcohol ingestion in North America and Europe,[43, 68] whereas ethanol is certainly not an etiologic factor in West and Southern Africa, and Asia. General experience would indicate that carcinoma arises most frequently in livers with large macro-nodules and a fine fibrosis in contrast to livers with small nodules and coarser fibrosis (Table 1).[56, 100] Our experience in Kansas was similar. The table indicates that

Table 1. Relation of Liver Carcinoma to Type of Cirrhosis

NODULE* TYPE	FIBROSIS†		
	Fine	Intermediate	Broad
Micro	$\frac{3‡}{22}$	$\frac{2}{19}$	$\frac{0}{8}$
Mixed	$\frac{4}{7}$	$\frac{1}{6}$	$\frac{0}{0}$
Macro	$\frac{19}{37}$	$\frac{3}{15}$	$\frac{0}{7}$

* *Nodule type: Micro* = liver in which the majority of the nodules are small, i.e., with one or less portal triad. *Macro* = liver in which the majority of the nodules contain two or more portal triads. *Mixed* = liver between the above degrees.
† *Fibrosis: Fine* = narrow fibrous bands, usually less than 0.2 cm wide. *Broad* = many bands more than 0.5 cm wide. *Intermediate* = liver between the above degrees.
‡ *Numerator* = carcinoma; *denominator* = total livers.
The livers indicated in this Table were from areas of both high and low incidence.

the high proportion of cirrhotic livers which are reported to show malignant change in Africa may in fact only indicate that the types of cirrhosis in both areas are different and that livers with fine fibrosis and large nodules undergo malignant change with equal frequency. This observation was also confirmed by the international liver group, of which one of the authors was secretary, which compared the pathology of cirrhosis in several geographical areas (unpublished).

It is possible that the combination of two parameters is only an indication of the regenerative capacity of the liver, large nodular regeneration leading to narrowing of the fibrous tissues. It has been reported that the proportion of cirrhotic livers showing neoplastic change is increasing in Western countries,[46, 68, 93] possibly due to an increased life expectancy associated with improved treatment. In Africa, cirrhosis and carcinoma appear to occur simultaneously, the cancer being observed in an advanced stage at the time of the first admission to hospital, in contrast to North America where a long history of cirrhosis may sometimes precede the onset of neoplasia. It would thus appear desirable to determine whether this difference in presentation is indicative of variations in the malignant potential of hyperplastic nodules in cirrhotic lesions in various parts of the world.

The use of the term "postnecrotic" referring to postviral hepatitis is no longer acceptable, since a similar morphologic picture may occur in livers due to either alcoholic indulgence or to diffuse indolent viral hepatitis. Moreover, the term "postnecrotic" suggests, inaccurately, a distinct type of cirrhosis while, from the point of view of ultimate pathogenesis, all types of cirrhosis follow necrosis—the gross and histologic features being dependent only upon the pattern and extent of the antecedent necrosis. The fact that in most neoplastic cases the fibrosis remains fine would suggest that in these the nodules are in a more active form. In contrast, bile-duct carcinomas arise relatively infrequently in cirrhotic livers.

EXPERIMENTAL ANIMALS. While spontaneous hepatocellular carcinomas in animals do not appear associated with cirrhosis, tumors induced with many chemical carcinogens are associated with cirrhosis and resemble histologically the situation seen in man. This fact may have etiologic implications in differentiating between "spontaneous" and induced tumors in each species.

However, experimental hepatocellular carcinomas produced by certain agents (e.g., aflatoxin), can arise in noncirrhotic livers. Such tumors can be related to small areas of cellular change which are of a clear cell nature (e.g., aflatoxin) or hyperbasophilic (e.g., DAB),[37, 63, 94, 96] and the coexistence of cirrhosis is to a large extent a dose response.

Cholangiocellular tumors are less frequently associated with cirrhosis. Their origin would appear to be from the intrahepatic bile ducts corresponding to cholangiofibrotic tumors following DAB.

The diagnosis of liver cell neoplasms in experimental animals, especially those of a spontaneous nature among mice, may provide diagnostic problems in association with large-scale carcinogen testing. The pathologist constantly carrying out such studies should familiarize himself with the nature of the nodules in each species, their histology, biology, and transplantability, etc., since some well-differentiated nodules may transplant although otherwise appearing benign. Thus, their differentiation from hyperplastic nodules may prove very difficult, since biologic behavior does not necessarily correlate with the histologic appearances.

Significance of the Hyperplastic Nodule

It is clear that cirrhosis *per se* is not necessarily precancerous but rather that the hyperplastic nodule plays a primary role.

There is now evidence that the hyperplastic nodule is the site of eventual malignant transformation in the experimental animal. A similar sequence may be suggested by the appearance of many nodules in human cirrhosis. This sequence has been carefully studied by Reuber[77] in rats where the change from hyperplastic non-transplantable nodules to carcinoma with increasing ease of transplantability has been followed carefully. Transplantability also appeared directly related to the degree of differentiation of the cells comprising the nodules.

In experimental cirrhosis in mice, whereas fibrosis and bile-duct proliferation are reversible lesions, some nodules continue to progress after removal of the hepatocarcinogen. It is in these that carcinomas arise.[75] In contrast, cirrhosis in man is essentially irreversible. Thus, an understanding of the nature of the process of the hyperplastic nodule will be essential to determine the nature of hepatocarcinogenesis.

To date, it has not been possible to determine meaningful biochemical differences between normal liver, hyperplastic nodules, and early carcinoma. That the basic metabolism is deranged is obvious,[52] but the relevant abnormalities have not been determined. For example, extensive analyses of the biochemical changes in hyperplastic nodules induced by FAA showed that either the glycogen or its response to metabolic controls differs from that of the surrounding liver.[20] Epstein and co-workers[19] reported persistent binding of metabolites of 2-fluorenylacetamide to glycogen and to DNA in hyperplastic nodules and to glycogen in liver cancer cells, in contrast to surrounding liver. Since the carcinogen or derivative was present originally in liver cells, this suggested that there was a direct lineage from liver cells to cancer via the hyperplastic nodules. However, it is of interest to note that in mice and hamsters, the hyperplastic nodule produced by carbon tetrachloride frequently undergoes neoplastic change, whereas similar nodules in rats do not.[27, 88]

Ultrastructural Studies

The use of ultrastructural techniques to investigate cellular changes involved in hepatocarcinogenesis is now common among many experimental pathologists. To provide a baseline for future studies in humans, an extensive ultrastructural investigation on the hepatic parenchymal cell was carried out to determine whether individual carcinogens of different chemical structure produced similar or specific ultrastructural alterations.[96, 99] It was further intended that such a study might distinguish irreversible cellular responses essential to neoplasia from epiphenomena and also provide a morphologic basis for known biochemical changes. The responses of liver cells were studied in acute and chronic conditions and following reversal. The carcinogens included aflatoxin B_1, DEN, DMN, ethionine, lasiocarpine, 3'-Me-DAB, tannic acid and thioacetamide.

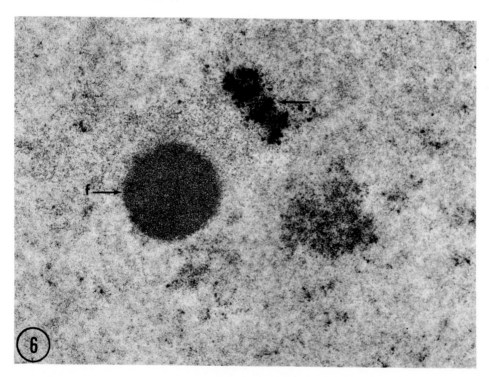

Fig. 6. Nucleolus of rat liver cell 12 hours after a single dose of aflatoxin B_1 (0.2 mg/kg, i. p.). The fibrillar component of the nucleolus is present as a circular condensation (f). The granular portion of the nucleolus is markedly reduced, although dense granular aggregates (resembling nucleolar granules) are present at the unmarked arrow. This pattern of complete separation of fibrillar and granular elements has been termed "macrosegregation" and typically occurs during acute stages (up to 72 hours) after administration of aflatoxin, 3'-Me-DAB, lasiocarpine, and tannic acid. X20,000.

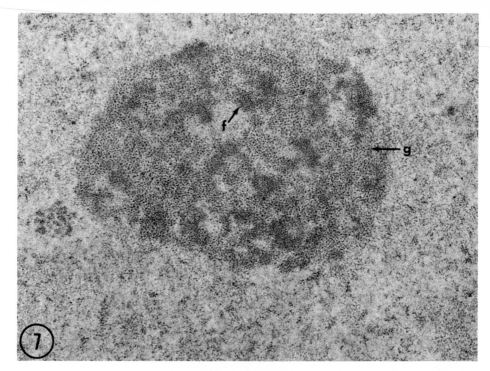

Fig. 7. In chronic stages of aflatoxin B_1 carcinogenesis, few liver cell nucleoli show partial separation of fibrillar and granular elements, while in most the fibrillar (f) and granular (g) components remain intimately mixed. X20,000.

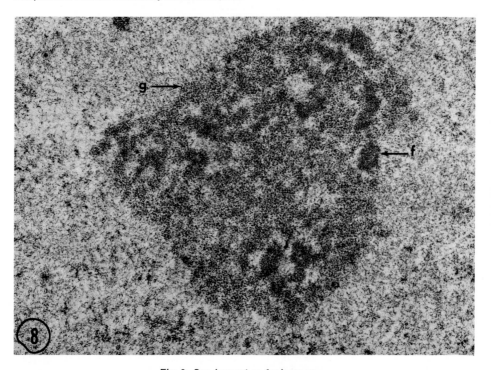

Fig. 8. See legend on facing page.

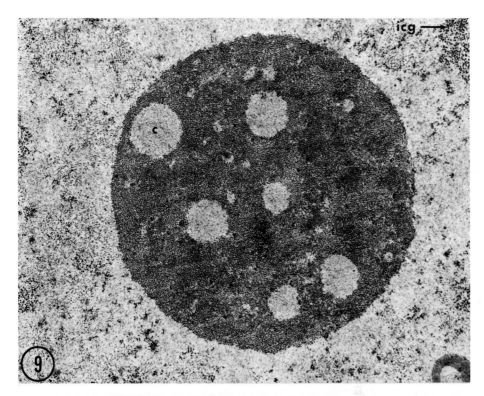

Fig. 9. Nucleolus of rat liver cell after 24 weeks of administration of thioacetamide (0.032 percent in the diet). There is marked enlargement of the nucleolus due principally to an increase in the granular component. Several cavities (c) are also present in the nucleolus, while in the nucleoplasm there is an increase in the number of interchromatin granules (icg). X14,000.

The observations indicated no correlation between acute and chronic liver damage and later tumor development. With the exception of DEN, all agents produced nuclear and nucleolar abnormalities in both acute and chronic stages (Figs. 6 to 9). Rearrangement and segregation of the nucleolar constituents with consequent decrease in RNA synthesis are generally regarded as indicative of DNA binding, but the full significance of the varied and individual patterns of nucleolar responses remains to be elucidated. In chronic phases, typical "macrosegregation" was not seen although "microsegregation" did persist, especially with DEN, and to a lesser extent with aflatoxin B_1 and 3'-Me-DAB. A wide variety of cytoplasmic changes involving endoplasmic reticulum, glycogen, and mitochondria was also observed. These lesions were highly variable and differed in degree from carcinogen to carcinogen. With the exception of hyperplasia of the smooth endoplasmic reticulum and some increase in

Fig. 8. In acute thioacetamide poisoning (60 mg/kg, 24 hours prior to sacrifice), there is partial separation of the fibrillar (f) and granular (g) elements of the nucleolus. The fibrils are present in small condensations; there is a moderate increase in the granules. This incomplete separation of the granular and fibrillar constituents has been termed "microsegregation" and is a characteristic alteration in the acute stages after administration of thioacetamide, dimethylnitrosamine, ethionine, and, to a lesser extent, lasiocarpine. X28,000.

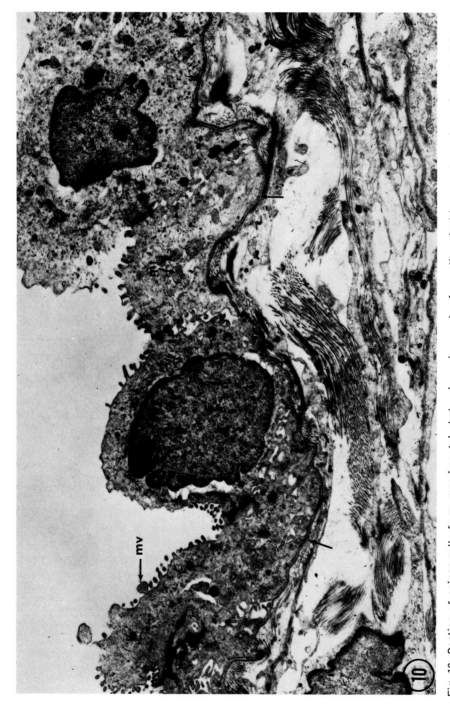

Fig. 10. Section of acinar cells from experimental cholangiocarcinoma showing well-marked basement membrane (arrows), which is not seen in hepatocellular carcinoma. Microvilli (mv) and mitochondria (mt) are identified.

free ribosomes, no changes persisted after withdrawal of the carcinogen. The theoretical consequences of these changes, placing the basic defect in the ergastoplasm ("membron") have been discussed by Pitot.[69, 70]

TUMORS.   No carcinogen produced tumors with ultrastructural features sufficiently characteristic to distinguish them from those produced by other carcinogens, but their origin from liver cells was clearly apparent. In general, mitochondria tended to be fewer and smaller than in normal cells, while profiles of granular endoplasmic reticulum were few, short, and often dilated. In broad terms, the tumor cells bore a superficial resemblance to those of embryonic liver. In the tumors, nucleolar enlargement persisted with thioacetamide and 3'-Me-DAB, while dense plaques in the nucleoli were present with aflatoxin. Reports on the ultrastructure of experimental cholangiocarcinoma are rare, but the derivation of these tumors from bile duct cells, rather than from hepatic parenchymal cells, is clear (Fig. 10).

MAN.   Unfortunately, the number of human tumors and precancerous cirrhoses which have been investigated with the electron microscope is limited and generalizations are not possible.[24, 80, 102]

In Africa the most extensive studies on human hepatocellular carcinoma and its preceding cirrhosis have been made by Theron[101] to whom we are indebted for the following description and Figures 11 to 14:

The nuclei show pronounced variation in size and shape with prominent nucleoli and invaginations of the cytoplasm into the nucleus. Some of the enlarged nucleoli show evidence of microsegregation not unlike the picture observed in experimental thioacetamide poisoning. Others show segregation into elongated linear dense clumps apparently composed of both fibrillar and granular elements giving the appearance of "Chinese characters." There is frequent communication in the space between the inner and outer nuclear membranes and dilated ER cisternae, the latter sometimes showing large electron dense material. Similar appearances have been seen in protein deficiency in rats. [97] The mitochondria show a variety of lesions, including swelling and loss of cristae. There are also alterations in the ER with detachment of the ribosomes. In precancerous cirrhosis nucleolar enlargement is also present. The cytoplasm tends to show crowding of the mitochondria and swelling of ER.

Misugi and co-workers[54] have shown that the liver cells in hepatoblastoma have few organelles and are unlike neoplastic and nonneoplastic parenchymal cells in the adult liver.

There is a paucity of data on the changes in acute toxic hepatic necrosis in man in different geographical regions. A study of the nuclei would appear useful in determining the type of agent which might be involved. No reports on the ultrastructure of human cholangiocarcinomas are available.

Factors Influencing Hepatocarcinogenesis

Effect of Age

The plateau curve in Africa in areas of high cancer frequency suggests the possibility that the carcinogenic stimulus is more intense in early life. While studies in young animals show an increased susceptibility to carcinogens under certain circum-

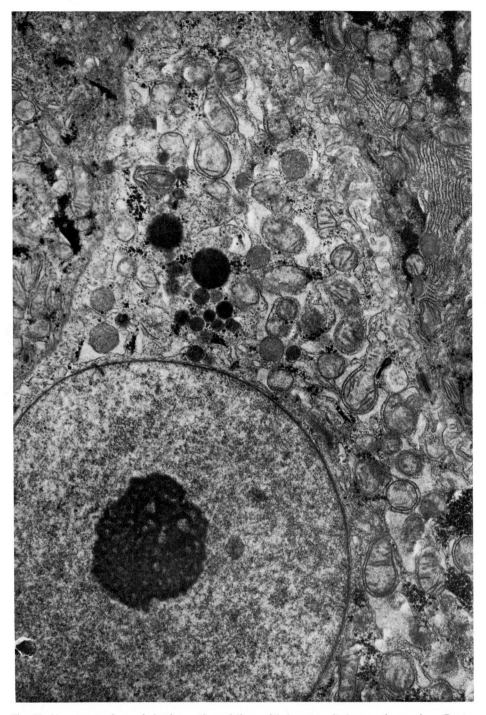

Fig. 11. Hepatocyte from cirrhotic portion of liver with hepatocellular carcinoma in a Bantu patient. Note mitochondrial alterations and enlargement of the nucleolus. (Courtesy of Dr. J. J. Theron.) X16,000; reduced 25%.

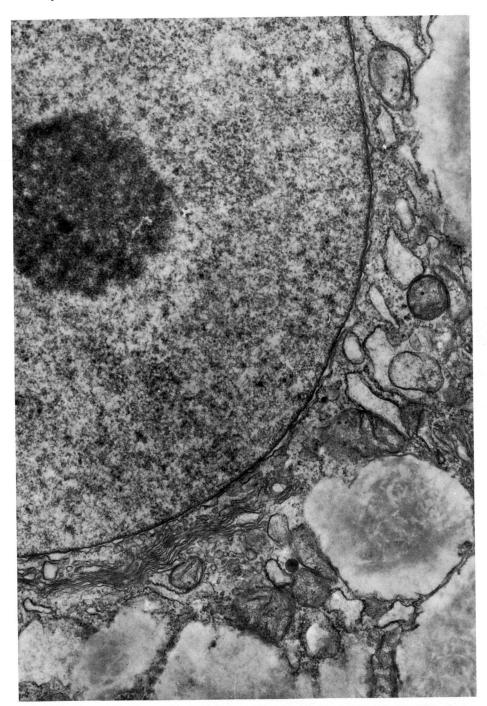

Fig. 12. Slight nucleolar enlargement in tumor cell in hepatoma from a Bantu patient showing marked vacuolation of the cytoplasm. Note also disorganization of the cytoplasmic organelles, including dilation of the ER system. (Courtesy of Dr. J. J. Theron.) X29,000; reduced 25%.

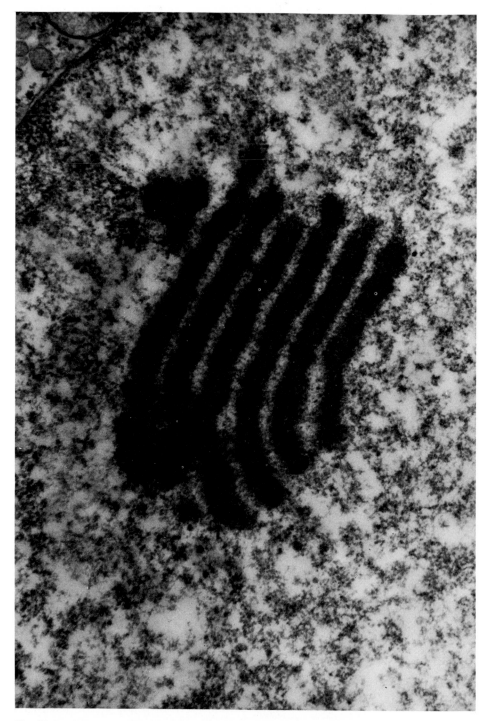

Fig. 13. Marked nucleolar abnormality with segregation in hepatocellular carcinoma from a Bantu patient. (Courtesy of Dr. J. J. Theron.) X90,000; reduced 25%.

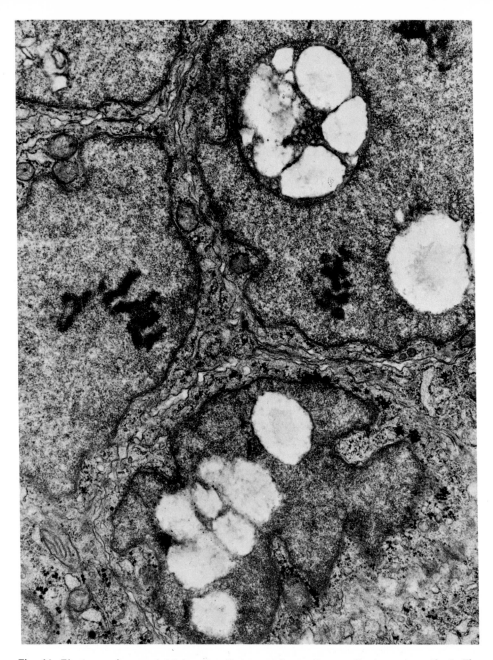

Fig. 14. Electron micrograph of hepatocellular carcinoma from a Bantu male patient. The tumor cells are clearly of liver cell origin, and the wide range of ultrastructural changes is apparent. The nuclei show variations in shape with prominent cytoplasmic invagination. There is significant segregation of the nucleoli which have a "Chinese character" appearance (see text). The general pattern would indicate that in man the nucleolar changes produced by the unknown carcinogenic stimulus persist in the tumor. They are of little value in indicating the etiologic agent concerned, being essentially nonspecific. The appearances are not inconsistent, however, with a stimulus of the aflatoxin type. (Courtesy of Dr. J. J. Theron.) X24,000; reduced 25%.

375

stances,[104] no such susceptibility has yet been demonstrated in man. Doll[15] has rather tended to equate aging with increased susceptibility. However, it should be noted that human studies refer not to the neonatal period but rather to youth and young adult life. The demonstration of aflatoxin M in mothers' milk may be of particular importance in this context. Shanmugaratnam[87] has shown evidence indicating that the causal stimulus for liver cancer may be more potent in young than in older Chinese. However, more recent studies by this author have indicated that this difference may not be so great as originally believed.[87a]

Genetic Factors

In contrast to experimental animals, there is no evidence of a racial susceptibility in man. However, a case has been reported of well-differentiated hepatomas occurring in three siblings, suggesting a genetic factor. Hepatoblastomas have also shown a relationship to congenital defects.[22] If the studies by Blumberg and associates[6] on the Australia antigen can be extrapolated to other lesions, indirect variations in susceptibility to liver cancer could occur which might not be easily identified.

Sex

In man, males are more frequently affected. Furthermore, most experimental studies have indicated susceptibility among males. Goodall[26] has shown that severe manipulation of the hormonal milieu, notably the sex, pituitary, and thyroid hormones, may have significant effects, but not all carcinogens react in the same way. These studies, which require the employment of extensive hormonal modifications of the host, would seem most unlikely to explain geographic differences. They cannot be applied uncritically to a healthy man in Africa in whom hormonal changes of such a degree are rare. Cirrhosis of the liver itself may lead to some degree of hyperestrogenism.

Dietary Deficiency

Historically, the role of nutrition in hepatocarcinogenesis received a great deal of emphasis following the demonstration of the importance of riboflavin deficiency in DAB hepatocarcinogenesis.[53] This, however, was a specific case related to detoxification of the carcinogen and has little relevance to other carcinogens or to man. Later, choline and protein deficiencies were found also to modify the action of DAB. Since they are both associated with fatty liver, it was assumed that kwashiorkor, a protein deficiency disease in Africa, was the basis of liver cirrhosis and carcinoma in that region. This is a concept still perpetuated in student pathology text books. However, follow-up of kwashiorkor patients has shown no significant sequelae.[12, 28]

Possible Hepatocarcinogens

Synthetic Chemical Agents

The observation that azo dyes caused liver cancer opened a wide field of investigation. The list of synthetic chemical hepatocarcinogens has expanded markedly during the last two decades. However, while man is most likely to be exposed to the majority of such chemicals in Western countries, the incidence of liver cancer in these areas is low. Most experimental hepatocarcinogens tend to produce a specific spectrum of tumors at other sites as well as the liver. Accordingly, if pertinent to man, these are not present at doses sufficient to affect other organs, since such an association with liver cancer is not found, with the possible exception of liver and esophageal carcinoma in alcoholics. Liver cancer has not been reported as an occupational hazard. The aromatic amines which produce hepatomas in mice, for example, cause cancer of the bladder in man.[7] Thus, it is possible to say that the induction of neoplasms in the laboratory does not necessarily imply that the same agents will do so in man. However, when a carcinogen has been shown to be metabolized to a proximate carcinogen in the human liver like in the experimental animal, such as is the case with 2 FAA where N-hydroxylation is of importance, elimination of exposure hazard would appear obligatory.

Alcoholic Beverages

There is evidence that the incidence of neoplastic change is increasing in cirrhotic livers of alcoholic origin in North America and Western Europe. This is possibly due to the longer survival associated with better treatment.[93] While the excessive use of alcoholic beverages is thus implicated as a possible carcinogenic stimulus, it is unknown whether ethanol or other constituents of the drink are the significant factors. Ethanol has a definite toxic effect on the liver.[78, 79, 98] However, in experimental studies, ethanol has not yet been known to cause hepatomas. In *Mastomys natalensis* given ethanol at 20 to 25 percent in the drinking water for periods up to 3 years, a total of 4 hepatomas was seen in 52 animals compared to 7 in 300 controls. This is of doubtful significance. A recent report from Zambia[48] has shown that local beverages in that area contain dimethylnitrosamine, a known liver carcinogen.

Naturally Occurring Carcinogens

SENECIO ALKALOIDS. These alkaloids, notably retronecine, retrorsine, and lasiocarpine, are well-known experimental carcinogens.[85] They have been ingested by man and have produced severe liver disease (veno-occlusive disease). Their role in man has been given careful consideration, but they do not appear to be associated with a significantly increased incidence of liver cancer in the Caribbean area where they are most prevalent.[8]

CYCASIN. This substance is the aglycone of methylazoxymethanol and produces tumors of the rat liver and kidney.[42] In Guam, where it has been considered of importance, no definitive evidence of increased liver cancer has been observed.[10] In Japan the contamination of yellow rice by *Penicillium islandicum Sopp III* which occurred during the war is no longer considered to be or to have been of significance.

MYCOTOXINS. At present, there is a great interest in the possible role of mycotoxins, especialy aflatoxin, as carcinogens in man.[1] These toxins are produced by fungi, primarily *Aspergillus flavus,* and are profusely distributed in many foodstuffs, notably peanuts, in areas where liver cancer is common. While they are powerful experimental carcinogens[61, 62, 109] and there is widespread acceptance that they are an important etiologic agent in human cancer,[40] much of the evidence is circumstantial and of doubtful validity.[74] Today, the ingestion of aflatoxins in any individual population group is unknown.

Confirmation of reports indicating a high level of aflatoxin in local diets from Thailand and India is urgent, as a high frequency of liver cancer does not occur in these areas. Such a lack of correlation might indicate that aflatoxins are not important in man. Rats fed aflatoxin at a carcinogenic level show no evidence of cirrhosis,[63, 94] whereas in man cirrhosis is a common lesion accompanying liver cell carcinomas. The fetuin test (see below) is negative in aflatoxin-induced tumors, although it is positive in tumors produced by nitrosamines and DAB in rats.[90]

To date, aflatoxin has not yet produced tumors in primates fed the substance up to 3 years,[66a] but this period is insufficient to exclude carcinogenic activity. A series of other fungal hepatotoxic metabolites have been discovered (e.g., ochratoxin), but their hepatocarcinogenic potential in man remains to be investigated.

VIRUSES. In the forties, workers in West Africa[3, 21] suggested that the type of cirrhosis in which cancer arose was similar to that caused by viral hepatitis. The transition of hepatitis to cirrhosis has been observed in biopsy. The cirrhosis would appear to be of the same type as that seen in cancer cases, but to date no case of unequivocal sequence of hepatitis, cirrhosis, and cancer has been reported. It has also been stated that in Africa hepatitis is very common and that sequelae may be more prevalent.[17, 58] The plateau in age incidence curves would be consistent with a viral origin, indicating that the more susceptible population is affected in early life and that, in later life, only the less susceptible population was at risk.

While the possible diagnostic value of Australia 2 antigen in viral hepatitis is under investigation,[44, 45] a search for an increased frequency of Australia antigen in a large number of cases of hepatocellular carcinoma has so far proven unsuccessful.[6a] The problem of the role of hepatitis is further compounded by the fact that certain cases of jaundice originally ascribed to viral hepatitis could be due to a hepatotoxin, such as aflatoxin. The authors have demonstrated significant histologic differences between the acute damage patterns following aflatoxin ingestion in rats and those in Rhesus monkeys.[94] In the latter, vacuolation and necrosis of liver cells and cellular infiltration were observed similar to that reported with toxic hepatitis in Africa, and the well-marked periportal necrosis that occurs typically in rats was not observed. These observations have been confirmed more recently by Linsell and Peers[44a] in baboons. The seeming contradiction between those supporting a viral etiology and those supporting naturally occurring carcinogens may be resolved if it is proven that the morphologic diagnostic base of the former has been inaccurate in the African continent. The identification of the etiology of icterus and hepatic necrosis in the African region would appear to have a high priority in determining the possible etiology of liver cirrhosis and carcinoma.

In conclusion, it cannot be stated with certainty that liver cancer in man is due to any of the above factors, and further critical analysis is necessary. Too often the subject has been bedeviled by undue enthusiasm for a new etiologic hypothesis developed without adequate testing in the field.

Miscellaneous Etiologic Agents

Whereas hemochromatosis is associated with a slightly increased frequency of liver cell carcinoma, studies from Southern Africa where hemosiderin deposition in the liver is prominent would indicate that it is not an important carcinogenic factor.[34] The injection of Thorotrast for diagnostic purposes has been associated largely with an increase in hemangioendotheliomas of the liver.[10] Several of the more familiar carcinogenic stimuli in animals and their possible relationship to human liver cancer are summarized in Table 2. These observations indicate the caution with which the experimental pathologist involved in drug testing must approach the problem of extrapolation from animals to man when expressing an opinion on the carcinogenic potential of a new chemical, not only for the liver itself but also as an index for other organs.

Table 2. Hepatocarcinogenic Agents and Their Possible Significance in Man and Animals

	Mouse	Rat	Nonhuman Primates*	Human Exposure	Liver Tumors in Man
Aflatoxin	H	H	—	+	?
Azo dyes	H	H & C	—	+	O
Carbon tetrachloride	H	O	—	+	O
Chlorinated hydrocarbons	H	H	—	+	?
Cycasin	H	H	—	—	O
Ethanol	O	O	—	+	+
Griseofulvin	H	—	—	+	O
Hepatitis virus†	O	O	O	+	O
Iron excess	O	O	—	+	O
Nitrosamines	H	H	H	Susp.	?
Polycyclic aromatic hydrocarbons	H	H	O	+	O
Protein deficiency	O	O	—	+	O
Selenium	H	O	—	+	O
Senecio alkaloids	—	H	—	+	O
Tannic acid	—	H	—	+	O
Urethan	H	O	—	+	O

H = Hepatoma. C = Cholangioma. O = Probably negative or very rare. — = Not or inadequately tested. + = Definite known exposure in man. Susp. = Suspected exposure in man. ? = Unknown.

* In most cases exposure time has been inadequate to exclude carcinogenic effects.
† Refers to virus indigenous to the species.

Multifactorial Origin of Liver Carcinoma

While most cancers in man have been related to a single predominant carcinogenic stimulus, it is generally accepted that a multifactorial origin should be considered for many human tumors. Workers in Africa have suggested that primary cancer of the liver is related to the presence of a second stimulus such as a virus or toxin acting on a liver already damaged, possibly by protein deficiency or by hepatitis. In studies on the ultrastructural changes in the monkey[76] or the rat liver,[95] we have been unable to demonstrate any evidence of continuing abnormality following protein deficiency, although an abnormality cannot be excluded completely at the metabolic level. In man, it has long been considered that the abnormal albumin/globulin ratios reported from Africa might be related to previous malnutrition.[17] It should be noted, however, that while protein deficiency tends to potentiate the acute effects of aflatoxin, it also tends to diminish the carcinogenic effects.[49, 50] Theoretically it would appear possible, however, that with severe protein deficiency in childhood, the detoxifying capacity of the liver might be diminished because of decreased ability to synthesize enzymes necessary to detoxify carcinogens. In such circumstance, carcinogens excreted in the milk might be more potent than in the healthy child.

Experimental evidence on synergism or cocarcinogenesis is somewhat limited. Some of the published reports in rats are indicated in Table 3. It should be noted that an increase in carcinogenic activity has been observed both with carcinogens of dissimilar chemical composition as well as with stimuli, one of which is noncarcinogenic. Other combinations, however, have lead to a decrease. In our studies, when carbon tetrachloride was given sometime before DAB (Table 4) there was a reduction

Table 3. Synergism in Experimental Hepatocarcinogenesis

STIMULUS 1	STIMULUS 2	EFFECT ON TUMOR PRODUCTION	REFERENCE
2 FAA	3'Me DAB*	Increased	47
2 FAA	Tannic acid*	Increased	59
CCl₄	DAB	Increased	51
CCl₄	Ethionine 2 FAA	Decreased	67
CCl₄	DEN*	Increased	84
DAB	Hepatectomy	Decreased	25
DEN	DAB*	Increased	83
DEN	4 DAB*	Increased	81
DEN	DAST*	Increased	82
DMN	MCA*	None	32
Ethanol	DEN	None	84
Ethionine	DAB*	Increased	55
Ethionine	3'Me DAB*	None	23
2'Me DAB	2'Me O DAB*	Increased	60
X-ray	DAB	None	31, 41

* Simultaneous.

**Table 4. Effect of Pretreatment by CCl₄ and Partial Hepatectomy
on DAB Liver Tumors**

GROUP	NO. OF ANIMALS	NO. OF LIVERS WITH TUMORS	TOTAL NO. TUMORS	GRADE OF CIRRHOSIS
DAB (120 days)	25	13 (52%)	19	5
CCl₄–Rest–DAB	21	12 (57%)	19	6
CCl₄–DAB*	18	7 (39%)	14	6
Hepatectomy–DAB	24	7 (29%)	7	1.6
Ethionine–Rest–DAB	26	14 (54%)	21	5

* CCl₄ every 2 weeks for 3 months.

rather than an increase in the incidence of tumors, contrary to the observations of Maltoni.[51] This may indicate that the regenerative cell may be more resistant to the action of DAB. It is also possible that the metabolizing enzymes are deficient or lacking in this case.

Diagnosis

Biopsy

Although numerous studies have been made on the role of liver function tests in detecting carcinoma,[5] the liver biopsy still remains the most accurate method. The failure to obtain a satisfactory core occurs frequently in primary carcinoma of the liver, in which necrosis of the tumor tissue is common. Sections of such fragmented scraps may often indicate viable neoplastic cells which would be missed otherwise.

Liver Function Tests

Liver function tests have been widely used in the past to diagnose the onset of carcinoma. They tend to be nonspecific and are largely being replaced by the fetuin test.

Fetuin Test

Recently the demonstration that many hepatocellular carcinomas contain an alpha 1 fetoprotein has proved useful for diagnosis. In Dakar[105] approximately 70 to 80 percent of all tumors contained this serum antigen. However, more recent results from East Africa[106] and Europe indicate that the proportion of positive results in that area is at a lower level. While this may limit the test as a perfect diagnostic tool, it yet remains of great potential value, as false positives would appear exceedingly rare, and a positive test thus can obviate a liver biopsy. It is possible that variations in positivity in different areas may indicate different etiologic stimuli. Data to date have not yet permitted the identification of alpha 1 fetoprotein production with any single histologic pattern.[107] Similar feto-specific serum proteins have also been observed experimentally in rats, where tumors produced by DAB and DMN are positive and those produced by aflatoxin are negative.[90]

Minimal Deviation Hepatomas

Recent biochemical studies on the nature of hepatic malignancy have concentrated largely on the so-called minimal deviation hepatoma.[57] Potter in 1961 introduced the term "minimal deviation"[71] postulating that there would be a theoretical minimal deviation tumor which would closely approximate normal liver and thus assist in distinguishing the essential biochemical differences between benign and malignant cells. Among the criteria for such experimental hepatomas which have been derived from rats were the following: 1) that the biochemistry showed few nonessential changes, i.e., that the majority of normal liver enzymes were present; and 2) that the histology showed a high degree of differentiation and had a karyotype that is normal diploid for the rat liver. While many bear a close morphologic similarity to hyperplastic nodules, only 2 of 41 hepatomas reported to 1968 showed normal number and morphology of chromosomes.[72] Moreover, the karyotype bears little relation to the degree of differentiation. Wu indicated that in most instances no correlation exists between enzyme activity and growth rate or chromosome number of these hepatomas.[110] He also found a wide degree of heteroploidy in the mouse hepatomas derived from a common strain. Thus, while from a theoretical point of view the term "minimal deviation" has had considerable value in the introduction of new concepts in the study of minimal biochemical changes in cancer, the term itself should be used with considerable discrimination when applied morphologically to experimental hepatomas.

Conclusions

The above discussion would indicate that the geographical pathology of primary cancer of the liver and its biologic characteristics in man have been considerably extended in recent years. However, no definite etiologic agent has as yet been implicated. Experimental work would indicate that the relationship of liver cancer in man and animals to cirrhosis is essentially a function of the hyperplastic nodular regeneration which occurs in this condition. In North America and Europe liver cancer can be regarded as definitely associated with excessive alcoholic ingestion, but in such countries liver cancer is comparatively rare. The presence of a positive "fetuin test" can now be regarded as diagnostic for the condition.

References

1. Alpert, M. E. Mycotoxins. A possible cause of primary carcinoma of the liver. Amer. J. Med., 46:325, 1969.
2. Ashley, L. M., and Halver, J. E. Dimethylnitrosamine-induced hepatic cell carcinoma in rainbow trout. J. Nat. Cancer Inst., 41:531, 1968.
3. Bergeret, C., and Roulet, F. Au sujet des ictères graves de la cirrhose et du cancer primitif chez le noir d'Afrique. Acta Trop., 4:210, 1947.
4. Berman, C. Primary Carcinoma of the Liver. A study in incidence, clinical manifestations, pathology and aetiology. London, H. K. Lewis and Co. Ltd., 1951.
5. Bersohn, I. Liver function tests in primary carcinoma of the liver in South Africa. S. Afr. Med. J., 31:828, 1957.

6. Blumberg, B. S., Sutnick, A. I., and London, W. T. Hepatitis and leukemia: Their relation to Australian antigen. Bull. N.Y. Acad. Med., 44:1566, 1968.
6a. ——— Personal communication.
7. Bonser, G. M. Factors concerned in the location of human and experimental tumours. Brit. Med. J., 2:655, 1967.
8. Bras, G. Nutritional aspects of cirrhosis and carcinoma of the liver. Fed. Proc., 20:353, 1961.
9. Bull, L. B., Culvenor, C. C. J., and Dick, A. T. The Pyrrolizidine Alkaloids. Amsterdam, North Holland Publishing Co., 1968.
10. Burdette, W. J., ed. Primary Hepatoma. Salt Lake City, Univ. Utah Press, 1965.
11. Carnaghan, R. B. Hepatic tumors in ducks fed a low level of toxic groundnut meal. Nature, 208:308, 1965.
12. Cook, G. C., and Hutt, M. S. The liver after kwashiorkor. Brit. Med. J., 3:454, 1967.
13. Cotchin, E. Neoplasms of the domesticated mammals. Review series No. 4 of the Commonwealth Bureau of Animal Health. England, Lamport Gilbert and Co. Ltd., 1956.
14. Crisler, C., Rapp, H. J., Weintraub, R. M., and Borsos, T. Forssman antigen content of guinea pig hepatomas induced by diethylnitrosamine: A quantitative approach to the search for tumor-specific antibodies. J. Nat. Cancer Inst., 36:529, 1966.
15. Doll, R. Age distribution of cancer in man. *In* Thule International Symposia, 1967: Cancer and Aging. Stockholm, Nordiska Bokhandelns Förlag, 1968.
16. ——— Payne, P., and Waterhouse, J., eds. Cancer Incidence in Five Continents: A Technical Report. Berlin, Springer Verlag, 1966.
17. Edington, G. M., and Gilles, H. M. Pathology in the Tropics. London, Edward Arnold, 1969.
18. Edmundson, H. Tumors of the Liver and Intrahepatic Bile Ducts. Washington, D.C., Armed Forces Institute of Pathology, 1958.
19. Epstein, S., McNary, J., Bartus, B., and Farber, E. Chemical carcinogenesis: Persistence of bound forms of 2-fluorenylacetamide. Science, 162:907, 1968.
20. Farber, E. Biochemistry of carcinogenesis. Cancer Res., 28:1859, 1968.
21. Findlay, G. M. Observations on primary liver carcinoma in West African soldiers. J. Roy. Micr. Soc., 70:166, 1950.
22. Fraumeni, J. F., and Miller, R. W. Primary carcinoma of the liver in childhood: An epidemiological study. J. Nat. Cancer Inst., 40:1087, 1968.
23. Gelboin, H. V., Miller, J. A., and Miller, E. C. Studies on hepatic protein-bound dye formation in rats given single large doses of 3'-methyl-4-dimethylaminobenzene. Cancer Res., 18:608, 1958.
24. Ghadially, F. N., and Parry, E. W. Ultrastructure of a human hepatocellular carcinoma and surrounding non-neoplastic liver. Cancer, 19:1989, 1966.
25. Glinos, A. D., Bucher, N. L. R., and Aub, J. C. The effect of liver regeneration on tumor formation in rats fed 4-dimethylaminoazobenzene. J. Exp. Med., 93:313, 1951.
26. Goodall, C. Endocrine factors as determinants of the susceptibility of the liver to carcinogenic agents. New Zeal. Med. J., 67:32, 1968.
27. Hartwell, J. L., and Shubik, P. Survey of Compounds Which Have Been Tested for Carcinogenic Activity, 2nd ed. Washington, D.C., U.S. Printing Office, 1951. Federal Security Agency: PHS No. 149, National Cancer Institute, National Institutes of Health, Bethesda, Maryland.
28. Higginson, J. The geographical pathology of primary liver cancer. Cancer Res., 23:1624, 1963.
29. ——— The definition of kwashiorkor, fatty change, necrosis, cirrhosis and cancer of the liver. Acta Union Internationale Contre le Cancer 13:525, 1957.

30. ———— and Steiner, P. E. Definition and classification of malignant epithelial neoplasms of the liver. Acta Un. Int. Canc., 17:593, 1961.
31. ———— and Svoboda, D. Unpublished results.
32. Hoch-Ligeti, C., Argus, M. F., and Arcos, J. C. Combined carcinogenic effect of dimethylnitrosamine and 3-methylcholanthrene in the rat. J. Nat. Cancer Inst., 40:535, 1968.
33. Hou, P. C. Relationship between primary carcinoma of the liver and infestation with *Clonorchis sinensis*. J. Path. Bact., 72:239, 1956.
34. Isaacson, C., Seftel, H. C., Keeley, K. J., and Bothwell, T. H. Siderosis in the Bantu: The relationship between iron overload and cirrhosis. J. Lab. Clin. Med., 58:845, 1961.
35. Ishak, K. G., and Glunz, P. R. Hepatoblastoma and hepatocarcinoma in infancy and childhood. Cancer, 20:396, 1967.
36. Jackson, E. W., Wolf, H., and Sinnhuber, R. O. The relationship of hepatoma in rainbow trout to aflatoxin contamination and cottonseed meal. Cancer Res., 28:987, 1968.
37. Karasaki, S. The fine structure of proliferating cells in pre-neoplastic rat livers during azo-dye carcinogenesis. J. Cell Biol., 40:322, 1969.
38. Kelly, M. G., O'Gara, R. W., Adamson, R. H., Gadekar, K., Botkin, C. C., Reese, W. H., and Kerber, W. T. Induction of hepatic cell carcinomas in monkeys with n-nitrosodiethylamine. J. Nat. Cancer Inst., 36:323, 1966.
39. Klein, G. Tumor-specific transplantation antigens. Cancer Res., 28:625, 1968.
40. Kraybill, H., and Shimkin, M. Carcinogenesis related to foods contaminated by processing and fungal metabolites. *In* Haddow, A., and Weinhouse, S., eds. Advances in Cancer Research. New York and London, Academic Press, Inc., 1964, Vol. 8.
41. Lacassagne, A., and Hurst, L. Effects of the combined action of roentgen rays and a chemical carcinogen (DAB) on the rat's liver. Amer. J. Roentgen., 87:536, 1962.
42. Laqueur, G. L., and Spatz, M. Toxicology of cycasin. Cancer Res., 28:2262, 1968.
43. Leevy, C. M., Gellene, R., and Ning, M. Primary liver cancer in cirrhosis of the alcoholic. Ann. N.Y. Acad. Sci., 114:1026, 1964.
44. Levene, C., and Blumberg, B. S. Additional specificities of Australia antigen and the possible identification of hepatitis carriers. Nature, 221:195, 1969.
44a. Linsell, C. A., and Peers, F. Personal communication.
45. London, W. T., Sutnick, A. I., and Blumberg, B. S. Australia antigen and acute viral hepatitis. Ann. Intern. Med., 70:55, 1969.
46. MacDonald, R. A. Cirrhosis and primary carcinoma of the liver; changes in their occurrence at the Boston City Hospital, 1897-1954. New Eng. J. Med., 255:1179, 1956.
47. MacDonald, J. C., Miller, E. C., Miller, J. A., and Rusch, H. P. The synergistic action of mixtures of certain hepatic carcinogens. Cancer Res., 12:50, 1952.
48. McGlashan, N. D., Walters, C. L., and McLean, A. E. M. Nitrosamines in African alcoholic spirits and oesophageal cancer. Lancet, 2:1017, 1968.
49. Madhavan, T., and Gopalan, C. Effect of dietary protein on aflatoxin liver injury in weanling rats. Arch. Path., 80:123, 1965.
50. ———— and Gopalan, C. The effect of dietary protein on carcinogenesis of aflatoxin. Arch. Path., 85:133, 1968.
51. Maltoni, C., and Prodi, G. The behaviour of connective tissues in the genesis and development of tumors. *In* Bucalossi, P., and Veronesi, U., eds. Recent Contributions to Cancer Research in Italy. Milan, Casa Editrice Ambrosana, 1960.
52. Merkow, L. P., Epstein, S. M., Caito, J., and Bartus, B. The cellular analysis of liver carcinogenesis: Ultrastructural alterations within hyperplastic liver nodules induced by 2-fluorenylacetamide. Cancer Res., 27:1712, 1967.
53. Miller, J. A., and Miller, E. C. The carcinogenic aminoazo dyes. *In* Greenstein,

J., and Haddow, A., eds. Advances in Cancer Research. New York, Academic Press, Inc., 1953, Vol. 1.

54. Misugi, K., Okajima, H., Misugi, N., and Newton, W. A. Classification of primary malignant tumors of liver in infancy and childhood. Cancer, 20:1760, 1967.

55. Miyaji, H., Nishi, H., Watanabe, S., Koyama, K., Tamura, K., Nasu, K., Kusaka, H., and Ishihama, S. Carcinogenic effect of ethionine on the DAB-carcinogenesis in rats. Gann, 48:585, 1957.

56. Mori, W. Cirrhosis and primary cancer of the liver. Comparative study in Tokyo and Cincinnati. Cancer, 20:627, 1967.

57. Morris, H. P., Sidransky, H., Wagner, B. P., and Dyer, H. M. Some characteristics of transplantable rat hepatoma No. 5123 induced by ingestion of N-(2-fluorenyl)-phthalmic acid. Cancer Res., 20:1252, 1960.

58. Morrow, R. H., Jr., Smetana, H. F., Sai, F. T., and Edgcomb, J. H. Unusual features of viral hepatitis in Accra, Ghana. Ann. Int. Med., 68:1250, 1968.

59. Mosonyi, M., and Korpassy, B. Rapid production of malignant hepatomas by simultaneous administration of tannic acid and 2-acetylaminofluorene. Nature, 171:791, 1953.

60. Neish, W. J. P., Parry, E. W., and Ghadhially, F. N. Tumour induction in the rat by a mixture of two non-carcinogenic aminoazo dyes. Oncology, 21:229, 1967.

61. Newberne, P., and Butler, W. Acute and chronic effects of aflatoxin on the liver of domestic and laboratory animals. A review. Cancer Res., 29:236, 1969.

62. ——— Hunt, C. E., and Wogan, G. N. Neoplasms in the rat associated with administration of urethan and aflatoxin. Exp. Molec. Path., 6:285, 1967.

63. ——— and Wogan, G. N. Sequential morphologic changes in aflatoxin B_1 carcinogenesis in the rat. Cancer Res., 28:770, 1968.

64. Ninard, B. Tumeurs du Foie. Paris, Librairie le François, 1950.

65. Norkin, S. A., and Campagna-Pinto, D. Cytoplasmic hyaline inclusions in hepatoma. Arch. Path., 86:25, 1968.

66. Nowell, P. C., Morris, H. P., and Potter, V. R. Chromosomes of "minimal deviation" hepatomas and some other transplantable rat tumors. Cancer Res., 27:1565, 1967.

66a. O'Gara, R. Personal communication.

67. Oyasu, R. Effect of pretreatment with hepatotoxic substances on 2-acetamidofluorene and indole tumorigenesis in rat; effect of carbon tetrachloride and dl-ethionine. Gann, 54:339, 1963.

68. Péquignot, H., Etienne, J. P., Delavierre, Ph., and Petite, J.-P. Cancers primitifs du foie sur cirrhose: Augmentation de fréquence et observation chez des cirrhotiques connus et suivis. Presse Méd., 75:2595, 1967.

69. Pitot, H. C. Some aspects of the developmental biology of neoplasia. Cancer Res., 28:1880, 1968.

70. ——— Endoplasmic reticulum and phenotypic variability in normal and neoplastic liver. Arch. Path., 87:212, 1969.

71. Potter, V. R. Transplantable animal cancer, the primary standard. Cancer Res., 21:1331, 1961.

72. ——— Summary of discussion on neoplasms. Symposium, "The Developmental Biology of Neoplasia," September, 1967. Cancer Res., 28:1901, 1968.

73. Prehn, R. T. Cancer antigens in tumors induced by chemicals. Fed. Proc., 24:1018, 1965.

74. Purchase, I. F. Fungal metabolites as potential carcinogens, with particular reference to their role in the etiology of hepatoma. S. Afr. Med. J., 41:406, 1967.

75. Quinn, P. S., and Higginson, J. Reversible and irreversible changes in experimental cirrhosis. Amer. J. Path., 47:353, 1965.

76. Racela, A. S., Grady, H. J., Higginson, J., and Svoboda, D. J. Protein deficiency in Rhesus monkeys. Amer. J. Path., 49:419, 1966.

77. Reuber, M. D. Histopathology of transplantable hepatic carcinomas induced by chemical carcinogens in rats. Gann, Monograph 1, page 43, 1966.

78. Rubin, E., Krus, S., and Popper, H. Pathogenesis of post-necrotic cirrhosis in alcoholics. Arch. Path., 73:288, 1962.
79. ——— and Lieber, C. S. Effect of alcohol on liver. New Eng. J. Med., 279:46, 1968.
80. Ruebner, B. H., Gonzalez-Licea, A., and Slusser, R. J. Electron microscopy of some human hepatomas. Gastroenterology, 53:18, 1967.
81. Schmähl, D. Synkarzinogenese. Dtsch. Med. Wschr., 91:1799, 1966.
82. ——— and Thomas, C. Experimentelle Untersuchungen zur "Syncarcinogenese." IV. Versuche zur Krebserzeugung an Ratten bei gleichzeitiger oraler Gabe von Diäthylnitrosamin und 4-Dimethylamino-Stilben. Z. Krebsforsch., 67:135, 1965.
83. ——— Thomas, C., and Konig, K. Experimental studies on "Syncarcinogenesis." I. Experiments on cancer induction in rats with simultaneous application of diethylnitrosamine and 4-dimethylamino-azobenzene. Z. Krebsforsch., 65:342, 1963.
84. ——— Thomas, C., Sattler, W., and Scheld, G. F. Experimentelle Untersuchungen zur Syncarcinogenese. III. Versuche zur Krebserzeugung bei Ratten bei gleichzeitiger Gabe von Diäthylnitrosamin und Tetrachlorkohlenstoff bzw. Athylalkohol; zugleich ein experimenteller Beitrag zur Frage der "Alkoholcirrhose." Z. Krebsforsch., 66:526, 1965.
85. Schoental, R. Toxicology and carcinogenic action of pyrrolizidine alkaloids. Cancer Res., 28:2237, 1968.
86. Segi, M., and Kurihara, M. Cancer mortality for selected sites in 24 countries. Sendai, Japan, Dept. of Public Health, Tohoku Univ. School of Med., 1962.
87. Shanmugaratnam, K. Primary carcinoma of the liver and biliary tract. Brit. J. Cancer, 10:232, 1956.
87a. ——— and Tye. Personal communication.
88. Shubik, P., and Hartwell, J. L. Survey of compounds which have been tested for carcinogenic activity. Washington, D.C., U.S. Department of Health, Education, and Welfare, Suppl. 1, PHS Publication No. 149, 1957.
89. Sinnhuber, R. O., Wales, J. H., Ayres, J. L., Engebrecht, R. H., and Amend, D. L. Dietary factors and hepatoma in rainbow trout (*Salmo gairdmeri*). I. Aflatoxins in vegetable protein foodstuffs. J. Nat. Cancer Inst., 41:711, 1968.
90. Stanislawski-Birencwajg, M., Uriel, J., and Grabar, P. Association of embryonic antigens with experimentally induced hepatic lesions in the rat. Cancer Res., 27:1990, 1967.
91. Steiner, P. E. Cancer of the liver and cirrhosis and trans-Saharan Africa and the United States of America. Cancer, 13:1085, 1960.
92. Stewart, H. L., and Snell, K. C. The histopathology of experimental tumors of the liver of the rat. A critical review of the histopathogenesis. *In* Homburger, F., ed. The Physiopathology of Cancer, 2nd ed. New York, Hoeber Division, Harper & Row, Publishers, 1959.
93. Stone, W. D., Islam, N. R. K., and Paton, A. The natural history of cirrhosis: Experience with an unselected group of patients. Quart. J. Med. (N. S.), 37:119, 1968.
94. Svoboda, D., Grady, H., and Higginson, J. Aflatoxin B$_1$ injury in rats and monkeys. Amer. J. Path., 49:1023, 1966.
95. ——— Grady, H., and Higginson, J. The effects of chronic protein deficiency in rats. II. Biochemical and ultrastructural changes. Lab. Invest., 15:731, 1966.
96. ——— and Higginson, J. A comparison of ultrastructural changes in rat liver due to chemical carcinogens. Cancer Res., 28:1703, 1968.
97. ——— and Higginson, J. Ultrastructural changes produced by protein and related differences in the rat liver. Amer. J. Path., 45:353, 1964.
98. ——— and Manning, R. Chronic alcoholism with fatty metamorphosis of the liver, mitochondrial alterations in hepatic cells. Amer. J. Path., 44:645, 1964.
99. ——— Racela, A., and Higginson, J. Variations in ultrastructural nuclear changes in hepatocarcinogenesis. Biochem. Pharm., 16:651, 1967.

100. Takahashi, T., Orii, T., and Kaneda, M. Precancerous condition of the human liver. Tohoku J. Exp. Med., 94:203, 1968.
101. Theron, J. J. Hydrolytic enzymes and fine structure of human hepatic cancer. *In* Burdette, W. J., ed. Primary Hepatoma. Salt Lake City, Univ. Utah Press, 1965.
102. Toker, C., and Trevino, N. Ultrastructure of human primary hepatic carcinoma. Cancer, 19:1594, 1966.
103. Tomatis, L., Magee, P., and Shubik, P. Induction of liver tumors in the Syrian golden hamster by feeding dimethylnitrosamine. J. Nat. Cancer Inst., 33:341, 1964.
104. Toth, B. Critical review of experiments in chemical carcinogenesis using newborn animals. Cancer Res., 28:727, 1968.
105. Uriel, J., and de Nechaud, B. Association d'antigenes embryonnaires avec l'hepatome primaire chez l'homme et les animaux de laboratoire. Rev. Méd. Franc., 43:47, 1968.
106. ———— de Nechaud, B., Stanislawski-Birencwajg, M., Masseyeff, R., Leblanc, L., Quenum, C., Loissillier, F., and Grabar, P. Les diagnostics du cancer primaire du foie par des methodes immunologiques. Presse Méd., 76:1415, 1968.
107. ———— Transitory liver antigens and primary hepatoma in men and rats. In press.
108. Weisburger, J. H., and Weisburger, E. K. Tests for chemical carcinogens. *In* Busch, H., ed. Methods in Cancer Research. New York, Academic Press, Inc., 1967, Vol. 1.
109. Wogan, G. Biochemical responses to aflatoxins. Cancer Res., 28:2282, 1968.
110. Wu, C. "Minimal deviation" hepatomas: A critical review of the terminology, indicating a commentary on the correlation of enzyme activity with growth rate of hepatomas. J. Nat. Cancer Inst., 39:1149, 1967.

Addendum

Since the preparation of this chapter, the following additional reports have appeared and may be of interest.

Alcoholic Beverages

Further epidemiologic studies in Nordic countries and in the United Kingdom would confirm the causal role of certain alcoholic beverages in cirrhosis and liver cell carcinoma. The latter is being observed more frequently in parts of Europe than previously anticipated. However, alcoholic beverages may vary in their cirrhogenic and carcinogenic potential, and ethanol per se may not be the only factor involved. These tumors show a lower degree of positivity to alpha-fetoprotein and Hepatitis B antigen.

Mycotoxins

Human exposure to aflatoxin undoubtedly occurs on a wide scale, especially in tropical countries. An association between the number of contaminated samples and the incidence of liver cancer has been shown by Alpert et al [1] in Uganda and in Swaziland by Keene et al.[2] In Kenya, Peers and Linsell,[3] in a pilot sample study, showed a correlation between the average ingestion of aflatoxin and liver cancer. Occasional periods of excessive exposure may be more important than the average exposure. Epidemiologic evidence also supports a possible relationship between aflatoxin consumption and primary liver cancer in Thailand.[4, 5]

In view of the emerging implication of human ingestion of aflatoxins, experiments were carried out to assess the degree of aflatoxin-induced chronic liver damage in nonhuman primates. In long-term experiments in shrews given 2 parts per million (ppm) of aflatoxin B_1 in their diet, hepatic tumors occurred in some animals after several weeks. Some of the tumors were poorly differentiated.[6] In long-term experiments in marmosets (*Saguinus oedipomidas*) of both sexes in which there was hepatic injury due to aflatoxin B_1 alone and in combination with the GB strain of human viral hepatitis agent, cirrhosis occurred in both singly and doubly injured animals by the 15th week, and liver tumors were present in 3 out of 16 marmosets (1 given aflatoxin alone and 2 given aflatoxin plus the viral hepatitis agent) between 50 and 87 weeks.[7] In all three animals, each liver had two to four tumors. The tumors were composed of irregular trabeculae several cells in thickness. The cells were very pleomorphic with a wide range in nuclear and nucleolar size. By the time tumors occurred, portal cirrhosis and bile duct proliferation were severe.[8]

It is clear that, depending on dose and schedule, there are differences in the hepatic responses to aflatoxins among nonhuman primates. Probably of greater importance is the observation that in marmosets and shrews tumors occur when the liver is cirrhotic, while in rats hepatomas occur in livers that show little or no architectural distortion. This is especially interesting in view of the epidemiologic observations that in several populations in which liver cancer is of unusually high incidence and in whom aflatoxin consumption appears, at least circumstantially, to be a distinct possibility, hepatic cancer is far more common in cirrhotic livers than in noncirrhotic organs.

Hepatitis B Virus

Both Ag B positive hepatitis and symptomless carriers are more frequent in tropical countries and are relatively rare in Europe and North America, except in certain communities. Further, a higher proportion of patients with liver cell carcinomas in Africa are Ag B carriers in the former, although interpretation of the data is somewhat confused due to the effects of age and sex. The tests for hepatitis B Ag are not completely satisfactory, and the proportion of positives may be higher. Thus, the evidence for a role of hepatitis B virus in liver cancer remains circumstantial, and any of the following hypotheses may apply: (1) a genetic predisposition to infection with hepatitis B virus; (2) a general depression of the immune response in patients with liver disease; and (3) a specific immune effect allowing persistence of the virus in the liver resulting in low-grade continuing cell damage. In addition, recent reports of familial occurrence of hepatoma and Australia antigen suggest a further possibility of genetic predisposition to the development of hepatocarcinoma.[9]

Alpha-Fetoprotein (AFP)

It is now clear that alpha-fetoprotein (AFP) is produced by the fetal liver, but only trace levels are detectable at birth and afterwards. A high proportion of the tumors in Africa are AFP positive, but the diagnostic test in Europe and North America is much less satisfactory since the percentage of positive carcinomas is smaller. An association has been found between hepatitis B Ag and AFP production in areas with liver cell carcinoma.

It should be noted that AFP is present in the serum of patients with embryonal gonadal tumors and with primary cancer of the stomach, esophagus, or prostate and in patients with nonneoplastic liver disease.[10] AFP has been reported in viral hepatitis,[11, 12] in cancer of the pancreas, and in normal people.[13] Despite the decrease in specificity of serum AFP with increased sensitivity of methods used for its detection, the evidence thus far indicates that high levels of AFP are more suggestive of hepatoma than of other nonhepatic neoplasms or nonneoplastic liver disease. The use of quantitative assays should further elucidate this matter. AFP is present in the serums of monkeys with chemically-induced hepatomas [14, 15] and appears early during chemical induction of hepatocarcinomas in rats.[16, 17]

Of special interest is the recent report of a new antigen, termed PN or preneoplastic, that is present in regenerative and hyperplastic liver nodules and in hepatomas in rats given a variety of hepatocarcinogens but that is not present in any normal tissue or fluid or in the serums of regenerating or fetal liver.[18]

Contraceptives

A number of vascular benign liver tumors have been reported in females using oral steroid contraceptives for prolonged periods.[19–21] These have been classified as adenomas, hepatomas, or hamartomas. The tumors are composed of well-differentiated hepatic cells with vacuolated cytoplasm and have many ultrastructural features that have been observed in nontumorous livers of women on oral contraceptives. The tumors may cause severe hemorrhage clinically and can be detected by hepatic angiography.[19] Similar tumors have also been reported in individuals on anabolic steroids.

Occupational Cancers

Angiosarcomas of the liver have been found in individuals exposed to high levels of vinyl chloride, but no unequivocal epithelial tumors have been recorded.

Evaluation of Experimental Hepatomas

Tomatis et al [22] have recently reviewed the literature on the value of the mouse hepatoma as an index of potential carcinogenic risk to other species in view of its frequency in test systems.

References

1. Alpert ME, Hutt MSR, Wogan GN, Davidson CS: Association between aflatoxin content of food and hepatoma frequency in Uganda. Cancer 28:253, 1971
2. Keen P, Martin P: Is aflatoxin carcinogenic in man? The evidence in Switzerland. Trop Geogr Med 23:44, 1971
3. Peers FG, Linsell CA: Dietary aflatoxins and liver cancers—a population based study in Kenya. Br J Cancer 27:473, 1973
4. Shank R, Wogan G, Gibson J, Nondasuta A: Dietary aflatoxin and human liver cancer. II. Aflatoxin in market foods and foodstuffs of Thailand and Hong Kong. Food Cosmet Toxicol 10:61, 1972
5. Shank R, Gordon T, Wogan G, Nondasuta A, Subhamani V: Dietary aflatoxin and human liver cancer. III. Field survey of rural Thai families for ingested aflatoxins. Food Cosmet Toxicol 10:71, 1972
6. Reddy J: Personal communication
7. Deinhardt F, Holmes A, Capps R, Popper H: Studies on the transmission of human viral hepatitis to marmoset monkeys. I. Transmission of disease, serial passages, and description of liver lesions. J Exp Med 125:673, 1967
8. Lin J, Liu C, Svoboda D: Long term effects of aflatoxin B_1 and viral hepatitis on marmoset liver: a preliminary report. Lab Invest 30:267, 1974
9. Sutnick A: Association of Australia antigen with diseases other than hepatitis. In Prier J, Friedman H (eds): Australia Antigen. Baltimore, University Park Press, 1973, pp 163–89
10. For review, see Zawadski Z, Kraj M: Alpha-fetoprotein in hepatocellular disease and neoplastic disorders. Am J Gastroenterol 61:45, 1974
11. Smith J, Barker L: α_1-fetoprotein and liver-specific antigen in viral hepatitis type B. Arch Intern Med 133:437, 1974
12. Hulbert K, Devault J, Gold P, et al: The detection of α_1-fetoprotein in patients with viral hepatitis. Cancer Res 34:244, 1974
13. Purves L, Branch W, Geddes E, et al: Serum alpha-fetoprotein VII: the range of apparent serum values in normal people, pregnant woman, and primary liver cancer high risk populations. Cancer 31:578, 1973
14. Adamson R, Correa P, Smith C, et al: Induction of tumors in monkeys by chemical carcinogens—correlation of serum alpha-fetoprotein and appearance of liver tumors. Proc Am Assoc Cancer Res, 114:42, 1973
15. McIntire K, Princler G, Adamson R: Quantitation of serum alpha-fetoprotein in monkeys with primary liver tumors. Proc Am Assoc Cancer Res 114:104, 1973
16. Watabe H: Early appearance of embryonic globulin in rat serum during carcinogenesis with 4-dimethyl-aminoazobenzene. Cancer Res 31:1192, 1971
17. Kroes R, Williams G, Weisburger T: Early appearance of serum fetoprotein as a function of dosage of various hepatocarcinogens. Cancer Res 33:613, 1973
18. Farber E: Pathogenesis of liver cancer. Arch Pathol 98:145, 1974
19. Baum J, Bookstein J, Holtz F, Klein E: Possible association between benign hepatomas and oral contraceptives. Lancet 926, 1973
20. Tountas C, Paraskevas G, Deligeorgi H: Benign hepatoma and oral contraceptives. Lancet I:1351, 1974
21. Horvath E, Kovacs K, Ross R: Benign hepatoma in a young woman on contraceptive steroids. Lancet I:357, 1974
22. Tomatis L, Partensky C, Montesano R: The predictive value of mouse liver tumor induction in carcinogenicity testing: a literature survey. Int J Cancer, 12:1, 1973

TUMORS OF THE EXTRAHEPATIC BILIARY SYSTEM

GEORGE F. GRAY, JR.
ROBERT W. McDIVITT

Tumors of the gallbladder and bile ducts present numerous problems to clinicians and pathologists. The close proximity of the biliary tract to the liver, pancreas, and ampulla and the nearly identical histology of cancers arising in these organs often makes identification of the source of tumors difficult. Furthermore, benign neoplasms and various tumor-like conditions may be confused with cancer. Finally, the difficulties in making early diagnoses and the limitations of present methods of therapy are reflected by high mortality rates of biliary carcinomas.

The biliary duct system, liver, and pancreas develop from the *hepatic diverticulum,* a ventral outgrowth of gut endoderm. Although anomalies of development are fairly common, the extrahepatic biliary system usually consists of a right and left hepatic duct which emerge from the liver, join, and form the *common hepatic duct.* The common hepatic duct is about 4 cm in length and 0.5 cm wide. The *gallbladder,* a sac 7 to 10 cm long, about 2.5 cm in greatest diameter, with a capacity of about 30 to 35 cc, is connected to the common hepatic duct by a narrow and somewhat tortuous 4 cm long *cystic duct.* The cystic and common hepatic ducts join to form the *common bile duct,* a structure 7 cm in length, which in turn empties into the duodenum. The distal common duct passes immediately posterior to the head of the pancreas and may be joined by the pancreatic ducts just proximal to the ampulla.

The epithelium of the entire biliary system is of tall columnar type, usually thrown into folds and ridges, particularly in the gallbladder (Fig. 1). These mucosal folds become accentuated by edema. A rather thin muscularis normally surrounds the ducts and gallbladder, but it may become markedly thickened in chronic inflammatory disorders or with calculi. A dense connective tissue layer forms an

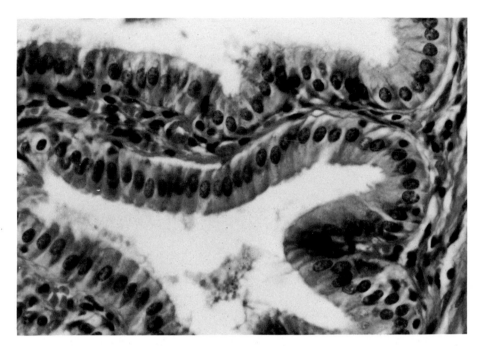

Fig. 1. Normal biliary mucosa. The epithelium is tall columnar with uniform basally located nuclei. H&E. X400.

adventitia external to the muscularis. Since the function of the biliary system is transport of bile from liver to duodenum, disturbance of this function by such abnormalities as tumor, calculus, or stricture may cause jaundice, pain, or alteration of alimentary function.

Cancer of the Gallbladder and Bile Ducts

INCIDENCE. Most clinically significant tumors of the biliary tract are carcinomas. Biliary cancer is less common than carcinoma of the colon, stomach, esophagus, or pancreas, but it is more frequent than primary cancer of the small intestine or liver.[33] The incidence is more difficult to determine than that of tumors in many other sites because of the nonspecific morphology and difficulty of separation from cancers originating in the pancreas, ampulla, pylorus, or even other parts of the gastrointestinal tract; however, published reports include more than 4,000 biliary cancers.

From a group of 4,821 patients who had biliary operations, Thorbjarnarson and Glenn[69] reported 147 cancers, including 26 ampullary carcinomas and 90 (1.9 percent of cases) carcinomas of the gallbladder. Ochsner and Ochsner[49] found 20 gallbladder cancers in 1,523 cholecystectomies (1.3 percent of cases); Balagero[5] reported an identical incidence, 11 biliary tract cancers in 789 operations. Earlier, Strauch,[65] from reports by various authors, collected 482 gallbladder carcinomas in 34,242 biliary operations (1.4 percent of cases). Tumors may occur in all parts of the gallbladder but are most frequently in the largest part, the fundus.[69]

Bile duct carcinomas appear to be less frequent than gallbladder carcinomas. Thorbjarnarson and Glenn[69] found only 31 (0.6 percent of cases) in 4,821 biliary operations, as opposed to 90 gallbladder carcinomas. Salmon[57] found 83 cholecystic cancers, but only 60 duct cancers among 586 malignant tumors of the pancreas and biliary tree. While primary carcinomas occur throughout the duct system, there appears to be a slight predilection for the bifurcation of the right and left hepatic ducts and for the junction of the cystic, hepatic, and common bile ducts. In some instances, however, tumors do not appear to be well localized.[35] Thus, in 173 bile duct tumors, Braasch[10] and his associates found 57 in the hepatic ducts, 62 in the distal common bile duct, 27 at the junction of the cystic, hepatic, and common bile ducts, and 27 which were spread throughout the entire system. A similar distribution has been observed by others.[12] Tumors of the distal common duct are easily confused with tumors arising in the head of the pancreas or ampulla.

AGE.   About half the patients with gallbladder cancer are in the seventh decade.[69] Although gallbladder cancer has been reported in the third[40] and fourth decades, it is infrequent before age 50 and after age 80.[65] The age distribution of patients with bile duct carcinoma is similar. Pallette[51] found the average age for gallbladder cancer was 65.3 years, for duct cancer 67.5 years.

SEX.   Gallbladder carcinomas are three times more common in women than in men. For example, Strauch[65] found, in a review of 1,016 cases, 75.3 percent in women and only 24.7 percent in men. However, there is little sex difference in incidence of biliary duct carcinomas.[57, 66]

Clinical Presentation

The similarity in presentation of cancer and calculus has been repeatedly emphasized.[9, 10, 17, 33, 40, 65] Pain is the most frequent symptom of cholecystic carcinoma. Weight loss and jaundice are the next most common complaints, followed by symptoms of digestive dysfunction such as bloating, flatulence, anorexia, and food intolerance. Abdominal swelling or a mass is an uncommon initial symptom, but a palpable gallbladder or a right upper quadrant mass is frequently found with advanced tumors. Hydrops of the gallbladder may result from cystic duct tumors.[50] Mild icterus detected chemically is more frequent than marked jaundice.[69] Patients with gallbladder cancers, particularly those associated with gallstones, frequently have a long history of symptoms of cholecystic disease. Persistence of symptoms referable to the biliary tract following cholecystectomy may indicate bile duct or pancreatic cancer.[7, 18, 54] On the other hand, gallbladder carcinoma presented as acute cholecystitis[68] in 11 percent of 90 cases, presumably because of obstruction of the gallbladder neck or cystic duct. One cystic duct cancer presented as gallbladder perforation.[52] Rapid onset of jaundice is more commonly a symptom of bile duct carcinoma, since these ducts may be obstructed by relatively small tumors. Of 76 patients with duct cancers, 62 percent presented with jaundice and 58 percent complained of pain.[68] Radiographic changes diagnostic of carcinoma are infrequent, since in many cases the findings are indistinguishable from those of other forms of biliary tract disease.[16, 25, 44, 55] Gallbladders with calcification of the wall ("porcelain" gallbladder) are relatively frequent sites of carcinoma.[53]

Etiology and Pathogenesis

Calculus is frequently associated with biliary cancer, prompting speculation that stones may have a causative role in the development of cancer of the gallbladder and bile ducts. Stones are found much more consistently with cancers of the gallbladder than with carcinomas of the ducts, being associated with 72 to 90 percent of gallbladder cancers.[40, 65] Calculi tend to be found more frequently in females (90 percent) than in males (59 percent) with cholecystic cancer.[69] A study of 11,129 autopsies in Oslo,[70] 45 percent of the total deaths, revealed gallstone incidence of 19.5 percent—27.5 percent in women and 12.7 percent in men. In this group, there were 39 unequivocal and 7 probable cancers of gallbladder origin (0.4 percent of cases). Of the 39 definite cancers, 36 were in women and 34 had associated stones. Similar studies in the United States have suggested that a 45-year-old person with stones has a 1.4 percent chance of developing gallbladder cancer, and that a 65-year-old person with stones has a 0.44 percent chance.[47]

Although calculi are the most common disorder associated with bile duct carcinomas, they are found much less frequently than with gallbladder carcinoma. Although some[51] have found calculi in nearly half (46 percent) of duct cancers, others[71] have found them in as few as 18 percent. Since it is not always clear whether these stones were within the gallbladder or within the duct system, evidence of a possible etiologic relationship is slight.

There has been little attention given to the type of gallstones, i.e., bilirubin, cholesterol, mixed, etc., associated with cancer. Such a study might give clues to possible etiologic factors common to calculi and stones.

Carcinomas are reported to occur in approximately 2 percent of choledochal cysts.[4, 67] Although this cancer incidence is higher than in the general population, it is not so frequent as to suggest an etiologic relationship such as bile stasis.[42] No other disorders are regularly associated with biliary tract carcinoma. Liver disease may result from chronic obstruction but does not appear to predispose to the development of biliary tract cancer. Diabetes[71] was found in 10 percent of one group of patients with bile duct carcinoma, and cancers of other organs were present in 6 percent of one large group of patients with cholecystic carcinoma,[69] but these associations are not noted in other studies.

In India there is a higher incidence of biliary and hepatic cancers in the North than in the South; variations in diet have been suggested as the cause,[43] even though no specific agent has been implicated. Nutritional factors have also been suggested to explain the apparent rarity, not only of biliary cancer, but of biliary diseases among Negroes in Uganda, among whom only 22 cases of biliary tract disease including 6 cancers of the gallbladder (1 female, 5 males) were found in 61,000 hospital admissions.[60] Obviously, other social and economic factors besides diet could affect apparent differences in occurrence of biliary carcinoma in Africa, the United States, Norway, and various regions of India. We have not found evidence of racial or ethnic variations in biliary cancer in the United States; there is specifically no indication that formation of gallstones early in life in patients with hemolytic disorders, which are common in American Negroes, leads to either increased or early development of biliary cancer.

Experimental Carcinogenesis

Experimental induction of biliary cancers has chiefly resulted from application of known carcinogenic chemicals or implantation of gallstones into laboratory animals. Methylcholanthrene, which is carcinogenic in many sites in a variety of experimental animals, has caused carcinoma when implanted into the gallbladders of cats and dogs.[29, 30] The cats developed invasive carcinoma with metastases 23 to 32 months after implantation, and one of five dogs had papillary adenocarcinoma in multiple sites of the biliary tree after 58 months. Another dog which did not have frank cancer had a diffuse papillary hyperplasia of the biliary epithelium. Aramite, another experimental carcinogen, caused adenocarcinomas of the intrahepatic and extrahepatic bile ducts, gallbladder, and ampulla of Vater in 15 of 19 dogs given this material orally.[64] Carcinogenesis required 38 to 101 months. These dogs also developed cirrhosis but neither calculi nor hepatocellular carcinoma was observed.

Foreign bodies such as glass beads or cholesterol pellets failed to induce carcinoma when introduced into the gallbladders of guinea pigs; however, the guinea pig does not appear to be a particularly susceptible animal, since methylcholanthrene produced only moderate epithelial dysplasia but not carcinoma.[22]

Three of 186 cats that had gallstones from cancer patients implanted in the gallbladder eventually developed carcinoma. However, the lack of suitable controls and the rather low incidence of cancer make evaluation of these experiments difficult.[31, 32]

Pathology

Adenocarcinoma is the predominant histologic type, comprising 85 percent or more of gallbladder and duct carcinomas. Variant forms include epidermoid carcinomas, which make up to 10 percent in some reports, and anaplastic carcinomas. The typical adenocarcinoma is composed of acini or tubules, frequently with papillary processes, which are lined by columnar epithelium often closely resembling normal biliary tract mucosa (Figs. 2, 3). Varying degrees of nuclear atypia may be present (Figs. 4, 5), but most carcinomas are well differentiated and are not usually characterized by a predominance of bizarre cell forms or abundant mitotic figures. Less frequently, the glandular or tubular pattern is partially or completely lost and the tumor grows in solid sheets or strands (Fig. 6). Biliary tract carcinomas may have a mixture of glandular and epidermoid features, similar to the pattern frequently seen with bronchogenic carcinoma (Fig. 7). In our own material, a glandular pattern is seen in all instances, although some of the tumors have epidermoid foci. Intercellular bridges may be seen, but keratinization is uncommon in biliary carcinoma. Vascular and perineural involvement is common and, when present, is a useful diagnostic feature (Figs. 8, 9). Mucin is frequently seen in tumors but also may be prominent in cholecystitis (Fig. 10).

Although scarring and thickening of the wall with diminution of the lumen may be the only gross characteristics of gallbladder or bile duct carcinoma, some gallbladder cancers protrude into the lumen as a solid or papillary tumor. Rarely a papillary growth on the mucosal surface without evidence of gross infiltration of

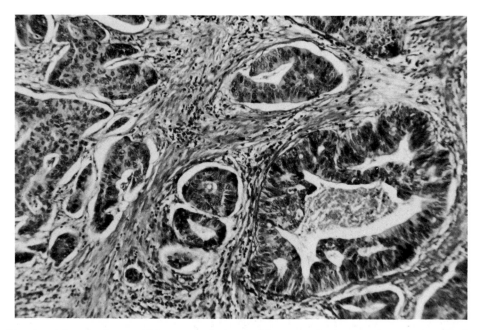

Fig. 2. Adenocarcinoma. This is a typical well-differentiated adenocarcinoma of gallbladder. There is infiltration of the muscularis. H&E. X100.

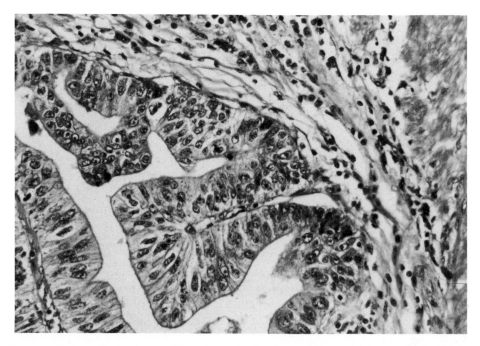

Fig. 3. Cholecystic carcinoma. There is moderate pleomorphism and loss of basal orientation of nuclei. In the upper left is a papillary projection of epithelium without stroma. H&E. X400.

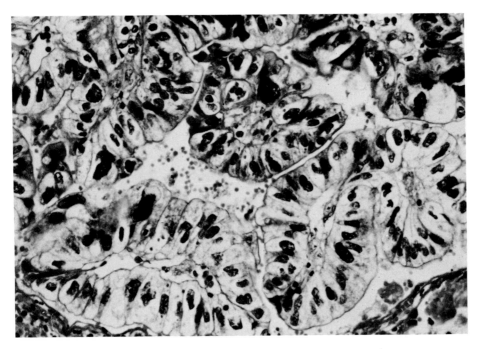

Fig. 4.   Adenocarcinoma. The columnar cell shape persists despite rather marked nuclear pleomorphism. There is focal mucin production. H&E. X400.

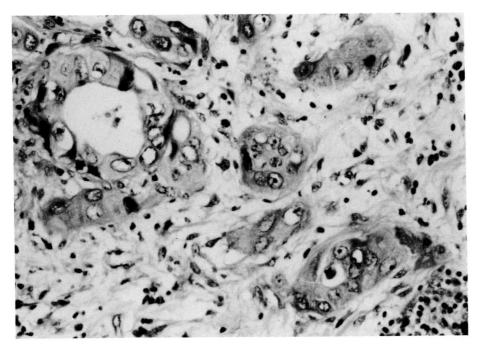

Fig. 5.   Adenocarcinoma of bile duct. Definite atypia distinguishes this from crypts of normal epithelium (Fig. 12), but an acinar pattern remains. H&E. X250.

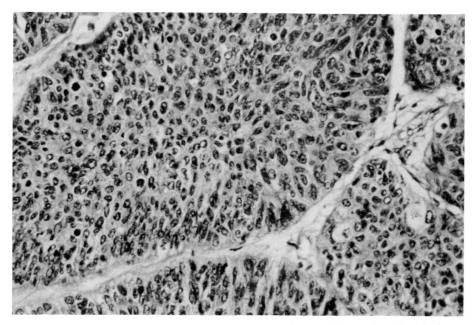

Fig. 6. Epidermoid carcinoma. Cholecystic carcinoma metastatic to a pericholedochal lymph node grows in sheets without formation of acini. Keratinization in biliary epidermoid carcinomas is uncommon. H&E. X250.

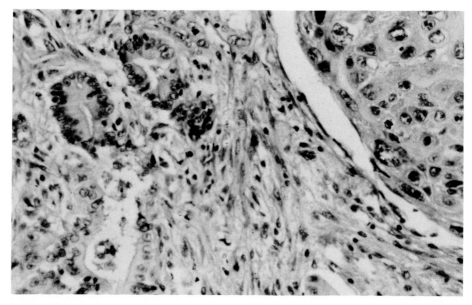

Fig. 7. Mixed pattern in biliary cancer. In the upper right, a solid nest of epidermoid carcinoma has intercellular bridges ("prickle cells"). On the left, the tumor grows in a glandular pattern. This mixture of epidermoid and glandular elements is more common than pure epidermoid carcinoma of biliary origin. In the metastases, the epidermoid pattern may predominate (Fig. 6). Mucicarmine. X250.

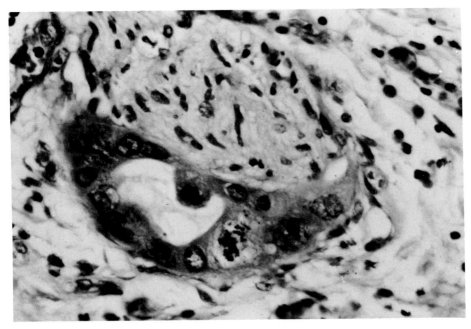

Fig. 8.   Poorly differentiated adenocarcinoma. The large bizarre nuclei and prominent mitotic figures seen in this example are relatively infrequent in biliary carcinomas. A glandular pattern persists, and there is perineural infiltration. H&E. X400.

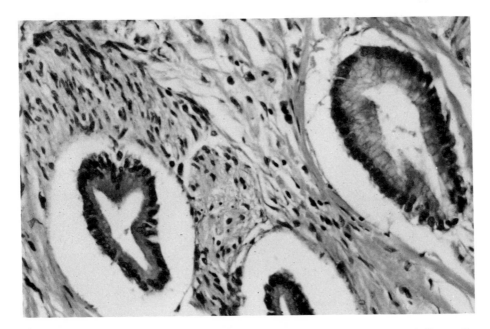

Fig. 9.   Well-differentiated carcinoma of common bile duct. This is a representative section from the deep part of a scirrhous mass involving the distal half of the common bile duct and extending into the pancreas and ampulla. The tumor resembles normal epithelium (Fig. 1), but there is infiltration of perineural spaces. H&E. X250.

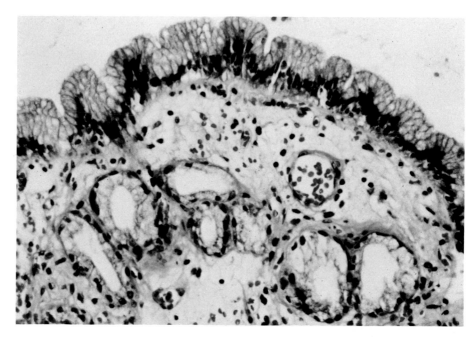

Fig. 10.   Mucin production in chronic cholecystitis. Mucin production may be markedly increased in inflammatory conditions. In this instance, there is mucin production in virtually all of the surface epithelium as well as in the small crypts below. H&E. X250.

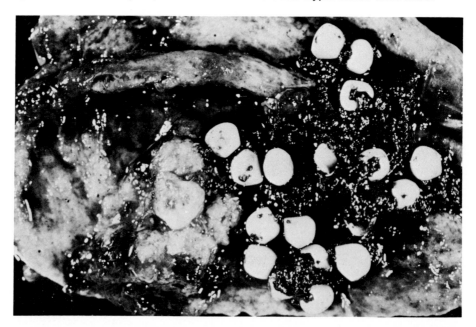

Fig. 11.   Papillary adenocarcinoma of gallbladder. A 78-year-old woman had a cholecystectomy for acute cholecystitis. In addition to calculi, a papillary tumor 3 cm in diameter was found in the fundus when the gallbladder was opened. There was superficial invasion of the muscularis by a well-differentiated adenocarcinoma, histologically identical to Figure 1.

the wall will prove to be superficial carcinoma, but there is no certain method to separate superficial carcinomas from adenomas by gross examination (Fig. 11).

Depth of tumor invasion is of greater prognostic significance than histologic variation. Discovery of cancer of the bile ducts in a preinvasive stage is most unlikely because symptomatic duct cancers are usually invasive, but in situ carcinoma of the gallbladder may be found incidentally after cholecystectomy for clinically benign disease. Approximately 3 percent of gallbladder cancers are reported as preinvasive.[2, 26, 69]

Most carcinomas have invaded the wall of the gallbladder or duct system, and more than half have metastasized or invaded adjacent structures by the time of diagnosis. Fahim[27] and associates found hepatic involvement in 34 percent of 151 patients with gallbladder cancer, mostly in the form of a local mass near the primary. Smaller but equal numbers had satellite nodules or disseminated liver metastases. One patient in four had metastasis to pericholedochal and pancreaticoduodenal lymph nodes but *not* to the lymph nodes of the hilum of the liver. Although local venous spread was found in 13 percent and perineural involvement in 24 percent of cases, these findings were not associated with apparent systemic disease. Direct peritoneal seeding was not found, and involvement of other abdominal organs was attributed to lymphatic spread. Extension along the duct system was identified in only 4 percent of cases, and it was a less frequent cause of jaundice than compression by metastases to periductal lymph nodes. Litwin[40] found a higher percentage of hepatic (63 percent) and lymph node (24 percent) involvement and also a higher incidence of omental (26 percent) and peritoneal (12 percent) involvement. Spread to the porta hepatis was observed in 12 percent, and 9 percent had lung metastasis. The apparent discrepancies between the findings of Litwin and Fahim, et al. are due to differences in the clinical stage of disease at examination.

Although no distant metastases were found in 60 percent of 22 cases of duct carcinoma studied by Coulter,[7] there were no survivors. Van Heerden[71] and associates found spread of disease beyond the primary site, but not necessarily distant metastases, in 71 percent of biliary cancers. The mode of spread of duct cancer is similar to that of cholecystic carcinoma except that the pancreas and ampulla are more likely to be involved by tumors of the distal common duct.

Differential Diagnosis

Adenomas may be distinguished from adenocarcinomas by lack of epithelial atypia and absence of invasion. Since careful orientation of tissue sections facilitates evaluation of invasion, a gallbladder with a suspected neoplasm should be carefully opened, gently washed free of bile and fixed for a few hours before taking sections. With the exception of extremely large lesions, which should be generously sampled, papillary lesions should be examined in their entirety to exclude invasion. Even with good tissue preparation, noninvasive carcinoma may be extremely difficult to distinguish from adenoma (Fig. 12). The histologic features of *nonneoplastic polyps* are quite different from carcinoma and should cause no confusion.

Chronic cholecystitis, particularly when associated with numerous stones, frequently results in thickening of muscularis with mucosal outpouchings deep into

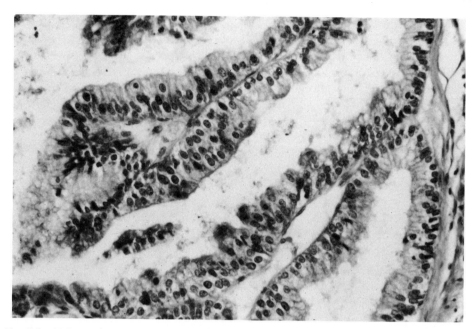

Fig. 12. Adenoma versus noninvasive adenocarcinoma. This papillary tumor was dis-covered in the gallbladder of a 75-year-old woman after cholecystectomy for chronic cholecystitis and cholelithiasis. There was only slight nuclear atypia and no demonstrable invasion. The patient had no evidence of cancer three years postoperatively. This illustrates the difficulty in distinguishing adenomas from low-grade, noninfiltrating carcinomas. H&E. X250.

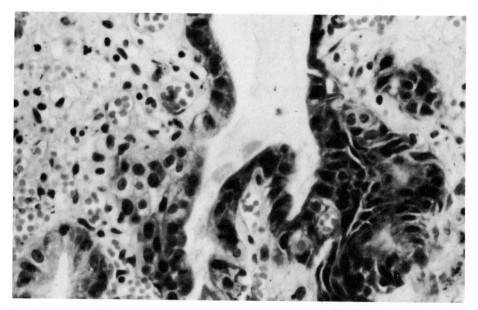

Fig. 13. Atypia in chronic cholecystitis. The epithelial cells are flattened or cuboidal. The nuclei appear large and hyperchromatic. Atypia of this degree is frequently seen with mucosal erosion due to stones. There is no evidence that this type change progresses to malignancy. H&E. X400.

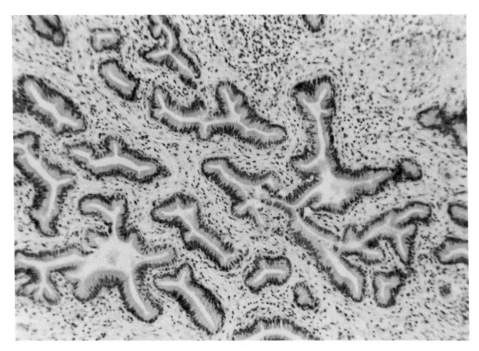

Fig. 14.   Mucosal crypts. Branching nests of normal epithelium extend deep into the wall. This is a normal finding in the neck of the gallbladder, the cystic duct and the distal common duct; it may be seen throughout the entire duct system with choledocholithiasis or following cholecystectomy. H&E. X100.

the wall (Rokitansky-Aschoff sinuses). These changes are usually diffuse but may be localized. Reactive epithelial atypia (Fig. 13) may be confused with cancer, particularly when it occurs in epithelial nests deep in the muscularis. Careful orientation of the specimen will help prevent error, and it must be remembered that epithelial crypts are common in the neck of the gallbladder and biliary ducts (Fig. 14).

Primary sclerosing cholangitis may be most difficult to distinguish from bile duct carcinoma, clinically and morphologically. Approximately 30 instances of this disorder have been recorded. Scarring with occlusion of the ducts following biliary tract surgery is far more common than primary sclerosis. The disease is characterized by either generalized or focal sclerosis of the extrahepatic biliary ducts with reduction or obliteration of the lumen. There is occasionally cholecystic involvement. A relationship to other sclerosing diseases, such as idiopathic retroperitoneal fibrosis or Riedel's struma, has been suggested,[6] but association with these disorders has been unusual. The symptoms, as with cancer, are usually those of chronic cholecystic disease. Jaundice is frequently the presenting complaint. At operation, a thickened sclerotic duct system which may closely resemble the gross appearance of duct cancer is found. Indeed, Altemeier[1] and associates believe that most patients who initially appear to have sclerosing cholangitis eventually will be shown to have scirrhous carcinoma of the bile ducts. The process may extend to the *intrahepatic duct;* in some instances, the bulk of the tumor may be within the liver and thus not recognized until autopsy. On the other hand, Glenn

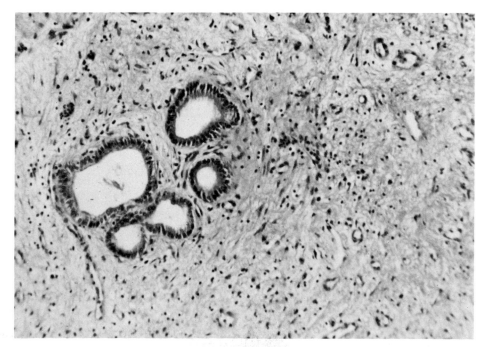

Fig. 15. Sclerosing cholangitis. Dense scar tissue replaces the wall of a bile duct. Only a few mucosal nests remain. At times it may be difficult to distinguish sclerosing cholangitis from well-differentiated adenocarcinoma (Fig. 9). H&E. X100.

and Whitsell[34] have reported seven instances of duct sclerosis with no antecedent biliary surgery and in which no tumor was found at biopsy. One of these patients was alive seven years after biliary diversion, a longer survival than would be expected with an unresected carcinoma. Autopsy follow-up in all proposed cases of this kind will ultimately determine whether this entity is different than sclerosing carcinoma. In the cases which have been accepted as sclerosing cholangitis, the most prominent histologic change has been scarring of the walls and ducts (Fig. 15). Since small islands of biliary mucosa may remain and focally resemble a well-differentiated biliary adenocarcinoma, it is imperative to examine as much tissue as can be obtained to get an overall picture of the disease process. Most surgeons understand that definitive diagnosis based on a single frozen section may not always be possible.

Other Malignant Tumors

A single *lymphoma* of the gallbladder was included in a group of 31 cancers.[48] The finding of lymphoma in the gallbladder should be regarded as evidence of systemic lymphoma until proven otherwise. *Malignant melanoma* in the biliary tract should also be regarded as metastatic until a careful search has excluded other primary sites. Six percent of patients with disseminated melanoma had involvement of the biliary tract,[19] but a few primary biliary melanomas have been reported, including one found at autopsy without tumor elsewhere.[56, 61] A few *leiomyosar-*

comas[10, 72] have been included in reports of gallbladder cancer. Since carcinoma may assume a spindly appearance, an erroneous diagnosis of sarcoma may result from inadequate examination. *Embryonal rhabdomyosarcoma*[20, 36] (sarcoma botryoides) has been recorded approximately a dozen times. All were in children ages 2 to 11, who presented with obstruction of the biliary system.

Prognosis

The poor prognosis of biliary carcinomas is exemplified by a follow-up study of 526 such patients. The five-year survival was 31 percent for ampullary cancer, 26 percent for pancreatic cancer, and zero for both gallbladder and bile duct cancer.[57] Nonetheless, an occasional patient with gallbladder cancer may be cured. Three of 90 (3.3 percent) patients of Thorbjarnarson and Glenn[69] lived seven years without disease; two of these, however, were not known to have carcinoma until the gallbladder was opened. Two of 76 (2.6 percent) patients of Van Heerden[71] and associates lived five years. The even higher five-year survival rate, 8 of 151 (5.9 percent), found by Fahim[26] and associates, was principally related to finding the tumors in an early stage, either in situ or with only superficial infiltration. In all eight instances, the discovery of the tumors was incidental to cholecystectomy for clinically benign disease. Although seven of the survivors had been treated by cholecystectomy alone, one also had wedge resection of the liver. The authors felt that radical surgery might have been beneficial to some of the 43 patients who had residual tumor following cholecystectomy. Appleman[2] and associates studied 21 long-term survivors of gallbladder cancer, and in all the diagnosis was unsuspected until the gallbladder was opened. Two solitary tumors were under 1.0 cm in diameter, 12 were multifocal, and 10 others were superficially invading the wall but not the liver. This histologic type of cancer among long-term survivors is the same as that seen in the fatal cases. The highest survival rates are reported from general hospitals where carcinomas are found in carefully examined gallbladders removed for clinically benign disease. Cancer hospitals treating patients referred for known or suspected cancer have fewer survivors.[63]

The prognosis of biliary duct cancer is even worse; only occasional long-term survivals are noted.[39, 45] Only 1 percent of 218 bile duct carcinomas reported by Den Besten and Leichty lived five years.[21] Other large studies include no long-term survivors.[57, 63]

Treatment

Long-term survival of biliary cancer has been associated only with complete surgical removal of localized disease. Although few gallbladder cancers are in situ when discovered, many more appear confined to the gallbladder and adjacent liver at the time of diagnosis. In this circumstance, right hepatic lobectomy has been proposed as a feasible method of treatment. One author estimated that as many as 15 percent of such patients might profit from this procedure.[15] The five-year cure of a patient with *invasive* carcinoma of the gallbladder treated by hepatic lobectomy[11] has stimulated interest in more radical surgery for this disease.

Palliation has been the primary goal in management of biliary duct cancers, since surgical resection of the tumor has been feasible only in rare instances; however, some believe that about 10 percent of patients with biliary cancer might benefit from more aggressive surgical procedures.[21, 39, 45] Radiation and chemotherapy usually have been used only for palliation. Cure of biliary carcinoma then depends on early, even fortuitous diagnosis, except in rare instances in which radical surgery has proved beneficial. The long history of biliary symptoms in many patients with carcinoma suggests that more cancers might have been found at a curative stage with earlier operation. Since carcinomas often cannot be distinguished from benign tumors by x-ray, any tumor demonstrated radiographically should be removed without delay. Furthermore, the relatively frequent association of carcinoma with acute cholecystitis suggests that when primary cholecystectomy is contraindicated, the gallbladder should be removed and the duct system explored as soon as is feasible to rule out carcinoma. Finally, since scirrhous carcinoma may masquerade as sclerosing cholangitis, resectable sclerotic lesions should be removed.

Benign Tumors of the Biliary Tract

The incidence of benign tumors of the biliary tract is difficult to determine because of inconsistent terminology in many reports; however, benign neoplasms seem to be rare, whereas non-neoplastic tumors are common. Small benign tumors of the gallbladder are likely to be asymptomatic and are frequently discovered only during surgery for cholelithiasis or at autopsy. Tiny tumors of the duct system may also be found only at autopsy, but even relatively small tumors may become symptomatic because of obstruction, especially when in the cystic duct.

Although radiographic studies may demonstrate tumors,[49] ordinarily they cannot be relied upon to distinguish the type. However, adenomas are more likely to be large, single and lobulated, whereas cholesterol polyps are usually small and multiple.[8] Of 52 polypoid lesions discovered on x-rays, 26 were cholesterolosis, 6 calculi, 4 inflammatory polyps, 8 Rokitansky-Aschoff sinuses (adenomyosis), and only 3 true adenomas.[48]

Inflammatory Lesions and Hyperplastic Conditions

Small focal mucosal or mural lesions are so frequent in gallbladders removed for stone or inflammation that little attention is given to these lesions. Most are of no clinical significance.

Cholesterol polyps result from focal subepithelial accumulation of cholesterol-containing macrophages, usually in association with diffuse cholesterolosis (Fig. 16). The polyps are usually multiple and small, only occasionally exceeding 5 mm in diameter. There is no constant relation to serum cholesterol levels or cholelithiasis.[58]

Inflammatory polyps are focal masses resulting from edema or granulation tissue and ordinarily are caused by local irritation by stones (Fig. 17).

Adenomyosis (adenomyomatosis)[28] is the proliferation of epithelium with outpouching of mucosa into or through a thickened muscularis. Some degree of

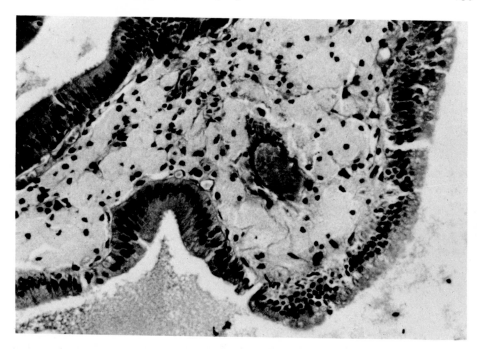

Fig. 16. Cholesterol polyp. Foamy macrophages filled with cholesterol infiltrate the lamina propria. Epithelium is normal. H&E. X250.

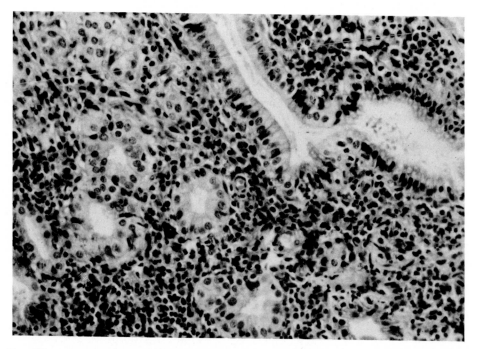

Fig. 17. Inflammatory polyp. There is a dense stromal infiltrate of chronic inflammatory cells and non-neoplastic epithelial proliferation. Lesions of this sort commonly accompany cholecystitis. H&E. X250.

adenomyosis is in all gallbladders with calculi. The entire gallbladder wall is usually involved, but, when focal, the lesions may be mistaken for tumor, both radiographically and at gross examination. Focal involvement is most common in the fundus. Synonyms of this condition include adenoma, adenomyoma, cystadenoma, fibromyoadenoma, cholecystitis glandularis proliferans, cholecystitis cystica, diverticulosis, and myoepithelial anomaly. The first three imply neoplasia and should be avoided. As an alternative designation for the time-honored Rokitansky-Aschoff sinuses, adenomyosis is likely to have greatest appeal to determined opponents of eponyms.

Papillomas are benign tumors of an epithelial surface. The term has been applied to both neoplasms and to non-neoplastic lesions, such as focal epithelial hyperplasia, which is seen frequently in inflammatory diseases of the biliary tract, or normal mucosal folds accentuated by edema or underlying connective tissue proliferation. All of the foregoing have been termed "hyperplastic cholecystoses."[41] We prefer *adenoma* for the designation of neoplastic polyps of the biliary system, even though this term has also been erroneously applied to non-neoplastic conditions in some reports.

Adenoma

The lack of consistent nomenclature hinders estimation of the true incidence of adenomas, but their relative rarity may be judged from a study of 3,024 gallbladders in which 32 cancers and only 6 adenomas were found.[48] Adenomas occur less frequently in the ducts than in the gallbladder, but are nonetheless the most common benign ductal neoplasms.[3, 23, 46] Multiple biliary adenomas[13] and one chloride-secreting adenoma have been reported.[38] Adenomas are distinguished from carcinomas by the absence of epithelial atypia, infrequent mitotic figures, preservation of polarity of cells, and, most important, absence of invasion. The importance of careful orientation of specimens and adequate sampling of lesions for microscopic examination cannot be overemphasized; however, at times definitive diagnosis may not be possible (see Fig. 12).

Miscellaneous Conditions

Amputation *neuroma* of the ducts following cholecystectomy may cause obstruction of the ducts or persistence of symptoms of cholecystic disease.[14,37] Proliferation of nerves, unnecessarily termed "neuromatosis"[41] is common in cholecystitis. A single instance of *granular cell myoblastoma*[59] in the cystic duct resulted in acute cholecystitis. Six instances of *heterotopic pancreas*[24] in the wall of the gallbladder are recorded. Lipomas, lymphangiomas, hemangiomas,[3] and other soft tissue tumors may involve the biliary tract. *Diverticula* of the gallbladder and *choledochal cysts* also may be a source of confusion in diagnosis of biliary masses.

References

1. Altemeier, W.A., Gall, E.A., Zinninger, M.M., and Hoxworth, P. Sclerosing carcinoma of the intrahepatic bile ducts. Arch. Surg., 75:450, 1967.
2. Appleman, R.M., Morlock, C.G., Dahlin, D.C., and Adson, M.A. Long-term survival in carcinoma of the gallbladder. Surg. Gynec. Obstet., 117:459, 1963.

3. Arbab, A.A., and Brasfield, R.D. Benign tumors of the gallbladder. Surgery, 61:535, 1967.
4. Ashby, B.S. Carcinoma in a choledochal cyst. Brit. J. Surg., 51:493, 1964.
5. Balangero, E.P. Surgical treatment of the biliary tract: Review of 787 cases. J. Int. Coll. Surg., 41:142, 1964.
6. Bartholomew, L.G., Cain, J.C., Woolner, L.G., Utz, D.C., and Ferris, D.O. Sclerosing cholangitis; its possible association with Riedel's struma and fibrous retroperitonitis: Report of two cases. New Eng. J. Med., 269:8, 1963.
7. Berk, J.E. Persistence of symptoms following gallbladder surgery. Amer. J. Dig. Dis., 9:295, 1964.
8. Borgerson, R.J., Delbeccaro, E.J., and Callaghan, P.J. Polypoid lesions of the gallbladder. Arch. Surg., 85:234, 1962.
9. Bossart, P.A., Patterson, A.H., and Zintel, H.A. Carcinoma of the gallbladder: A report of 76 cases. Amer. J. Surg., 103:366, 1962.
10. Braasch, J.W., Warren, K.W., and Kune, G.A. Malignant neoplasms of the bile ducts. Surg. Clin. N. Amer., 47:627, 1967.
11. Brasfield, R.D. Right hepatic lobectomy for carcinoma of the gallbladder. Ann. Surg., 153:563, 1961.
12. Brown, D.B., Strang, R., Gordon, J., and Hendry, E.B. Primary carcinoma of the extrahepatic ducts. Brit. J. Surg., 49:22, 1961.
13. Cattell, R.B., Braasch, J.W., and Kahn, F. Polypoid epithelial tumors of the bile ducts. New Eng. J. Med., 266:57, 1962.
14. ———— and St. Ville, J. Amputation neuromas of the biliary tract. Arch. Surg., 83:242, 1961.
15. Chandler, J.J., and Fletcher, W.S. A clinical study of primary carcinoma of the gallbladder. Surg. Gynec. Obstet., 117:297, 1963.
16. Clemett, A.R. Carcinoma of the major bile ducts. Radiology, 84:894, 1965.
17. Coulter, E. Primary carcinoma of extrahepatic bile ducts: Review of 22 cases. Amer. Surg., 32:565, 1966.
18. Cowley, L.L., and Wood, V. Carcinoma developing in a remnant of the gallbladder. Ann. Surg., 159:465, 1964.
19. Das Gupta, T., and Brasfield, R. Metastatic melanoma: A clinicopathological study. Cancer, 17:1323, 1964.
20. Delany, H.M., Driscoll, P.J., and Ainsworth, H. Sarcoma botryoides of the common bile duct: Report of a case and review of the literature. J. Pediat. Surg., 1:571, 1966.
21. Den Besten, L., and Liechty, R.D. Cancer of the biliary tree. Amer. J. Surg., 109:587, 1965.
22. DesForges, G., DesForges, J., and Robbins, S.L. Carcinoma of the gallbladder: An attempt at experimental production. Cancer, 3:1088, 1950.
23. Dowdy, G.S., Jr., Olin, W.G., Jr., Shelton, E.L., Jr., and Waldron, G.W. Benign tumors of the extrahepatic bile ducts: Report of three cases and review of the literature. Arch. Surg., 85:503, 1962.
24. Elving, G. Heterotopic pancreatic tissue in the gallbladder wall: Report of a case. Acta Chir. Scand., 118:32, 1959.
25. Evans, J.A. Biliary tract problems in the aged. Radiol. Clin. N. Amer., 3:305, 1965.
26. Fahim, R.B., Ferris, D.O., and McDonald, J.R. Carcinoma of the gallbladder: An appraisal of its surgical treatment. Arch. Surg., 86:334, 1963.
27. ———— McDonald, J.R., Richards, J.C., and Ferris, D.O. Carcinoma of the gallbladder: A study of its modes of spread. Ann. Surg., 156:114, 1962.
28. Fotopoulos, J.P., and Crampton, A.M. Adenomyomatosis of the gallbladder. Med. Clin. N. Amer., 48:9, 1964.
29. Fortner, J.G. The experimental induction of primary carcinoma of the gallbladder. Cancer, 8:689, 1955.
30. ———— and Leffal, L.D. Carcinoma of the gallbladder in dogs. Cancer, 14:1127, 1961.

31. ——— and Randall, H.T. On the carcinogenicity of human gallstones. Surg. Forum, 12:155, 1961.

32. ——— and Randall, H.T. Endogenous carcinogens for the extrahepatic biliary tree. Acta Un. Int. Cancer, 19:629, 1963.

33. Glenn, F., and McSherry, C.K. Cholecystic disease in the aged. Geriatrics, 22:106, 1967.

34. ——— and Whitsell, J.C. II. Primary sclerosing cholangitis. Surg. Gynec. Obstet., 123:1037, 1967.

35. Ham, J.M., and Mackenzie, D.C. Primary carcinoma of the extrahepatic biliary ducts. Surg. Gynec. Obstet., 118:977, 1964.

36. Hays, D.M., and Snyder, W.H., Jr. Botryoid sarcoma (rhabdomyosarcoma) of the bile ducts. Amer. J. Dis. Child, 110:595, 1965.

37. Joske, B.A., and Finlay Jones, L.R. Amputation neuroma of the cystic duct stump. Brit. J. Surg., 53:766, 1966.

38. Kerr, A.B., and Lendrum, A.C. A chloride-secreting papilloma of the gallbladder. Brit. J. Surg., 23:615, 1936.

39. Lippmann, H.N., McDonald, L.C., and Longmire, W.P., Jr. Carcinoma of the extrahepatic bile ducts. Amer. Surg., 25:819, 1959.

40. Litwin, M.S. Primary carcinoma of the gallbladder: A review of 78 patients. Arch. Surg., 95:236, 1967.

41. Lubera, R.J., Climie, A.R.W., and Kling, G.E. Cholecystitis and the hyperplastic cholecystoses: A clinical, radiologic and pathology study. Amer. J. Dig. Dis., 12:696, 1967.

42. Macfarlane, J.R., and Glenn, F. Carcinoma in a choledochal cyst. J. Amer. Med. Assoc., 202:1003, 1967.

43. Malhortra, S.L. Geographical distribution of gastrointestinal cancers in India with special reference to causation. Gut, 8:361, 1967.

44. McNulty, J.G. Preoperative diagnosis of carcinoma of the gallbladder by percutaneous transhepatic cholangiography. Amer. J. Roentgenol., 101:605, 1967.

45. Monge, J.J., and Rudie, P.S. Segmental resection of the common hepatic duct for carcinoma: A report of three cases. Arch. Surg., 93:1015, 1966.

46. Moore, S.W., McElwee, R.S., and Romiti, C. Benign tumors of the biliary tract. J.A.M.A., 150:999, 1952.

47. Newman, H.F., and Northrup, J.D. Gallbladder carcinoma in cholelithiasis: A study of probability. Geriatrics 19:453, 1964.

48. Nugent, F.W., Meissner, W.A., and Hoelscher, F.E. The significance of gallbladder polyps. J.A.M.A., 178:426, 1961.

49. Ochsner, S.F., and Ochsner, A. Benign neoplasms of the gallbladder: Diagnosis and surgical implications. Ann. Surg., 151:630, 1960.

50. Pack, G.T., and Teng, P.K. Carcinoma of cystic duct leading to hydrops of gallbladder. J.A.M.A., 203:153, 1968.

51. Pallette, E.M., Harrington, R.W., and Pallette, E.C. Carcinomas of the extrahepatic biliary system. Amer. Surg., 29:719, 1963.

52. Parker, R.H. Carcinoma of the cystic duct with gallbladder perforation. Ann. Intern. Med., 63:475, 1965.

53. Polk, H.C., Jr. Carcinoma and the calcified gallbladder. Gastroenterology, 50:582, 1966.

54. Quattlebaum, J.K., and Quattlebaum, J.K., Jr. Malignant obstruction of the major hepatic ducts. Ann. Surg., 161:876, 1965.

55. Rabinov, K. Primary carcinoma in a functioning gallbladder. Gastroenterology, 50:808, 1966.

56. Raffensberger, E.C., Brason, F.W., and Triano, G. Primary melanoma of the gallbladder. Amer. J. Dig. Dis., 8:356, 1963.

57. Salmon, P.A. Carcinoma of the pancreas and extrahepatic biliary system. Surgery, 60:554, 1966.

58. Seltzer, D.W., Dockerty, M.B., Stauffer, M.H., and Priestly, J.T. Papillomas (so-called) in the non-calculous gallbladder. Amer. J. Surg., 103:472, 1962.
59. Serpe, S.J., Todd, D., and Baruch, H. Cholecystitis due to granular cell myoblastoma of the cystic duct. Amer. J. Dig. Dis., 5:824, 1960.
60. Shaper, A.G. Diseases of the biliary tract in Africans in Uganda. E. African Med. J., 41:246, 1964.
61. Simard, C., George, P., Caulet, T., and Diebold, J. Les melanomes malins de la vesicule biliaire. Rapport de deux cas. J. Chir. (Paris), 92:51, 1966.
62. Smith, V.M., Feldman, M., Sr., and Warner, C.G. Neoplasms of the cystic and hepatic ducts, Amer. J. Dig. Dis., 7:804, 1962.
63. Statistical Report of End Results, 1949-1957. New York, Memorial Hospital for Cancer and Allied Diseases and the James Ewing Hospital of the City of New York, 1965.
64. Sternberg, S.S., Popper, H., Oser, B.L., and Oser, M. Gallbladder and bile duct carcinomas in dogs after long-term feeding of aramite. Cancer, 13:780, 1960.
65. Strauch, G.O. Primary carcinoma of the gallbladder: Presentation of 70 cases from the Rhode Island Hospital and a cumulative review of the last ten years of the American literature. Surgery, 47:368, 1960.
66. Strohl, E.L., Reed, W.H., Diffenbaugh, W.G., and Anderson, R.E. Carcinoma of the bile ducts. Arch. Surg., 87:567, 1963.
67. Thistlethwaite, J.R., and Horwitz, A. Choledochal cyst followed by carcinoma of the hepatic duct. Southern Med. J., 60:872, 1967.
68. Thorbjarnarson, B. Carcinoma of the gallbladder and acute cholecystitis. Ann. Surg., 151:241, 1960.
69. ———— and Glenn, F. Carcinoma of the gallbladder. Cancer, 12:1009, 1959.
70. Torvik, A., and Hoivik, B. Gallstones in an autopsy series. Incidence, complications and correlation with carcinoma of the gallbladder. Acta Chir. Scand., 120:168, 1960.
71. Van Heerden, J.A., Judd, E.S., and Dockerty, M.B. Carcinoma of the extrahepatic bile ducts: A clinicopathologic study. Amer. J. Surg., 113:49, 1967.
72. Whitcomb, F.F., Jr., Corley, G.J., Babigian, D.N., and Colcock, B.P. Leiomyosarcoma of the bile ducts. Gastroenterology, 52:94, 1967.

Addendum

Biliary Carcinoma

An interesting observation, confirmed in several reports,[1-3] is the development of biliary tract carcinoma in patients with long-standing ulcerative colitis. The coexistence of these conditions appears to be too frequent to be explained by chance alone. Many of the patients have been younger than the usual age for appearance of biliary carcinoma, and most carcinomas have occurred in the setting of active ulcerative colitis of many years' duration. Chronic inflammation of the biliary tract seen in these patients is a possible basis for the development of carcinoma.

A well-documented instance of malignant mixed tumor of the gallbladder was reported by Higgs et al.[4] In addition to elements of adenocarcinoma, the tumor contained fibrosarcoma, chondrosarcoma, and osteoid. However, the pleomorphic spindly carcinomas described by Appleman and Coopersmith[5] demonstrate that most sarcomatous appearing biliary tumors are carcinomas.

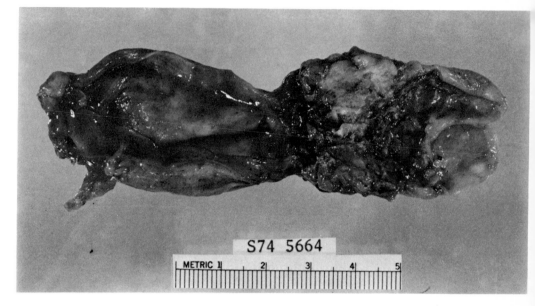

Fig. 1. Adenomyoma of gallbladder. The large mass in the wall of the distal fundus consists of hypertrophic muscularis with mucosal outpouchings containing inspissated bile. Although this patient had cholelithiasis and microscopic changes of chronic cholecystitis in the remaining gallbladder, in many instances of adenomyoma there are no calculi, and only a fixed defect in the wall is found.[11]

Benign Conditions

Specific radiographic findings are seen in many instances of localized adenomyoma of gallbladder, and recognition of this entity as being different from the diffuse muscular hyperplasia with Rokitansky-Aschoff sinuses seen in chronic cholecystitis seems justified.[2] Many of the patients with adenomyoma have symptoms of biliary tract disease but do not have calculi. Some adenomyomas may attain striking size (Fig. 1).

Heterotopic tissues in the gallbladder may occasionally simulate tumors. The subject was reviewed by Curtis and Sheahan.[6]

Other Tumors

Among the recently documented rarer tumors of the biliary system are instances of lymphosarcoma,[7] reticulum cell sarcoma,[8] embryonal rhabdomyosarcoma,[9] and granular cell tumor (granular cell myoblastoma).[10]

References

1. Converse CF, Reagan JW, DeCosse JJ: Ulcerative colitis and carcinoma of the bile ducts. Am J Surg 121:39, 1971

2. Morowitz DA, Glagor S, Dordal E, Kirsner JB: Carcinoma of the biliary tract complicating chronic ulcerative colitis. Cancer 27:356, 1971
3. Ross AP, Braasch JW: Ulcerative colitis and carcinoma of the proximal bile ducts. Gut 14:94, 1973
4. Higgs WR, Morcega EE, Jordan PH Jr: Malignant mixed tumor of the gallbladder. Cancer 32:47, 1973
5. Appleman HD, Coopersmith N: Pleomorphic spindle-cell carcinoma of the gallbladder. Relation to sarcoma of the gallbladder. Cancer 25:535, 1970
6. Curtis LE, Sheahan DG: Heterotopic tissues in the gallbladder. Arch Pathol 88:677, 1969
7. Van Slyck EJ, Schuman BM: Lymphosarcoma of gallbladder. Cancer 30:810, 1973
8. Carpenter Y, Lambilliote JP: Primary sarcoma of the gallbladder. Cancer 32:493, 1973
9. Davis GL, Kissane GM, Ishak KG: Embryonal rhabdomyosarcoma (sarcoma botryoides) of the biliary tree; report of five cases and review of the literature. Cancer 24:333, 1969
10. Whitmore JT, Whitley JP, LaVerde P, Cerda JJ: Granular cell myoblastoma of the common bile duct. Am J Dig Dis 14:516, 1969
11. Shapiro R: Fixed defects of the gallbladder wall adenomyosis. Surg Gynecol Obstet 136:745, 1973

INDEX

415